...oratory
Procedures

Medical
Laboratory
Procedures
2nd Edition

Mary Ellen Wedding, MEd, MT(ASCP), CMA

Professor of Health and Human Services
Director of Medical Assisting Technology
University of Toledo
Community and Technical College
Toledo, Ohio

Sally A. Toenjes, MA, MT(ASCP), CMA

Professor Emerita of Health and Human Services
Former Director of Medical Assistant Program
Macomb Community College
Clinton Township, Michigan

 F. A. DAVIS COMPANY ▪ Philadelphia

F. A. Davis Company
1915 Arch Street
Philadelphia, PA 19103

Printed in the United States of America

Last digit indicates print number: 10 9 8 7 6 5 4

Publisher: Jean-François Vilain
Developmental Editors: Ralph Zickgraf and Marianne Fithian
Production Editor: Stephen D. Johnson
Cover Designer: Louis J. Forgione

As new scientific information becomes available through basic and clinical research, recommended treatments and drug therapies undergo changes. The authors and publisher have done everything possible to make this book accurate, up to date, and in accord with accepted standards at the time of publication. The authors, editors, and publisher are not responsible for errors or omissions or for consequences from application of the book, and make no warranty, expressed or implied, in regard to the contents of the book. Any practice described in this book should be applied by the reader in accordance with professional standards of care used in regard to the unique circumstances that may apply in each situation. The reader is advised always to check product information (package inserts) for changes and new information regarding dose and contraindications before administering any drug. Caution is especially urged when using new or infrequently ordered drugs.

Library of Congress Cataloging-in-Publication Data

Wedding, Mary Ellen.
    Medical laboratory procedures   / Mary Ellen Wedding, Sally A.
Toenjes. — Ed. 2.
       p. cm.
    Includes index.
    ISBN 0-8036-0052-6 (alk. paper)
    1. Diagnosis, Laboratory.   2. Physicians' assistants.
  I. Toenjes, Sally A. II. Title.
    [DNLM: 1. Diagnosis, Laboratory—programmed instruction. QY 18.2
W388m 1997]
RB37.W42 1998
616.07′5′078—dc21
DNLM/DLC
for Library of Congress
                                                                97-984
                                                                  CIP

To my husband, Don, and my children, Carol Ann, Don K., II, M.E. Victoria, and Daniel; and in loving memory of my father, Arthur Anthony Karwacki.

M.E.W.

To my loving husband, Richard, for his support and contribution to this endeavor, and my children, Sandie and Tim.

S.A.T.

Preface

Medical Laboratory Procedures, 2nd Edition, is a competency-based textbook/workbook that explains the fundamentals of laboratory procedures for personnel working in a clinical laboratory or physician's office laboratory (POL). The textbook leads the student through the most frequently used tests and up-to-date methods by means of procedural steps with rationales that reinforce the learning process. After completing the tests, students will have mastered the principles and techniques necessary to:

- Demonstrate laboratory safety and quality assurance when performing laboratory tests.
- Perform urinalysis on specimens using proper collection techniques.
- Perform a venipuncture and calibrate and maintain laboratory instruments for blood chemistry analysis.
- Perform a capillary puncture and carry out a complete blood count and other hematology studies.
- Perform serology tests, using antigen-antibody reactions for demonstrating end results.
- Prepare bacterial smears and Gram stain smears and perform throat and urine cultures for bacteriology studies.

Students learn the theory behind the specific tests and practice each test in a step-by-step format. Test selection is based on the 1990 DACUM Analysis of the Medical Assisting Profession. The DACUM (Developing a Curriculum) Analysis fulfills the American Association of Medical Assistants requirements for a competency-based curriculum. Each chapter includes:

- Learning Objectives
- Chapter Outline
- Theory
- Summary
- Patient Education
- Technical Considerations
- Sources of Error
- Procedure with Rationale
- Questions
- Terminal Performance Objective
- Instructor's Evaluation Form
- Illustrations
- Margin Definitions

We feel that laboratory personnel will benefit from the various test procedures presented and the illustrations provided. Our use of brand names and trademarks for the products and instruments used in some of the procedures is not meant as an endorsement; rather, we have tried to present a variety of choices for the many specific tests demonstrated and instruments used.

For instructors of medical assistants and clinical laboratory personnel, this text provides an opportunity to assess the student's skills by means of an evaluation form. All pages are perforated for the convenience of the instructor. The Instructor's Evaluation

Form stands alone and may be removed from the text without destroying the theory sections. This form provides the evaluation tools necessary for educators to assess entry-level competencies for medical assistants, clinical laboratorians, and medical technicians.

Mary Ellen Wedding
Sally A. Toenjes

Acknowledgments

The authors wish to thank the following professionals, who donated time and expertise to a project that could not have been completed without them. Their talents are apparent throughout the book.

Richard G. Toenjes, for the line drawings and photography that add so much to the text.

Daniel K. Wedding and his wife, Trisha Noel, for many of the drawings and illustrations.

Peggy Estes, BS, MT(ASCP), Program Director, School of Medical Technology, and Nancy Kovacs, BS, MT(ASCP), Educational Specialist, St. Charles Hospital, Oregon, Ohio for providing valuable ideas and resources.

Agnes Gray, BS, MT(ASCP), Program Director, David's House Compassion, Inc., a friend, colleague, and outstanding microbiologist, who provided helpful ideas for several chapters.

Nancy Gurney, SBB, MT(ASC), Technical Supervisor, Blood Services, American Red Cross, Northwest, Ohio.

Patricia Carroll, MT(ASCP), Medical Technologist, St. John Hospital and Medical Center, Detroit, Michigan.

Barbara A. Pendolino, MT(ASCP), Medical Technologist, St. John Hospital and Medical Center, Detroit, Michigan.

The reviewers, whose careful critiques were invaluable: Bonnie L. Deister, MS, BSN, MA, CMA-C, Assistant Professor and Chairperson, Medical Assisting Department, EMT/Paramedic Department, Broome Community College, Binghamton, New York; Patricia S. Hurlbut, MSED, MT, CLS, CMA, CPT, RPT, Instructor, Medical Assisting Department, Waukesha County Technical Institute, Pewaukee, Wisconsin; Beverly M. Kovanda, PhD, MT(ASCP) MS, Coordinator/Professor, Medical Technology Department, Columbus State Community College, Columbus, Ohio; Ursula J. Pennell, MT(ASCP) MED, Program Director, Medical Assisting Department, Northeast Career Schools, Manchester, New Hampshire; and Sharon L. Thatcher, EDS, MT(ASCP), Program Director, MLT/Phlebotomy Department, Dekalb Technical Institute, Clarkston, Georgia.

And finally, all the staff at F. A. Davis, in particular Jean-François Vilain, Publisher, for his constant support and encouragement; Marianne Fithian, Developmental Editor, for her editing skills; and Herbert J. Powell, Jr., Director of Production, for his patient help throughout the production process.

Contents

FUNDAMENTALS
OF LABORATORY
PRACTICE

Introduction to Laboratory Practice

1

LEARNING OBJECTIVES

On completing this chapter, you will be able to:

COGNITIVE OBJECTIVES
- Describe medical technology or clinical laboratory science and explain its relationship to laboratory testing.
- Describe laboratory testing and explain how test results are used by the physician.
- List the advantages of performing laboratory tests in a physician's office laboratory.
- List the various medical personnel employed in a clinical laboratory or physician's office laboratory.
- Describe the medical assistant's role in the physician's office.

Medical technology or clinical laboratory science is the health profession that specializes in performing medical laboratory tests in urinalysis, **hematology,** clinical chemistry, **microbiology,** and **immunology.** Large laboratories employ highly skilled professionals and perform complicated analyses. A small facility, such as a physician's office laboratory (POL), usually performs less complicated tests. Many different levels of skilled professionals staff these laboratories. The skill level of the laboratorian depends on educational background and training.

> **Hematology:** *the study of blood and blood-forming tissues*

> **Microbiology:** *scientific study of microorganisms*

> **Immunology:** *study of immunity to disease*

LABORATORY TESTING

Disease is a **pathological** condition of the body that is manifested by a group of clinical signs and symptoms. Diseases are confirmed by findings of laboratory tests related to the pathological condition. These findings set the condition apart as abnormal or differing from the normal state. When the results vary from normal values, a pathological condition may be present.

> **Pathological:** *diseased; due to disease*

3

Diagnose: *to evaluate the history of the disease process; to use the clinical signs and symptoms, laboratory findings, and special test results to arrive at the nature and cause of a person's disease*

Prognosis: *prediction of the course of disease*

Referral laboratory: *a laboratory that performs testing for other clinical laboratories and institutions*

Physicians use laboratory test results to **diagnose** and treat diseases and to maintain the health of patients. Laboratory testing plays a vital role in determining normal and abnormal conditions. A physician may decide that disease is present by comparing the results of the patient's tests with a range of normal values called the *reference range*. The clinical symptoms detected during physical examinations and the laboratory test results provide the data that assist the physician in the diagnosis, **prognosis,** and treatment of disease.

CLINICAL LABORATORY

Most clinical laboratories are located in hospitals, outpatient clinics, physicians' offices, industrial clinics, public health departments, and **referral laboratories**. Smaller laboratories, such as those in physicians' offices, may send some or all of their laboratory work to hospital-based, commercial, or referral laboratories. Often hospital laboratories send specialized testing, such as drug detection, to highly specialized laboratories.

PHYSICIAN'S OFFICE LABORATORY

In the past, few laboratory tests were performed in the physician's office. Today, however, new instrumentation has simplified testing procedures, and as a result, physicians, who depend more than ever on laboratory tests to provide effective medical care, may establish their own office laboratory.

One of the major benefits of laboratory testing in the physician's office is that it avoids sending the patient to another location. In addition, results are immediately available to the physician for diagnosis of the illness. This enables the physician to treat the patient at the time of the office visit.

CLINICAL LABORATORY PERSONNEL

The clinical laboratory staff may consist of pathologists, clinical science specialists, medical technologists or clinical laboratory scientists, medical laboratory technicians or clinical laboratory technicians, **phlebotomists,** and medical assistants.

Phlebotomist: *a person who collects blood by venipuncture*

Clinical Comment: Phlebotomists

Phlebotomists may be trained and/or certified by the following agencies:
- American Society of Phlebotomy Technicians (ASPT), Inc.; PO Box 1831, Hickory, NC 28603; (704) 322-1334
- American Society of Clinical Pathologists (ASCP); 2100 West Harrison St., Chicago, IL 60612; (800) 621-4142
- National Certification Agency for Medical Laboratory Personnel (NCA); PO Box 15945-289, Lenexa, KS 66285; (913) 438-5110, Fax (913) 541-0156

Medical Technologist

A *certified medical technologist* or *clinical laboratory scientist* usually has a baccalaureate degree and formal training in an accredited medical technology program that meets the criteria set forth by the National Accrediting Agency for Clinical Laboratory Sciences (NAACLS). To become certified, the technologist must pass an examination given by a national certifying agency. The titles awarded medical technologists and clinical laboratory scientists, with the appropriate certifying agency, follow:

- MT (ASCP) — Medical Technologist
  American Society of Clinical Pathologists
- CLS (NCA) — Clinical Laboratory Scientist
  National Certification Agency for Medical Laboratory Personnel
- MT (AMT) — Medical Technologist
  American Medical Technologists
- RMT (ISCLT) — Registered Medical Technologist
  International Society for Clinical Laboratory Technology

Medical Laboratory Technician

A *certified medical laboratory technician* or *clinical laboratory technician* usually has completed 2 years of formal training equivalent to an associate's degree in an accredited program that meets the criteria set forth by the NAACLS. After passing an examination administered by one of the national certifying agencies, the medical laboratory technician is certified. The titles awarded medical laboratory technicians and clinical laboratory technicians, with their appropriate certifying agency, follow:

- MLT (ASCP) — Medical Laboratory Technician
  American Society of Clinical Pathologists
- CLT (NCA) — Clinical Laboratory Technician
  National Certification Agency for Medical Laboratory Personnel
- MLT (AMT) — Medical Laboratory Technician
  American Medical Technologists
- RLT (ISCLT) — Registered Laboratory Technician
  International Society for Clinical Laboratory Technology

Two of the listed agencies also offer certificates for physician's office laboratory personnel who do not have formal laboratory training in an accredited program. A physician office laboratory technician (POLT) certificate is granted by the International Society for Clinical Laboratory Technology. A certified office laboratory technician (COLT) certificate is offered by the American Medical Technologists in conjunction with the American Association of Physician Office Laboratories (AAPOL). Both certificates require a minimum of a high school diploma, or equivalent, combined with 12 months' experience for the POLT and 6 months' experience for the COLT in a physician's office laboratory.

Medical Assistant

The *medical assistant* is a multiskilled allied health professional dedicated to assisting in patient-care management. This person performs administrative and clinical duties and basic laboratory tests, assists in certain aspects of emergency situations, and may manage facilities and personnel. Competence in the field requires that a medical assistant display professionalism and communicate effectively. Medical assistant programs are available in many community colleges, vocational-technical schools, and proprietary schools.

The Curriculum Review Board of the American Association of Medical Assistants Endowment and the Commission on Accreditation for Allied Health Education Programs (CAAHEP) cooperate to establish, maintain, and promote appropriate standards of quality for educational programs in medical assisting. These entities provide recognition for educational programs that meet or exceed those minimum standards.

MEDICAL ASSISTANT CERTIFICATION PROGRAMS

A *certified medical assistant* is a professional who has completed a minimum of 1 year of education in a program accredited by CAAHEP and has passed a national certifying examination administered by the American Association of Medical Assistants (AAMA).

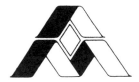

Figure 1-1 The CMA pin and logo. (Courtesy American Association of Medical Assistants.)

A *registered medical assistant* is a graduate of a medical assisting program accredited by the Accrediting Bureau of Health Education Schools (ABHES) and has passed an examination offered by the American Medical Technologists.

MEDICAL ASSISTANT PROFESSIONAL AFFILIATIONS

A professional person is one who has been trained to render a particular service that is governed by an organized body which regulates practice in the field of training by requiring adherence to a code of ethics and an assessment of competency.

The AAMA is a national professional organization for medical assistants. National membership in the AAMA includes state and local chapter memberships.

The AAMA conducts occupational analyses to develop entry-level competencies for the medical assistant profession. These competencies are used for *developing a curriculum* (DACUM). See Appendix E for the DACUM analysis of the medical assisting profession.

The AAMA retains the National Board of Medical Examiners as test consultants. They offer a national certifying examination twice each year, in January and June. Effective February 1, 1998, only graduates of medical assisting programs accredited by the Commission on Accreditation for Allied Health Education Programs will be eligible to take the national certification examination. The examination is designed to certify that a medical assistant has entry-level knowledge and skills needed to competently perform routine clinical and administrative duties in an ambulatory- or immediate-care setting. An individual who passes the certification examination is awarded the Certified Medical Assistant (CMA) credential and may wear the CMA pin (Fig. 1-1).

Recertification is mandatory every 5 years by accumulating continuing education units (CEU) or by examination. The national office at 1-800-ACT-AAMA provides information on dates of certifying examinations, CEU, and membership in the AAMA.

The American Medical Technologists also offer an examination for medical assistants. This examination is given by schools accredited by the ABHES. Applicants must be graduates of schools accredited by the ABHES or meet certain experience requirements. On successfully completing this examination, the title of Registered Medical Assistant (RMA) is awarded and members may wear the RMA insignia (Fig. 1-2).

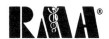

Figure 1-2 The RMA logo. (Courtesy Registered Medical Assistants Association.)

SUMMARY

Laboratory test results assist the physician in the diagnosis, prognosis, and treatment of disease conditions. Testing also provides parameters for patients to maintain health and prevent future diseased states. Without accurate and precise laboratory test results, physicians would find it difficult to determine the nature and cause of the disease.

Medical assistants, as multiskilled allied health professionals, have many opportunities for employment in the physician's office. Employment is also available in hospitals, clinical laboratories, medical centers, ambulatory- and immediate-care facilities, and various other health-related settings.

Questions

Name _____ Date _____

1. Explain laboratory testing and describe how test results are used by the physician.

2. Explain the advantage of performing laboratory tests in a physician's office.

3. Give a brief description of the educational requirements for the following: a medical technologist or clinical laboratory scientist; a medical laboratory technician or a clinical laboratory technician; and a medical assistant.

4. Describe the medical assistant's role in the physician's office.

5. Name two organizations that certify medical assistants.

6. Give a definition of a professional person and name two professional organizations associated with medical assistants.

Safety and Infection Control

2

LEARNING OBJECTIVES

On completing this chapter, you will be able to:

COGNITIVE OBJECTIVES

- Briefly describe OSHA's Hazard Communication Program.
- Briefly state some of the information required for Material Safety Data Sheets.
- Identify guidelines to protect against injury when using chemicals and electrical equipment.
- Describe the infectious process and relate this information to laboratory safety.
- Briefly explain the OSHA Bloodborne Pathogens Standard.
- List the specimens included in the Bloodborne Pathogens Standard.
- Tell when and what type of personal protective equipment is required for various laboratory activities involving bloodborne pathogens.

Maintaining a safe working environment is the responsibility of all medical office personnel, from physician to cleaning staff. Dangers exist in all work settings, but especially in a clinical laboratory. Chemicals, electrical equipment, patients, and clinical specimens pose special risks to everyone associated with the medical office. These risks may be minimized or eliminated by careful attention to safety rules.

Most safety rules are based on common sense. Unfortunately, they may be neglected, overlooked, or ignored in the interest of saving time. Shortcuts are tempting, but they often compromise safety and lead to disastrous consequences.

EMERGENCY INFORMATION

Emergency telephone numbers must be posted in plain view at or near the telephone. They should include:

- Emergency 911
- Fire department
- Poison control center
- Hospital burn unit
- Police department
- Supervisor or physician

Evacuation routes must be posted at all doors in case of fire or other emergencies. Aisles and doorways should be free of any obstructions and clutter. All laboratories must have fire extinguishers, fire blankets, eyewash stations, and broken-glass containers.

HEALTH AND SAFETY HAZARDS IN THE CLINICAL LABORATORY

The Occupational Safety and Health Administration (OSHA) is an agency of the Department of Labor. Its mission is to save lives, prevent injuries, and protect the health of workers in the United States. OSHA works in partnership with state agencies to ensure that employees are provided a safe workplace. OSHA establishes protective standards, enforces the standards, and assists employers by providing technical assistance and consultation programs. Fines are levied against employers who are not in compliance with OSHA Standards.

Chemical Hazards

Caustic: *burning or corrosive; destructive to tissue*

Carcinogenic: *cancer causing*

One of OSHA's charges is to maintain a safe working environment for those who produce and work with chemicals. To avoid injury, chemicals must be handled carefully. OSHA requires that safety regulations, procedures, and policies be accessible to all laboratory personnel. This information must be kept in a safety manual. OSHA also requires that every employer in the United States implement a federally defined "Hazard Communication Program" for its employees. This program must include both *warning* and *training* regarding hazardous chemicals in the workplace. Chemicals may be flammable, **caustic,** poisonous, **carcinogenic,** or explosive. (Figure 2–1 gives examples of warning symbols that are used to identify corrosive, toxic, and flammable materials.)

OSHA requires that vendors of hazardous chemicals provide their customers with Material Safety Data Sheets (MSDS), which give information on proper storage, han-

  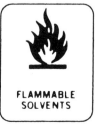

CORROSIVE MATERIALS

TOXIC CHEMICALS

FLAMMABLE SOLVENTS

Figure 2–1 Warning symbols for corrosive, toxic, and flammable materials.

dling, and disposal of the product. The MSDS also contain information on any health or safety risk associated with use or exposure.

Clinical Comment: The MSDS

The MSDS must answer the following questions regarding the hazardous substance:
- What is it?
- Who makes it or sells it?
- Where, in the laboratory, is it located?
- Why is it hazardous?
- What conditions could increase the hazard?
- How must it be handled?
- What protective equipment is required for safe use?
- What should you do if you are exposed to it?
- What do you do if there is a spill or an emergency?

All laboratories must maintain a notebook containing the MSDS for each chemical used in the laboratory. Table 2–1 lists safety guidelines that should be followed when working with chemicals.

HAZARDOUS CHEMICAL LABELING SYSTEM

National Fire Prevention Association (NFPA) warning labels must be affixed to chemical containers (Fig. 2–2). These color-coded signs identify the following hazards:
- Blue area for health hazards
- Yellow area for reactivity
- Red area for flammability
- White area for specific hazards, such as corrosiveness or radioactivity (This area can also be used to specify protective equipment for safe handling.)

A numeric listing provides the danger rating as follows:
- 0 = none
- 1 = minor
- 2 = moderate
- 3 = severe
- 4 = extreme

Table 2–1   *Safety Guidelines—Chemicals*

- Use a **hood** when you work with flammable and **volatile** substances.
- Store flammable and volatile chemicals in a well-ventilated area.
- Never mouth pipette any substances. Use an aspirator bulb, a mechanical pipette, or suction.
- When chemicals are spilled or come in contact with the skin or eyes, apply copious amounts of water to the affected area.
- Become familiar with all reagents used in the tests you perform, and follow all safety instructions provided by the manufacturer.
- Immediately recap all reagent bottles containing toxic substances when not in use.
- Label all reagent bottles and include the date of preparation and the initials of the preparer.
- Label hazardous chemicals and indicate proper storage, handling, and disposal

Hood: *specially enclosed and ventilated workstations used to direct poisonous fumes and airborne microbes away from the laboratorian*

Volatile: *easily vaporized or evaporated*

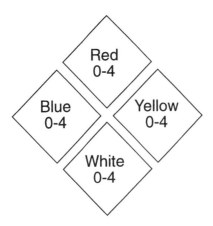

Figure 2-2 The NFPA system consists of four small, diamond-shaped symbols grouped into a larger diamond shape. (From Frew, MA, Lane, K, and Frew, D: Comprehensive Medical Assisting: Competencies for Administrative and Clinical Practice, ed 3, FA Davis, Philadelphia, 1995, p 737.)

Electrical Hazards

Electrical equipment may be a source of fire, burns, or electrical shocks. Care must be taken to minimize these risks. Observe the following when working with electrical equipment.

- Ground all electrical equipment and use three-pronged Underwriters Laboratories (UL) or Canadian Standards Association (CSA) approved plugs.
- Avoid using extension cords.
- Never overload electrical circuits.
- Inspect all cords and plugs periodically.
- Unplug electrical equipment before servicing, even if the service is as minor as replacing the light bulb in a microscope.
- Use electrical equipment in accordance with the manufacturer's directions.
- Use a surge protector on sensitive electronic equipment and computers to adjust for unexpected spikes in electrical power.
- Use signs and labels to indicate the presence of high-voltage equipment or other electrical hazards (Fig. 2-3).

Biologic Hazards

Pathogenic: *capable of causing disease*

Biologic specimens are a unique source of risk to health and safety. Specimens often contain **pathogenic** bacteria, viruses, fungi, and other parasites that can inadvertently infect the clinical laboratorian. All members of the health-care team, and especially clinical laboratorians, should understand the infectious process.

INFECTIOUS PROCESS

Five factors or links are included in the infectious cycle. If there is an interruption in the cycle at any link, the cycle is broken and the infectious process ends. All infection control is based on breaking at least one link of the cycle (Fig. 2-4).

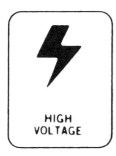

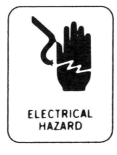

Figure 2-3 Warning symbols for electrical hazard.

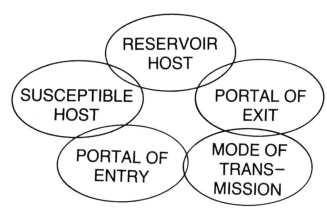

Figure 2-4 Links in the infectious cycle.

The Infectious Cycle

- *Reservoir host*—the individual who harbors the infectious organism
- *Portal of exit*—the place on the body (mouth, skin, rectum, wound, etc.) where the infectious organism leaves the reservoir host
- *Mode of transmission*—the method the infectious organism uses to go from the patient to the susceptible host (air, food, hands, body fluids, insects, etc.)
- *Portal of entry*—the place on the body of the susceptible host that the organism uses for an entry (mucous membrane, wound, mouth, nose, skin, vascular system, etc.)
- *Susceptible host*—the individual who, lacking body defenses against the pathogen, may develop the disease and become a new reservoir host

The analysis of body specimens—whole blood, plasma, **exudates**, stool (feces), and urine—is the focus of attention in a clinical laboratory. These specimens often contain pathogenic organisms. They serve as the mode of transmission of infection from the patient. If a pathogenic organism successfully enters a susceptible host, the infectious process continues.

Laboratorians and all who handle and process specimens must protect against exposure to the pathogenic organisms associated with clinical specimens by breaking one of the links in the chain of the infectious process. An understanding of the infectious process and especially the modes of transmission of various pathogens is the best defense against accidental exposure.

Exudates: *pathological fluids that collect in tissue spaces*

SPECIAL CONCERNS IN THE CLINICAL LABORATORY

Two dangerous diseases are a constant threat to the health and safety of the clinical laboratorian, hepatitis B and AIDS (acquired immune deficiency syndrome). Both of these potentially deadly diseases are transmitted through exposure to blood and body fluids. The infectious process for both diseases is similar. In the laboratory setting, these diseases are transmitted by way of blood and other potentially infectious material from the infected patient to the vascular system (breaks in skin, needlestick injuries, etc.) or to the mucous membranes (eyes, nose, or mouth) of the laboratorian.

Hepatitis B is a viral infection that attacks the liver. It is transmitted by the hepatitis B virus (HBV). Originally it was believed that HBV could be transmitted only through blood exposure (transfusions, contaminated needles, etc.). We now know that the disease is transmitted via other body fluids.

Clinical Comment: Hepatitis B Virus

About 10 percent of those infected with HBV become "carriers" and pose a risk to others, as well as being at risk themselves. Carriers often develop chronic hepatitis, cirrhosis of the liver, and a certain type of liver cancer. An HBV carrier has about 340 times the risk of developing primary liver cancer than does a person from the same environment who is not a carrier of the disease. Fortunately, an effective vaccine for HBV is now available, and all those who routinely work with body fluids should receive the vaccine. It is a three-dose series, and the physician-employer must offer the vaccine and defray its cost for employees engaged in activities that may expose them to this virus. There are about 8700 new cases yearly of HBV among workers in the health-care professions.

Compromised:
weakened

The causative organism of AIDS is the human immunodeficiency virus (HIV). In this disease the body's defense mechanisms are **compromised.** The patient with a weakened immune system contracts a host of diseases he or she could normally fight were it not for the deficient immune state. Diseases of this nature are called *opportunistic infections*. In other words, organisms that are normally "friendly" or "neutral" seize the opportunity provided when body defenses are low to invade areas where they are normally not present or to multiply to such a large number that they cause disease. Patients with AIDS (PWAs) usually die of opportunistic infections.

HISTORICAL PERSPECTIVE

In 1983 the Centers for Disease Control (CDC) published a document titled "Blood and Body Fluid Precautions." This publication listed precautions for health-care workers who come in contact with the blood and body fluids of patients known to be or suspected of being infected with a bloodborne pathogen, especially the HBV virus. It provided guidelines to protect against the spread of infections associated with exposure to blood and body fluids.

In 1987, responding to the concerns of health-care workers who are exposed to the HIV virus, the CDC published a document titled "Recommendations for Prevention of HIV Transmission in Health-Care Settings." This document directed that the blood and certain body fluids of *all patients* be considered potentially infectious. The guidelines extending blood and body fluid precautions to all patients are referred to as "universal blood and body fluid precautions" or, more simply, "universal precautions." The universal precautions guidelines are designed to minimize or prevent **parenteral,** mucous membrane, and nonintact skin exposures of health-care workers to bloodborne infections, especially HBV and HIV.

Parenteral: *denoting any route other than the alimentary canal; piercing mucous membranes or the skin barrier through such events as needlesticks, human bites, cuts, and abrasions*

OSHA'S BLOODBORNE PATHOGENS STANDARD

Because of public concern regarding HBV and HIV, OSHA mandated the Bloodborne Pathogens (BBP) Standard, which covers all employees who could be "reasonably anticipated as the result of performing their job duties to face contact with blood and other potentially infectious materials." The BBP Standard requires that employers prepare an exposure control plan. This plan requires that employers (1) identify tasks, procedures, and job classifications where occupational exposure to blood is likely to occur; (2) establish methods that protect employees and comply with OSHA regulations; (3) implement a vaccination program for HBV; (4) provide training regarding bloodborne pathogens and the proper use of protective equipment; and (5) maintain records to show compliance with the BBP Standard. (Table 2–2 gives symbols for OSHA bloodborne pathogen exposure controls.)

Table 2-2 *Symbols for OSHA Bloodborne Pathogen Exposure Controls Applicable to Clinical Procedures*

  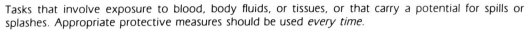 OSHA exposure categories applied to specific tasks as follows:

 Tasks that involve exposure to blood, body fluids, or tissues, or that carry a potential for spills or splashes. Appropriate protective measures should be used *every time.*

 Tasks that involve no exposure to blood, body fluids, or tissues in the normal work routine, but exposure or potential exposure may occur in certain situations. Appropriate protective measures should be used in these situations.

 Tasks that involve no exposure to blood, body fluids, or tissues. Appropriate protective measures are *not* necessary.

 Washing hands after a procedure.

  Washing hands before and after a procedure.

 Disposable sharp equipment that must not be bent, recapped, removed, sheared, or purposely broken. Equipment should be disposed of in a rigid, leakproof, puncture-resistant container that is color-coded orange or orange-red or labeled with the orange-red biohazard sign.

 Reusable sharp equipment that must be placed immediately, or as soon as possible, after use into appropriate sharps containers. The containers used to receive contaminated equipment must be puncture-resistant, leakproof, and color-coded orange or orange-red or labeled with the orange-red biohazard sign.

 Face shielding with masks and goggles is required as protection whenever splashes, spray, splatter, or droplets of blood or other potentially infectious materials may be generated and eye, nose, or mouth contamination can reasonably be anticipated.

 Protective clothing, such as laboratory coats, gowns, or aprons, is required as protection whenever splashes, spray, splatter, or droplets of blood or other potentially infectious materials may be generated and clothing contamination can reasonably be anticipated.

 Biohazard bags must be used to discard materials containing blood or other potentially infectious materials. The bags must be leakproof and color-coded orange or orange-red or labeled with the orange-red biohazard sign.

 Decontamination requires using a bleach solution or Environmental Protection Agency–registered germicide. All contaminated work surfaces must be decontaminated after completion of procedures and immediately, or as soon as feasible, after any spill of blood or other potentially infectious materials (as well as at the end of the work shift) if the surface may have become contaminated since the last cleaning.

 Gloves must be worn when it is reasonably anticipated that there will be hand contact with blood, other potentially infectious materials, nonintact skin, and mucous membranes. Gloves are not to be washed or decontaminated for reuse and are to be replaced as soon as practical when they become contaminated, or if they are torn or punctured or their ability to function as a barrier is compromised. *Utility* gloves may be decontaminated for reuse provided that the glove is intact and able to function as a barrier. *Examination* gloves are used for nonsterile procedures. *Sterile* gloves are used for minor surgery and other sterile procedures.

Source: Frew, MA, Lane, K, and Frew, DR: Comprehensive Medical Assisting: Competencies for Administrative and Clinical Practice, ed 3, FA Davis, Philadelphia, 1995, Table 17–1, with permission.

Methods of Compliance

OSHA compliance regulations regarding bloodborne pathogens are grouped into four areas:

- Adoption of universal precautions
- Engineering and work practice controls
- Personal protective equipment
- Housekeeping techniques

UNIVERSAL PRECAUTIONS

In addition to blood and blood products, the BBP Standard also applies to any "other potentially infectious materials" (OPIM). The only body fluid or material not specifically included in OSHA's BBP Standard is urine. However, because blood and blood elements are frequently associated with urine, it must be considered as a possible source of contamination.

OPIM include semen, vaginal secretions, cerebrospinal fluid, synovial fluid, pleural fluid, pericardial fluid, peritoneal fluid, amniotic fluid, saliva in dental procedures, any body fluid that is visibly contaminated with blood, and all body fluids in situations in which it is difficult or impossible to differentiate between body fluids. They also include any unfixed tissue or organ other than intact skin from a human (living or dead), human immunodeficiency virus (HIV)–containing cell or tissue cultures, organ cultures, and HIV or hepatitis B (HBV)–containing culture medium or other solutions as well as blood, organs, or other tissues from experimental animals infected with HIV or HBV.

(Bloodborne Pathogens Standard Number: 1910.1030.)

ENGINEERING AND WORK PRACTICE CONTROLS

Handwashing

Handwashing is a cornerstone in the prevention of infection. It is the single most effective way of preventing the spread of infection. Proper handwashing removes infectious organisms and protects you as well as the patients you serve. The following handwashing guide should be scrupulously observed:

- Wash hands on arriving at and before leaving the laboratory.
- Wash hands before and after each patient encounter.
- Wash hands after contact with blood and body fluids even when gloves are worn.
- Wash hands before and after eating.
- Wash hands before and after using the restroom.

Needles and Sharps

Use great care when handling needles and sharps. Avoid recapping. Use puncture-proof containers for sharps disposal (Fig. 2–5). If leaking of infectious material is anticipated, the container must be placed within a second container with directions for decontamination should leaking occur.

Personal Rules of Safety

Microorganisms: *organisms so small that they cannot be seen by the human eye (e.g., bacteria)*

Do not eat, drink, or smoke in the laboratory. Never store food or beverages in refrigerators containing chemicals, **microorganisms,** or clinical specimens. Do not apply cosmetics in the laboratory. Observe proper dress code. Laboratory coats, jackets, or aprons must be worn when engaged in laboratory duties. Be sure to remove them before leaving the laboratory.

Specimen Handling and Processing

Aerosol: *a solution that is dispensed in the form of a mist*

Use procedures that minimize splashing, spraying, or generating **aerosol** exposures. Keep specimens tightly covered whenever possible. Never mouth pipette.

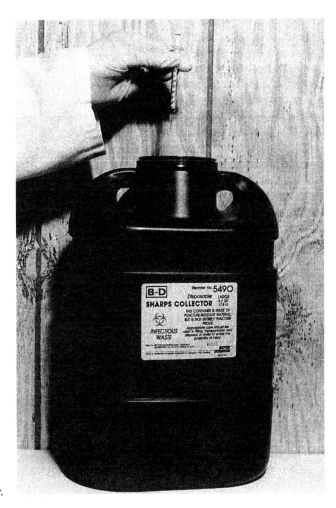

Figure 2-5 Sharps container.

Warning Labels

Use warning labels when equipment and instruments have become soiled with biologic material. Use labels that state the potential hazard and instructions for decontamination. The **biohazard** symbol (Fig. 2–6) indicates that the material within the container may contain *infectious organisms*. Infectious organisms are disease-causing bacteria, viruses, **protozoa,** or fungi that can be transmitted to others through exposure. The biohazard symbol is placed on containers that may harbor certain disease-causing organisms, especially HBV and HIV. It alerts others to take additional care when handling or

> **Biohazard:** *anything that is potentially hazardous to human beings, other species, or the environment*

> **Protozoa:** *single-celled organisms, some of which are pathogenic*

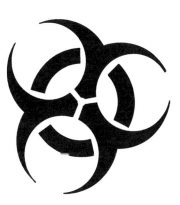

Figure 2-6 Biohazard symbol.

Incinerated: *burned*

Sterilized: *having been rendered totally free of all living microorganisms*

Autoclave: *laboratory instrument using steam under pressure to destroy microorganisms; sterilizer*

transporting the container. When the biohazard symbol appears on a container, the waste within the container must be **incinerated** or **sterilized** using an **autoclave** before disposal. See Table 2–3 for additional safety guidelines when working with OPIM.

PERSONAL PROTECTIVE EQUIPMENT

OSHA requires a personal protective equipment (PPE) program. The components of this program include:

- A workplace hazard assessment, with written hazard certification
- Proper equipment selection
- Employee information and training, with written competency certification
- Regular reassessment of work hazards

Use of Gloves for Phlebotomy

Gloves are required for all phlebotomy procedures, including fingersticks. They must be made available to all employees who collect blood. They are to be worn whenever there is even a remote possibility of blood or OPIM contact. They must be replaced between patients, after gross contamination, after extended wear, and when there is a break or tear.

Because gloves do not protect against penetration injuries, adhere to the following guidelines:

- Use care when handling needles, scalpels, and other sharp instruments or devices.
- Do not remove used needles from disposable syringes by hand.
- Do not break, bend, or otherwise manipulate needles or syringes.
- Place used disposable syringes and needles, scalpel blades, and other sharp items in a **sharps container** for disposal.
- Place the sharps container as close as practical to the area of use.

Sharps container: *puncture-resistant container for disposal of needles, scalpels, and so forth*

Clinical Comment: Double-Gloving

Although latex gloves do not protect against penetration injuries, they reduce the possibility of contracting disease. Most authorities believe that blood on the surface of the needle is wiped away, to a large extent, as the needle passes through the latex glove. Because of this, when drawing blood from a known HIV- or HBV-positive patient, many authorities recommend double-gloving.

Eye and Face Protection

Goggles, glasses, masks, face shields, and counter shields are required as barriers to mucous membrane exposure, when splashing, splattering, spraying, or aerosol exposure to blood or OPIM is anticipated.

Germicidal agent: *a substance that destroys microorganisms*

Disinfectant: *a substance that controls the spread of infection by destroying disease-causing organisms*

Table 2–3 *Safety Guidelines—OPIM*

- Handle and process all specimens as if they contained infectious material.
- Wipe the outside of specimen containers with a **germicidal agent.**
- Dispose of all infectious materials following federal and state laws.
- Clean up spills using a **disinfectant.** (An effective disinfectant for most routine cleanups can be prepared by mixing 1 part household bleach with 9 parts water. This should be made fresh weekly. Keep it within easy reach when working with blood or OPIM.)
- Immediately dispose of any chipped or broken glassware in a special disposable box. (Broken glass must not be discarded in a regular trash can since the cleaning staff may be injured when they collect trash containing broken glass.)

Body Clothing

Gowns, aprons, lab coats, surgical caps and scrubs, shoe covers, and disposable arm sleeves must be worn when there is the possibility of contamination to parts of the body or garments not covered by gloves, eye protection, or face guards.

HOUSEKEEPING

OSHA provides guidelines for the cleaning and decontamination of surfaces, equipment, and receptacles and for the handling of broken glassware. Institutions are required to have policies and procedures for all housekeeping tasks. They must be detailed and specific, including the type of disinfectant or sterilization method to be used for each cleaning or decontamination task.

Record Keeping

OSHA requires that accurate and complete medical records be maintained for all employees with occupational exposure. The records must be kept confidential and maintained for 30 years. The record must include:

- Employee name and social security number
- HBV status
- A copy of all results of examinations, medical testing, and follow-up necessitated by the exposure incident (The employee may elect to have this information remain with the examining health-care professional for confidentiality.)
- The employer's copy of the examining health-care professional's opinion if an exposure incident occurs

SUMMARY

Medical assistants and all who work in a clinical laboratory must be committed to safety in the workplace. Although it is impossible to anticipate every health and safety risk, common sense provides a basis for safe laboratory practices. When in doubt regarding the safety of a procedure, ask your supervisor or refer to the facility's Safety Manual. Learn the symbols used to indicate hazards in the laboratory, and use appropriate protection.

The BBP Standard specifically addresses the dangers associated with HIV and HBV. Use PPE and barrier protection when exposure is possible.

If you become aware of a safety hazard, tell someone in authority. Your welfare, and that of your coworkers and patients, depends on a commitment to safety by all members of the health-care team.

Questions

Name _____ Date _____

1. What is OSHA? Briefly describe OSHA's Hazard Communication Program.

2. What is an MSDS? What is its purpose? How are MSDS records maintained?

3. Describe the NFPA warning label as to color and number.

4. What are the five factors in the infectious cycle?

5. Give the two major bloodborne pathogens associated with clinical laboratory practice, and give their portal of entry.

6. What is the OSHA Bloodborne Pathogens Standard? On what document is this standard based?

7. List some of the specimens listed as "other potentially infectious material."

8. List several engineering and work practice controls designed to control the spread of bloodborne pathogens in the clinical laboratory.

9. List some personal protective equipment and tell when each is used.

10. Tell what records must be kept on employees who have occupational exposure to bloodborne pathogens.

Legal and Ethical Considerations

3

Learning Objectives
Cognitive Objectives

CLIA '88
Levels of Tests
Requirements for Testing Personnel
  ○ Personnel records
Proficiency Testing
Quality Control Procedures

Tort Law
Personal Liability
Elements of a Tort
  ○ Respondeat superior

○ Acts done outside the scope of
  authority
Malpractice
  ○ Standard of care documentation
Intentional Torts
  ○ Assault and battery
    Informed consent
  ○ Invasion of privacy
    Right to know

Ethics

Summary

Questions

LEARNING OBJECTIVES

On completing this chapter, you will be able to:

COGNITIVE OBJECTIVES
- Briefly explain the major areas of the CLIA '88 regulations.
- List the three levels of testing identified by CLIA and briefly explain each.
- List the elements of a tort and explain assault and battery as they relate to the medical laboratory.
- Explain the importance of proper documentation in the medical office.
- Identify the features that constitute informed consent.
- Explain the importance of privacy and confidentiality as they relate to laboratory testing.
- Relate some obligations identified in the Code of Ethics of the American Association of Medical Assistants.

Two important areas of law directly affect those who work in laboratory medicine. These are the Clinical Laboratory Improvement Act of 1988 (CLIA, CLIA '88) and a broad area of civil law known as **tort law.**

CLIA is a comprehensive set of regulations that became effective in February 1992. It addresses quality control, quality assurance, record keeping (see Chapter 4), and the educational and experiential qualifications of testing personnel. CLIA affects everyone who tests human specimens for the diagnosis, prevention, or treatment of disease.

Tort law is based on the premise that in a civilized society, people will conduct themselves so that they will not negligently or intentionally harm others. Patients have the same rights as all members of society to be free from harm. In fact, additional rights are afforded patients because of the special relationship they have with their physician.

Although they are not legally mandated, the principles associated with **professional ethics** are a third area of influence that regulates the interaction of patient and health-care professional. Professionals are expected and required to conduct themselves in

Tort law: *the area of civil law that involves breaches of duty that cause injury*

Professional ethics: *a written code of behavior designed to regulate the behavior of members of a professional organization*

25

their professional endeavors in a manner that represents the highest form of moral behavior. This includes the interactions of colleagues. Professional ethics are specific to each health-care occupation. Although there is also a philosophical area of influence involving **moral ethics** that examines questions of "right" and "wrong" and "good" and "bad" (e.g., abortion and right-to-die issues), this area is beyond the scope of this text.

Moral ethics: *the philosophy that deals with "good" and "evil"*

CLIA '88

The CLIA '88 provisions were not the first laws designed to ensure quality testing in clinical laboratories, but they were the first to bring the physician's office laboratory (POL) under federal scrutiny.

Prior to CLIA '88 it was not unusual to observe a variety of individuals, from the receptionist to the physician, performing at least some aspects of laboratory testing in POLs. Traditionally, only a few uncomplicated tests were performed in the physician's office. However, with the advent of automated equipment it became possible to perform a variety of tests in POLs that were previously performed only in hospital laboratories. Many POLs consequently expanded their testing menu to include more than just the simplest tests.

Methodology: *a sequence of steps that a skilled professional takes to achieve a specific result*

Levels of Tests

Three levels of tests are defined by CLIA and are categorized according to their complexity.

Waived tests are uncomplicated and require minimal quality control rigors and documentation. They are safe, cost-effective, and have demonstrated accuracy and precision. No special training or educational background is required to perform waived tests. The number and types of waived tests have been growing over the past few years. The general types of tests that are now included in the waived test menu are those that require minimum quality control and are simple to perform and those that have been approved for home use such as the Blood Glucose System and Blood Hemoglobin System manufactured by HemoCue, Inc. Even though these tests are easy to perform, the office physician must be able to validate that all results are accurate and precise and belong to the patient from whom the specimen was obtained.

Calibration: *procedure to make the results of a measuring instrument accurate by assessing a substance of a known value for the purpose of setting the instrument's output to match the substance's known value*

Moderate-complexity tests are more complicated to perform than waived tests and require understanding of test **methodology**, including quality control, reagent stability, and instrument **calibration.** Most testing procedures, approximately 7500 tests and analytes, fall into this category. Currently, personnel who perform moderate-complexity tests must have at least a minimum of a high school diploma and documentation of satisfactory completion of training appropriate to the testing performed in the specific office. The training may have been obtained either formally through schooling or informally on the job, depending on the particular state requirements.

Cytology: *the science that deals with the formation, structure, and function of cells*

Cytogenetics: *the study of cells in relation to genetics, especially as it relates to the diagnosis of fetal abnormalities*

High-complexity tests include sophisticated testing methodology, and they frequently require independent judgment for interpretation. Educational and experiential background for personnel who perform these tests are more stringent than for moderate-complexity tests. Included in this category are clinical **cytology, cytogenetics, histopathology,** and **histocompatibility.** High-complexity testing is usually not performed in POLs.

By 1997, changes in personnel qualifications are anticipated, and the reader is directed to become familiar with current standards that apply to testing personnel.

Histopathology: *study associated with tissue changes that accompany disease*

Requirements for Testing Personnel

Histocompatibility: *the study associated with tissue compatibility between donor and recipient in organ transplantation*

Testing personnel are employees whose main responsibility includes specimen processing, testing, and reporting results. The present CLIA minimum requirements include a high

Table 3–1 **Documentation for Personnel Files**

- Job application
- Résumé
- Copy of certificates, licenses, or registration numbers (if applicable)
- Copy of degrees, military laboratory training certificates, or technical school diplomas
- Documentation of any on-the-job training
- Documentation of any continuing hours of education
- Documentation of "right to know" and/or safety training
- Results of hepatitis B virus (HBV) prescreening test and/or HBV vaccine form
- Detailed job description
- Annual evaluation
- OSHA training on bloodborne pathogens

school diploma and appropriate training for most of the tests currently performed in POLs. Some states have additional experiential and educational requirements for laboratory testing. Also, some states do not allow medical assistants to perform invasive (venipuncture) procedures. Before undertaking any laboratory task, be sure that you have the proper education and experience as determined by your State Board of Medical Examiners.

PERSONNEL RECORDS

Because CLIA has identified qualifications for employees who do waived, moderate-complexity, and high-complexity testing, personnel files must document the educational training of POL staff. Complete personnel records are required and must be available for inspection (Table 3–1).

Personnel files are confidential documents and must be kept in a secured place, available only to the physician and office manager.

Proficiency Testing

Proficiency testing (PT) is an external evaluation of the quality of a laboratory's performance. Three times during the year the physician's office laboratory receives from an external PT laboratory five sample specimens for each analyte tested by the POL. These samples are tested with patient samples, and the results are returned to the PT laboratory for evaluation. With few exceptions, the passing score is 80 percent.

Quality Control Procedures

Quality control (QC) procedures are designed to ensure accuracy and precision for each of the analytes that are tested in the POL. At a minimum, manufacturer's instructions must be scrupulously followed. Calibration procedures for all instruments must be performed and documented at least once every 6 months. Two levels of controls must be run daily. A procedures manual must be developed that includes all relevant information regarding each test. It should cover specimen collection, handling, and processing. The conditions that cause the specimen to be rejected must be identified. The procedures manual must also document remedial action to be taken when errors occur in specimen testing (see Chapter 4).

TORT LAW

Personal Liability

In our society, when one member causes injury or harm to another, the injuring party is responsible and must make restitution to the injured party. We know that when we drive a car and have an accident, we must pay for the harm we cause. It doesn't matter whether we were driving recklessly or carefully—if we cause injury, we must make restitution. It is of little consequence in the eyes of the law that the car skidded on a patch of ice, or that our brakes failed, we are still **liable** for the injury. This same legal theory holds true in the delivery of health care. When medical personnel cause injury to patients, they are responsible to the patient for the injury. The branch of civil law that deals with behavior that causes injury to others is called *tort law*.

Elements of a Tort

For liability to exist, the following elements or components that identify a tort must be present:

- A duty owed by the health-care provider to the injured party (patient)
- A breach of this duty
- A loss of something valuable by the injured party
- A direct connection between the failure in the duty of the health-care provider and the resulting loss (damages) by the injured party

In a health-care setting, the duty owed to the patient arises from the expressed or implied medical contract that exists between the physician and the patient. A breach of this duty can be any act that causes injury or loss, or it can be any failure to act that causes injury or loss. The act or failure to act must directly cause the injury to the patient. Finally, there must be a direct cause or causal connection between the breach of duty and the damages sustained by the patient. When all of these elements are met, a tort action by the patient against the physician or health-care provider is possible.

RESPONDEAT SUPERIOR

Others may share liability with the individual who has committed a tort. Under the legal doctrine of *respondeat superior*, the physician-employer is fully liable for all testing he or she authorizes to be performed in the POL. Courts have traditionally recognized that when an employee causes injury to a third party, the employer is often in a better financial position to compensate the injured party than is the employee. Therefore, the courts have imputed (assigned) liability to the employer for injuries to others caused by the careless behavior of the employee. The legal theory of *respondeat superior* holds that the employer, in the normal course of operating a business, is in a position to control the acts of the employee. If injuries caused by the careless behavior of the employee occur, the employer is not "properly controlling" the employee, and therefore is legally responsible for the injury. The doctrine of *respondeat superior* does not remove liability from the employee, however. The employee is always responsible for his or her careless behavior. The doctrine allows the injured party to seek compensation from both the employer and the employee.

ACTS DONE OUTSIDE THE SCOPE OF AUTHORITY

If, however, the employee disregards the directions of the employer, and acts outside the scope of authority, and in doing so, causes injury to another, the employee may be held fully and solely responsible for any injury sustained by the patient. For example, if the employee performs laboratory tests not authorized by the physician and in violation of CLIA guidelines, any injury sustained by the patient may result in liability only for the employee.

Malpractice

Malpractice is a term that generally relates to professional negligence. It applies to any action by a member of a profession who fails to meet the *standard of care* of that profession. To meet the required standard of care, physicians must treat their patients as other physicians who are similarly trained and with like experience normally treat their patients. In other words, when a patient presents with a "strep throat," one should expect that physicians with similar training and experience would treat this condition in a similar manner. A failure to act according to established practice is malpractice. It is the failure to meet the standard of care, or a deviation from the standard of care, that forms the basis of a malpractice suit.

Clinical Comment: Malpractice Prevention

- State medical practice acts define your scope of practice. Be sure you know and follow these laws.
- Perform only the tasks that you have been trained to perform.
- Document all aspects of your interactions with the patient:
  Patient education
  Specimen collections and processing
  Test reports and results
  Consent forms
  Verbal requests
- Advise the physician or office manager when patients have complaints or concerns.
- Maintain a professional demeanor in all professional encounters.

It is imperative that all health-care providers have the knowledge, skill, and expertise required of their specific profession and that they act accordingly. It is of little consequence in a court of law to say, "I didn't mean for this to happen." If you cause injury through negligence, you are liable for that injury. Intent is not a part of malpractice.

Because most allied health professionals, especially in a physician's office, work directly under the authority of a physician-employer, they must carefully follow all orders and directions of the physician-employer. Medical assistants must not assume tasks that they are not trained to do. When you take it upon yourself to do things that you are not authorized or trained to do, additional liability may result as a consequence of your behavior.

STANDARD OF CARE DOCUMENTATION

The best way to establish that you acted in accordance with the appropriate standard of care and that you did not violate any of your professional responsibilities is by carefully and completely documenting all interactions with the patient. In law, "If it is not recorded, it is not done!"

Documentation is necessary any time patient education is undertaken, specimens are collected, and test results are received and reported. Medical records are business records. As such, they can be subpoenaed as evidence in a court of law. They are used by the physician and the members of the medical office to establish:

- The type of care provided to the patient
- The level and type of visit (for the purpose of billing the carrier and/or the patient)
- That the treatment provided to the patient by the physician and the staff followed the accepted standard of practice

All medical records should be:

- Current
- Complete
- Concise
- Correct

- Confidential
- Clean

Because of our current medical-legal environment, the office visit should be appropriately documented to verify that accepted standards of practice were followed. In other words, the medical record must do more than document patient care. The medical record must also provide a "paper trail" that clearly documents that the care provided during the visit is the same care that would be provided in any other physician's office under similar circumstances.

Be sure that the patient's name is on each page of the medical record. Write in black ink. Record the date and time of all entries. Do not document for others. Make sure that all entries are factual. Record only objective data. (*Correct:* "The patient was crying uncontrollably." *Incorrect:* "The patient was very sad.")

Clinical Comment: The "SLIDE" Rule

> When mistakes occur in the medical record, the proper method of correction involves applying the "SLIDE" rule.
> Draw a Single Line through the mistake. Place your Initials and Date by the erroneous entry, and write the word "Error." Place the correct information as close as possible to the incorrect entry.

Intentional Torts

Patients have the same legal rights as the public in general. They do not lose these rights when they become patients. Some of the rights enjoyed by all members of society, including patients, are the right to be free from bodily harm, the right to own and dispose of property, the right to privacy, and the right to "one's good name."

A legal right places a corresponding duty on others not to violate or interfere with that right. Any time a duty owed to another is breached, the injury that results from the breach may be recoverable by the injured party.

ASSAULT AND BATTERY

Two important torts associated with the medical profession are *assault* and *battery*. Legally, assault is defined as putting a person in fear of life and limb, and battery is any unpermitted touching of another. Some of the procedures performed in the POL are "frightening" and may involve the actual touching of the patient, which may cause pain. As an example, even though a venipuncture is considered by most people as a routine procedure with a minimal amount of discomfort, some may consider it to be extremely frightening and painful. Experienced laboratorians can tell many tales about patients who faint at the sight of a needle. A simple venipuncture can, under certain circumstances, meet the legal definition of assault and battery. The defense to this allegation is *informed consent* by the patient. Once there is informed consent by the patient, the legal definition of battery is no longer present.

Informed Consent

Informed consent requires that you explain the procedure in simple terms and provide all the information a reasonably prudent person would need to decide whether to undergo the procedure. Patients do not have to be told about *all* risks. They should be told about those risks that are important for them to know and understand so that the consent is truly informed. Experienced laboratorians tell patients as much as possible, without unduly alarming them. Patients appreciate honesty. They lose trust if you say "moderate" pain and they experience "excruciating" pain.

For infants and young children, consent is given by parents or legal guardians. In an emergency situation, a court order can be sought when life-threatening conditions exist and parental consent cannot be obtained. Some jurisdictions allow minors to consent to reproductive services or drug treatment without the consent or notification of the parents. Health-care providers should know the law in their state.

When you are treating children who are old enough to understand the basic consequences of their actions (usually children about 12 years old), it is advisable to obtain their consent for treatment as well as that of their parents or guardians. This is referred to as the Doctrine of Mature Minors. States vary with respect to this doctrine, and it is always advisable to check with superiors if any doubt exists as to the validity of consent.

Any time a mature and mentally sound patient refuses a procedure, no matter how simple it is, the laboratorian must not proceed. Laboratorians must check with supervisors or physician-employers when such a refusal occurs.

INVASION OF PRIVACY

All laboratory test results are subject to the same requirements of confidentiality and privacy that are expected in the general practice of medicine. When health-care providers fail to protect the patient's right to privacy, they may be liable for any negative consequences that result. Unauthorized disclosure of medical information that you know as a result of your employment is not the only way to violate the patient's right to privacy. Leaving results of laboratory tests in areas where others can see them is also a violation of the patient's right to confidentiality and privacy. Even though no results are written on a test request slip, the disclosure of certain test orders may in itself violate the patient's right to confidentiality and privacy. For example, if a physician orders HIV testing for a patient, the laboratorian must never disclose this information to others. Test request slips must be kept away from the curious eyes of those who are in the physician's office.

If you are permitted and requested to give test results using the telephone, keep your voice low, or call from a private office so that patients in the waiting room do not overhear. Verify that the individual to whom information is given is the proper person to receive the information. Do not give the information to another individual and ask this person to give the "message" to the patient. If in doubt as to the identity of the person on the phone, do not give out the information—not even to parents or spouses—especially in the event of pregnancy, sexually transmitted diseases, or drug or alcohol dependence. Unless the medical information involves employment physicals, and the patient has signed a release form, do not give any information to the employer of the patient. Information cannot even be given to insurance companies without a release signed by the patient.

Right to Know

Laboratory results can be given only to those who have a right or a need to know. This right belongs first and foremost to the patient, and it is the physician's duty and prerogative to give laboratory results to the patient. The medical contract exists between the patient and the physician, not the patient and the laboratorian. As an employee of the physician, your duty is to provide information regarding test results to the physician. The physician then relays the information to the patient. When laboratorians give results to the patient without the authorization of the physician, the legal presumption may be that the laboratorian is "practicing medicine without a license."

If patients request information on "lab work," be sure you are authorized by the physician to give it to the patient, or refer the patient to the physician.

Some laboratory results can have both legal and medical implications. Do not give information to the employer of a patient, the spouse of a patient, the parent of a teenage patient, the insurance company of the patient, or any third party unless specifically directed to do so by the physician. You must also have the written permission of the patient. Your physician-employer must always be consulted when nonroutine requests for information on laboratory results are sought by others.

ETHICS

Laws involve minimum standards of behavior needed to keep society running smoothly. *Ethics* involve the highest standards of moral conduct. They challenge individuals to go above and beyond the "bare minimum" standards of behavior in their interactions with others. The goal of ethical behavior is to make the world a better place to live.

Character traits needed by all health-care professionals include compassion, sensitivity, a love of people, and a desire to serve. Those who choose a career in health care must have more than a love of the discipline. They must also love people. Skills can al-

```
                        CODE OF ETHICS
The Code of Ethics of AAMA shall set forth principles of

ethical and moral conduct as they relate to the medical

profession and the particular practice of medical assisting.


Members of the AAMA dedicated to the conscientious pursuit of

their profession, and thus desiring to merit the high regard

of the entire medical profession and the respect of the

general public which they serve, do pledge themselves to

strive always to:

    A. render service with full respect for the dignity of

    humanity;

    B. respect confidential information obtained through

    employment unless legally authorized or required by

    responsible performance of duty to divulge such

    information;

    C. uphold the honor and high principles of the profession

    and accept its disciplines;

    D. seek to continually improve the knowledge and skills

    of professional colleagues;

    E. participate in additional service activities aimed

    toward improving the health and well-being of the

    community.
```

Figure 3-1   Code of Ethics of the American Association of Medical Assistants.

ways be taught; love and concern cannot be taught. Before entering into any people-oriented profession, you should take a personal inventory that focuses on your relationships with others. Do you have a list of people you don't speak to anymore? What type of relationship do you have with the members of your family? What were your feelings toward classmates and teachers? In relationships, are you as willing to "give" as you are to "take"? Attention to detail is part and parcel of those who serve in the medical profession. If detail work is not your style, then a rewarding career in health care will not be possible.

Thoroughness, friendliness, neatness, and a commitment to duty are a must for all who choose a career in health care. A laboratorian must have a desire to improve and grow as a health-care professional and stay current in his or her area of expertise. Continuing education and training are essential.

Needless to say, working with others requires tact, manners, and consideration. A friendly "good morning," "please," and "thank you" should be the hallmark of those who care for others. Good personal hygiene is absolutely necessary. Hair and nails must be neat and groomed. Uniforms should be cleaned and pressed. Avoid heavy or gaudy makeup, perfumes, and colognes. Your voice should always be calm and quiet. Loud and boisterous laughing or talking is out of place in a medical office.

Health-care providers occasionally need to take a personal inventory to see how they measure up to the ethical standards of their profession. Medical assistants, medical technologists, physicians, nurses, and other health-care professionals all have codes of ethics that help clarify the obligations required of their specific discipline. The Code of Ethics of the American Association of Medical Assistants (Fig. 3–1) is based on the Code of Ethics of the American Medical Association. It parallels the **tenets** found in the ethics codes of the various health disciplines. The code of ethics for your health-care discipline should serve as a foundation for your professional life.

Tenets: *principles, dogmas, or opinions*

SUMMARY

The CLIA regulations were designed to ensure that laboratory testing produces accurate and reliable results. Several areas of clinical practice were placed under CLIA regulations, including personnel qualifications. Three levels of testing are identified by CLIA: waived, moderate-complexity, and high-complexity testing. Testing personnel must know the level of tests they are qualified to perform. Their educational and experiential training must meet the requirements established by CLIA.

A comprehensive set of civil law, known as tort law, impacts on clinical practice. The torts that may arise in laboratory testing include malpractice, also called professional negligence, and the intentional torts of assault, battery, and invasion of privacy.

Ethics are high standards of performance demanded by professional organizations. When health-care providers follow the code of ethics of their profession, it helps ensure that the best care possible is provided for all patients.

Questions

Name _____ Date _____

1. Briefly explain the purpose of CLIA '88.

2. What information should be kept in personnel files of those who do laboratory testing in a POL?

3. Name three levels of testing identified by CLIA and briefly explain each.

4. What is a tort? List the elements of a tort.

5. What is malpractice?

6. List some of the features required in documentation, and briefly explain the "SLIDE" rule.

7. What is informed consent? Why is it important to obtain informed consent prior to undertaking medical procedures?

8. List ways to protect the patient's right to privacy.

9. Briefly explain "need to know" as it relates to a medical setting.

10. Briefly describe the major areas included in professional ethics.

Quality Assurance and Quality Control

4

Learning Objectives
Cognitive Objectives

Quality Assurance

Quality Control
Standards and Controls
Systematic Error
Random Error
Specimen Collection

Laboratory Personnel Orientation
Laboratory Procedure Manual

Laboratory Documentation

Laboratory Instrumentation

Proficiency Testing

Summary

Questions

LEARNING OBJECTIVES

On completing this chapter, you will be able to:

COGNITIVE OBJECTIVES

- Describe quality assurance in the clinical laboratory and list five aspects of quality assurance.
- Describe quality control and explain why quality control procedures promote accuracy and precision.
- Explain systematic and random error of test results.
- List the guidelines for specimen collection and tell how they relate to quality control.
- Explain how personnel orientation and laboratory documentation are necessary for quality assurance.
- Explain the relationship of instrument calibration and maintenance to quality assurance.
- Describe proficiency testing as it relates to quality assurance.

Clinical laboratories must establish and follow policies and procedures that (1) monitor and evaluate quality, (2) identify and correct problems, (3) provide a competent staff through personnel orientation, and (4) ensure accurate and precise test results. The physician is responsible for overseeing these policies and procedures, and the laboratorian is responsible for reviewing quality control data, interpreting the proficiency testing program, and ensuring that quality assurance policies are implemented.

QUALITY ASSURANCE

Quality assurance (QA) is a comprehensive set of policies and procedures developed to ensure the accuracy and reliability of laboratory testing. It includes:

- Quality control
- Personnel orientation
- Laboratory documentation

- Knowledge of laboratory instrumentation
- Enrollment in a proficiency testing program

Quality assurance benefits the patient, the physician, and the laboratorian. QA benefits the patient by providing quality test results so that an accurate diagnosis can be determined. It benefits the physician by reducing the possibility that disease conditions might be undiagnosed because of the inaccurate reporting of test results. In order for the physician to diagnose a disease condition, he or she must compare laboratory test results with **reference values** established for the population in the physician's geographic area. Reference values or ranges may vary by region. Reference values may also vary according to age, sex, and physical conditions. Determining the reference values for the patients in a specific population is a necessary part of quality assurance.

QA benefits the laboratorian by providing guidelines for the performance of laboratory duties. QA allows the person performing the test to detect small but significant changes from the usual performance before erroneous patient test results are reported. At the same time, the QA program enables the laboratorian to assess, verify, and document the quality of laboratory test results.

> **Reference values (normal values, expected values):** *a range of values determined for each analyte that includes the expected results when performed on healthy people*

QUALITY CONTROL

Quality control (QC) procedures are designed to ensure that laboratory tests produce accurate and precise results. Laboratory results are used by the physician to diagnose disease conditions, prescribe treatment, and monitor a patient's progress. For laboratory test reports to be useful to the physician for these purposes, they must be accurate and precise. The fact that a laboratorian can perform a specific test does not guarantee that the test results will be accurate or precise.

Accuracy is how closely a measurement approximates the true value of an **analyte**. *Precision* refers to the reproducibility or closeness of results. A laboratory test result should be both accurate and precise. However, a test result can be precise and still not be accurate (Fig. 4–1).

For example, for a patient sample that has a true glucose value of 80 mg/dL, accurate test results may be 81, 80, 82, or 79 mg/dL, as determined by the manufacturer. An example of a precise but not an accurate result would be determinations of 90, 91, 92, and 94 mg/dL. The QC program helps to guarantee accuracy and precision by monitoring and detecting variations in the test system.

> **Analyte:** *the substance or constituent being measured*

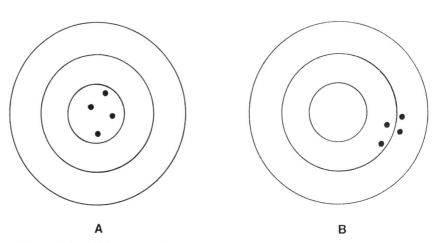

| A | B |

Figure 4–1 *(A)* Accuracy and precision demonstrated. *(B)* Precision without accuracy.

Standards and Controls

QC procedures involve using a **standard** or analyzing substances called **controls**. When the standard is reproduced and the control results are within the acceptable range provided by the manufacturer, the unknown value can be considered correct. Standards are used in the **calibration** of instruments to guarantee that the equipment is working properly so that results are accurate. *Controls* are used to check the equipment, the chemical reagents, and expertise of the laboratorian performing the analysis.

Sera are commercially prepared controls specific for the analyte being tested. Normal and abnormal controls are used before or along with each run of patient specimens. The normal control has normal quantities of an analyte, and the abnormal control has abnormally high or abnormally low quantities of an analyte. The control test results are checked against a **range** of acceptable values listed on an **assay sheet** provided by the manufacturer of the controls. When a test result is *out of control,* that is, does not fall within the control range, the results must be rejected. Steps must be taken to discover the reasons for an out-of-control situation. Look for discrepancies in the equipment, the reagents, and the procedure. When corrected, repeat the testing process. A patient's results should not be reported until the control tests fall within an acceptable range.

A **Levey-Jennings chart** is used to display control results, demonstrate the range of results obtained, and alert the laboratorian to an out-of-control situation (Fig. 4–2). To use the chart, the laboratorian needs to know the **mean** and the **standard deviation** of the control. These are provided by the manufacturer of the control. The horizontal axis represents the days on which the control is run. The vertical axis represents the values obtained when the control is run. A chart is used for each type of control. For most automated chemistry instruments, controls are run in the same batch as patient samples. Instructions for the smaller chemistry instruments and hematology instruments advise first running the controls and evaluating the results. If they are in the acceptable range, the patient samples can be tested and results reported. However, if the controls do not fall within the acceptable range, then the patient test results must be rejected.

Clinical Comment: CLIA '88

> The Clinical Laboratory Improvement Amendment of 1988 (CLIA '88) requires laboratories to have quality control programs. In addition, CLIA '88 requires that the laboratory maintain Levey-Jennings charts for each procedure performed. Most instruments have standards and controls for their analyzers. Some of the newer instruments have quality control programs built into their computer systems. Moreover, the laboratory must participate in a proficiency testing program.

The plotting of control results immediately demonstrates when results are out of control. The Levey-Jennings chart in Figure 4–3 shows a *"trend."* Figure 4–4 demonstrates a *"shift."* A *trend* exists when six or more consecutive control values increase or decrease by moving in one direction above or below the mean. A *shift* occurs when more than six consecutive control values maintain a constant level above or below the mean. A Levey-Jennings chart is used in the laboratory to monitor the laboratorian's performance, check instruments, evaluate any new procedures, and troubleshoot for errors. There are two types of errors in testing: systematic and random.

Systematic Error

Systematic errors are those errors introduced into the test method that create a **bias** in the instrument. Systematic errors affect the *accuracy* of the testing procedures. A systematic error will cause the test results to be either consistently higher or consistently

---

Standard: *a substance that is prepared with a known quantity of the analyte being tested*

Controls: *materials, solutions, or collections of human sera having known concentrations of the same analytes as those being measured in the patient sample*

Calibration: *determining the accuracy of an instrument by comparing information or a measurement provided with that of a known standard or an instrument known to be accurate*

Range: *allowable limits in which the control's value is acceptable and patients' samples may be tested*

Assay sheet: *a sheet provided by manufacturers of controls showing the acceptable range of values*

Levey-Jennings chart: *a quality control chart that demonstrates the precision of a method using the calculated mean and standard deviation results*

Mean: *average of calculated values attained by summing them and dividing the sum by the number of values*

Standard deviation: *a statistical term describing the amount of variance from the mean value in a set of values*

Bias: *a measure of the departure from accuracy*

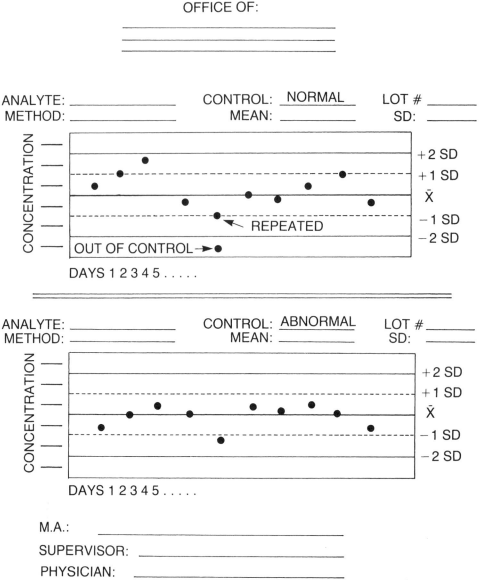

OFFICE OF:

ANALYTE: _____   CONTROL: <u>NORMAL</u>   LOT # _____
METHOD: _____   MEAN: _____   SD: _____

ANALYTE: _____   CONTROL: <u>ABNORMAL</u>   LOT # _____
METHOD: _____   MEAN: _____   SD: _____

M.A.: _____

SUPERVISOR: _____

PHYSICIAN: _____

Figure 4–2   Levey-Jennings quality control chart for normal and abnormal controls.

lower than the correct value. For example, the patient sample has a true glucose value of 96 mg/dL, but the laboratorian's results are 120, 125, 123, and 121 mg/dL when the sample is tested several times. Systematic errors are caused by incorrect instrument calibration or by using out-of-date or improperly prepared reagents. A function of the QC program is to detect systematic errors so that the laboratorian may be confident of the accuracy of test results being reported to the physician.

Random Error

Variance: *the amount by which results differ from each other in a set of values*

Random error appears as a slight **variance** in the test system each time the test is performed. Often these variances are due to human error. A temperature change within the instrument can cause a slightly different result when the test is repeated. The amount of

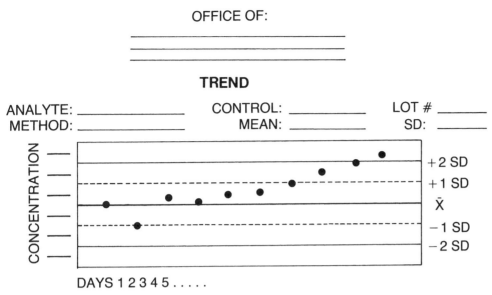

Figure 4–3 Levey-Jennings chart demonstrating a trend.

random error determines the *precision* or reproducibility of that test. For example, the patient sample has a true glucose value of 96 mg/dL, but random error produces results of 94, 98, 95, 91, and 99 mg/dL when the sample is tested several times.

Some variation in results is unavoidable. Because of these variations, CLIA '88 favors instrumentation with fewer steps in analysis rather than manual procedures where human error is more likely to occur. Random error may be introduced by the laboratorian if he or she does not perform the test procedure *exactly* the same way each time. Detection of a random error requires strict adherence to procedures. A good QC program monitors the testing of analytes for both systematic and random errors to be sure that reliable results are reported.

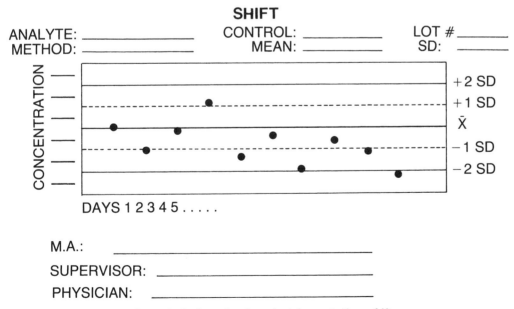

Figure 4–4 Levey-Jennings chart demonstrating a shift.

Specimen Collection

QC in the clinical laboratory includes the proper collection, handling, and processing of patient samples. Guidelines for specimen collection and handling are as follows:

- *Patient preparation.* Give the patient instructions regarding fasting, special diet, and ingestion of special preparations. Before administering the test, check to make sure the patient has followed the instructions.
- *Specimen collection.* Choose the proper containers, with **preservatives** if necessary.
- *Specimen labeling.* Label the container with the patient's name, age, sex, date, type of specimen, time of collection, physician's name, and the initials of the person responsible for the collection of the specimen.
- *Preparation of specimen for transport.* Follow any instructions specifically provided by the referral laboratory.
- *Procedure manual.* Consult the office manual for specific specimen collection instructions.

Preservative: *a substance used to inhibit or prevent changes in a specimen while not interfering with test results*

LABORATORY PERSONNEL ORIENTATION

A well-managed clinical laboratory provides new employees with clearly written instructions for each laboratory instrument. Every employee should be able to demonstrate proficiency in using the instrument. Orientation should include instruction in the proper use of QC materials and in the various test kits available for each instrument. A *laboratory procedure manual* is an excellent source for this material and is required by CLIA '88.

Laboratory Procedure Manual

The laboratory procedure manual should contain essential information for the performance of laboratory testing. The manual should also give up-to-date, step-by-step instructions for performing tests. A well-written procedure manual provides documentation of QA in your laboratory. The following information should be included in the laboratory procedure manual:

- Patient preparation and instructions for testing
- Requirements for specimen collection and processing, including criteria for rejection
- Step-by-step performance of test procedures, including calculation and interpretation of results
- Instrument calibration instructions and verification of procedures
- Test reference normal ranges with **panic values** as determined by your laboratory
- Limitations of test procedures, including interfering substances
- Sources of error
- QC procedures
- Remedial action to be taken when calibration or QC results fail to meet the criteria for acceptability as determined by your laboratory
- System for reporting test results established by your laboratory, including how panic values are handled
- Specimen preservation, storage, and transport required to insure specimen integrity until testing is completed
- Preparation of reagents, standards and controls, and other materials used in test performance
- Safety information for reagents, controls, and instruments
- Instrument maintenance instructions
- Literature references

Panic values: *levels of a substance that are considered life-threatening to the patient*

Manufacturers' product inserts may be included in the manual as a supplement but should not take the place of written instructions for each test performed. These inserts need to be monitored regularly for changes made by the manufacturer. All personnel performing tests should review the procedures periodically and document this review by initialing and dating on a special review page in the manual.

LABORATORY DOCUMENTATION

Documentation is an important aspect of QA in the laboratory. For proper documentation include the following elements:

- Log patient samples using an identification system that assigns a number to each specimen (Fig. 4–5).
- Record results on duplicate laboratory reports, one for charting and one for billing purposes.
- Establish protocol for reporting panic values.
- Establish a system for physician's review before charting reports.
- Indicate personnel who may release laboratory results and to whom they may be given.
- Maintain records of specimens sent to referral laboratories and results received.
- Establish guidelines for the security of records and confidentiality of reports.
- Set standards for reporting infectious diseases to the appropriate agencies when required by law.
- Maintain a test result log that records the actual test results for each instrument or test kit used (Fig. 4–6).
- Maintain a record of normal and abnormal control results (Fig. 4–7), proficiency testing results, instrument maintenance (Fig. 4–8), and time and temperature checks.

Patient Identification Log

DATE	PATIENT NAME	ID #	SPECIMEN	DATE/TIME COLLECTED	TEST ORDERED	RESULT	INITIALS

Figure 4–5   Sample of patient identification log.

Test Result Log

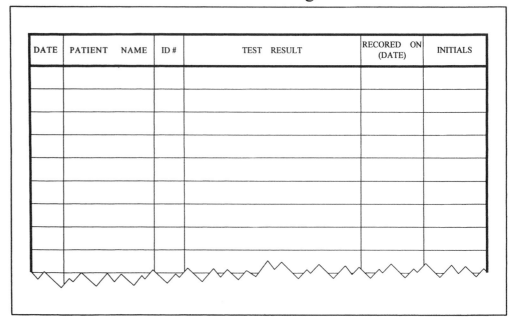

Figure 4–6 Sample of test result log.

LABORATORY INSTRUMENTATION

Continuous care of your instruments is important to ensure proper operation and accurate test results. Preventive maintenance prolongs the life of your instruments and reduces breakdowns. It includes daily cleaning and adjusting and replacing parts when necessary. Each instrument should have a log or worksheet on which to record all changes, including daily calibration readings. Modern instruments have quality control

Quality Control
Test Log

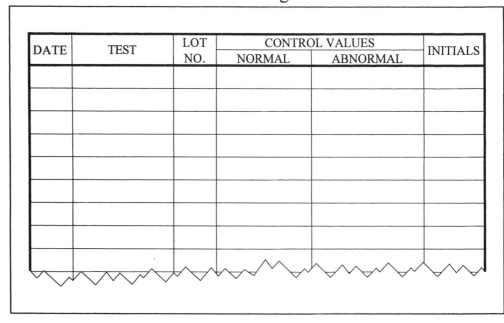

Figure 4–7 Sample of quality control test log.

```
┌─────────────────────────────────────────────────┐
│         INSTRUMENT MAINTENANCE RECORD             │
│                                                   │
│   INSTRUMENT  NAME: _____ │
│   MODEL  NUMBER: _____ SERIAL  NUMBER: ___│
│   PURCHASE  DATE: _____ PURCHASE  PRICE: _│
│                                                   │
│   MANUFACTURER: _____ │
│   CONTACT  PERSON: _____ │
│   WARRANTY  NUMBER: _____ │
│   PHONE: _____ FAX: _____ │
│   ADDRESS: _____ │
│           _____ │
│           _____ │
│                                                   │
│   DEALER: _____ │
│   CONTACT  PERSON: _____ │
│   WARRANTY  NUMBER: _____ │
│   PHONE: _____ FAX: _____ │
│   ADDRESS: _____ │
│           _____ │
│           _____ │
│                                                   │
│                 REPAIR RECORD                     │
│                                                   │
│  ┌──────┬──────────────┬────────────┬──────────┐ │
│  │      │              │ CORRECTIVE │PERFORMED BY│ │
│  │ DATE │ SERVICE CODE │ACTION TAKEN│ (INITIALS) │ │
│  ├──────┼──────────────┼────────────┼──────────┤ │
│  │      │              │            │          │ │
│  ├──────┼──────────────┼────────────┼──────────┤ │
│  │      │              │            │          │ │
│  └──────┴──────────────┴────────────┴──────────┘ │
└─────────────────────────────────────────────────┘
```

Figure 4–8   Sample of instrument maintenance record.

programs with a computerized printout already installed in the analyzer. The following guidelines are provided for a preventive maintenance program:

- Follow the manufacturers' instructions for calibration.
- Have personnel read and follow instructions for maintenance and routine care.
- Perform all preventive maintenance required by the manufacturer.
- Keep spare parts available for immediate use.
- Record the name, address, and phone number of a contact person for maintenance or repair.
- Create a maintenance form or use the one provided by the manufacturer.

PROFICIENCY TESTING

A clinical laboratory can further ensure the accuracy and precision of its test results by joining a *proficiency testing* (PT) program. CLIA '88 requires PT for any procedure other than a waived test. PT, which is a form of external QC, is the performance of tests on unknown specimens from an outside source. The program assesses the accuracy of the clinical laboratory results and compares the results to those of other laboratories performing the same tests using the same method and equipment. The program can help the clinical laboratory evaluate and improve its performance by providing an external quality check of test results. Every employee likely to run patients' samples must perform analyses in PT so that the evaluation reflects the true quality of laboratory performance.

Target value: *the expected value to be obtained when analyzing the control sample*

When the laboratory subscribes to such a program, specimens are received quarterly from an agency and tested as if they were patients' samples. The results are returned within a specified time to a computer center that compiles the results and compares them with peer laboratories. The computer center establishes **target values** and reference ranges of acceptable results based on values established by reference laboratories or by the means of the participants' values. Participants are then evaluated on the proximity of their results to within two standard deviations above and below the established mean for each analyte tested. The agency sends a written summary to the clinical laboratory. The laboratorian must review all proficiency test results, document the summary, and establish policies for out-of-control situations.

Under CLIA '88, clinical laboratories and physician's office laboratories are required to participate in a recognized proficiency testing program for the laboratory tests they perform. The following programs are available for proficiency testing:

- American Association of Bioanalysts: AAB Proficiency Testing Service
- American Academy of Family Physicians: AAFP-PT
- American Society of Internal Medicine: Medical Laboratory Evaluation (MLE)
- College of American Pathologists: External Comparative Evaluation for Laboratories (EXCEL)

SUMMARY

Maintaining a laboratory in the office increases the physician's liability. By testing patients' specimens in the office, the physician assumes responsibility for the interpretation and accuracy of the results. A quality assurance program for the physician's office laboratory (POL) may reduce the risks involved and still allow the patient to benefit from the convenience of office testing. Quality assurance is mandated by the government, and pressures are increasing to control POLs. Clinical laboratories that have established quality assurance programs, with written policies and procedures which ensure that those programs are implemented, will be in compliance.

Questions

Name _____ Date _____

1. Define quality assurance in the clinical laboratory and give five examples of quality assurance.

2. Define quality control and describe how its procedures promote accuracy and precision.

3. Describe systematic and random errors.

4. Give the definitions for standards, controls, and reference values and state the purpose of each within quality control.

5. Explain how personnel orientation is necessary for quality assurance.

6. List the contents of a complete laboratory procedure manual.

7. List the procedures involved in preventive maintenance of laboratory instruments.

8. Name two proficiency programs and explain how they relate to quality assurance.

Instrumentation

LEARNING OBJECTIVES

On completing this chapter, you will be able to:

COGNITIVE OBJECTIVES
- Explain the principles of colorimetry.
- State briefly Beer-Lambert's law.
- Describe a reflectance photometer and give an example of this instrument.
- Name two types of automated chemistry instruments and explain the technology used.
- Describe two automated hematology technologies.
- Identify the major components of a compound microscope.
- Describe the proper use and care of the microscope.

Physicians use **quantitative analyses** of various substances found in the blood and urine for laboratory testing. Laboratorians need to determine how much of each substance is present in the blood components or urine sample. To make these quantitative measurements, clinical laboratories use **colorimeters, photometers, and spectrophotometers.** These instruments indirectly measure analytes by measuring color changes that occur after adding **reagents.**

Quantitative analysis: *chemical analysis to determine the amount of a substance*

Colorimeter: *an instrument that measures the transmission of light through a solution to determine the concentration of light-absorbing material present using a colored filter or glass*

PRINCIPLES OF COLORIMETRY

When a reagent reacts with the analyte in a sample, the solution changes color. The color change occurs because the reagent reacts with the analyte in the sample to form a new chemical. The intensity of the color depends on the number of molecules of the new chemical present. The more molecules present in the solution, the more light is absorbed and the more intense the color. The intensity of the color is directly proportional

Photometer: *an instrument that measures the intensity of light*

Spectrophotometer: *a photometer that measures the light transmitted through a solution to determine the concentration of light-absorbing material present using light filters with a diffraction grating device or prism*

Reagent: *a substance that produces a chemical reaction in a sample that permits another substance to be detected and measured*

to the concentration of the analyte in the solution. Known as *Beer-Lambert's law,* this principle is basic to the operation of colorimeters and spectrophotometers.

These instruments measure either directly the amount of light that passes through the solution (*percent transmittance,* or % T) or indirectly the amount of light that the solution absorbs (absorbance). By comparing the % T or absorbance of the test solution to a known standard, the instrument determines the concentration of the analyte. This value is converted by the instrument to units of concentration of the analyte.

COLORIMETERS, SPECTROPHOTOMETERS, AND PHOTOMETERS

Clinical laboratories have used colorimetric principles for many years to make quantitative measurements of analytes in blood serum, plasma, or urine. The first instruments for this purpose allowed comparison of light transmittance between sample and standards by visual means. Next, instruments called *photometers,* which made comparisons electrically, were developed. Almost all instruments in use today measure analyte concentration electrically. Many are fully automated.

Photometers are used in POLs to determine the concentration of substances, such as hemoglobin and blood glucose. Two types of photometry are used in POLs. One type of photometry determines the percent transmission of light and includes colorimeters and spectrophotometers. The other type of photometer is the *reflectance photometer,* which measures the intensity of light reflected back from a reagent pad (Fig. 5–1). Blood glucose monitors and analyzers that automatically read urine reagent strips (see Chapter 12) are examples of reflectance photometers.

DRY CHEMISTRY ANALYZERS

Reflectance photometry is a modification of the principle used in colorimeters and spectrophotometers; it measures the intensity of reflected light and not the transmission of

Reflectance Photometry

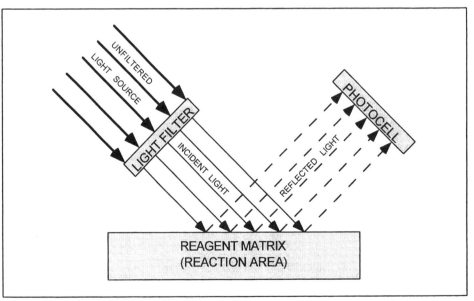

Figure 5–1   An illustration of the principle of a reflectance photometer, which measures the intensity of light reflected back from a reagent pad.

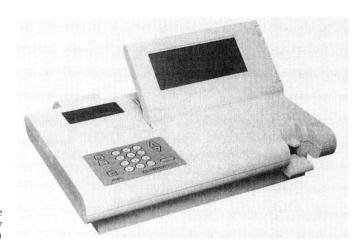

Figure 5–2 CliniTek 100 Urine Chemistry Analyzer. (Courtesy Bayer Corporation, Elkhart, Ind.)

light. Reflectance photometers were developed to be used in all dry-reagent chemistry where the light that reflects off the surface of the reagent strip measures the amount of blood or urine chemical analytes. Using this type of instrument eliminates inaccurate readings associated with the individual variations of visual interpretation. As with all tests, the accuracy of the test results depends on following manufacturer's directions.

The CliniTek 100 Urine Chemistry Analyzer from Bayer (Fig. 5–2) measures light reflected from the reagent strip that is manually dipped in a urine specimen. The instrument compares the amount of light reflection to that of a known concentration. It displays the results on a screen and prints them out. This instrument does not require special calibration because it calibrates itself when it is turned on and before each specimen is read.

Another example of reflectance photometry for reading urine specimen strips is the Chemstrip Mini UA Urine Analyzer from Boehringer Mannheim (Fig. 5–3). It also provides a visual display for positive and negative results and a printout of the results.

AUTOMATED CHEMISTRY ANALYZERS

Some chemistry analyzers used in POLs incorporate the principle of *discrete analysis,* a method in which the sample of each analyte is tested in its own separate container. Some discrete analysis instruments use **centrifugal analysis** in which the sample to be tested is first centrifuged with the test reagents. Another type of discrete analysis is solid-phase chemistry. In this type of analyzer the sample is added to a strip or slide that contains all the reagents for the analysis in dried form. The reagents are in multiple layers, with each

Centrifugal analysis: *a method using the centrifugation of reagents in liquid form for wet chemistry procedures*

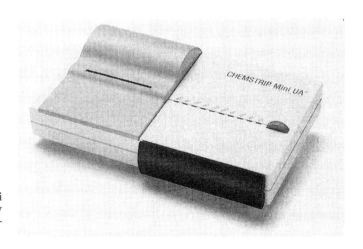

Figure 5–3 Chemstrip Mini Urine Analyzer. (Courtesy Boehringer Mannheim Corporation, Indianapolis, Ind.)

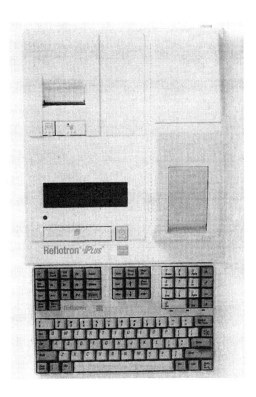

Figure 5–4 Reflotron Plus. (Courtesy Boehringer Mannheim Corporation, Indianapolis, Ind.)

layer having a specified function in the reaction. An example of this type of instrument is the Reflotron Plus from Boehringer Mannheim (Fig. 5–4) and the Vitros DT60 II Chemistry System from Johnson & Johnson Clinical Diagnostics (Fig. 5–5).

AUTOMATED HEMATOLOGY ANALYZERS

Hematology: *the study of blood and blood-forming tissues*

There are two types of blood cell counters in **hematology** that use diluted samples. They are aperture-impedance cell counters and light-scattering cell counters.

The aperture-impedance method of cell counting requires the blood cells to be diluted with an *electrolyte,* a solution that conducts electricity. When the blood cells, which are poor conductors of electricity, pass through the opening *(aperture)* of the instrument, the nonconducting blood cells cause a pulse or interruption *(impedance)* of the electrical circuit. These pulses are counted as cells. The Cell-Dyn 1700 from Abbott Diagnostics is an example of an automated analyzer that uses electrical impedance (Fig. 5–6).

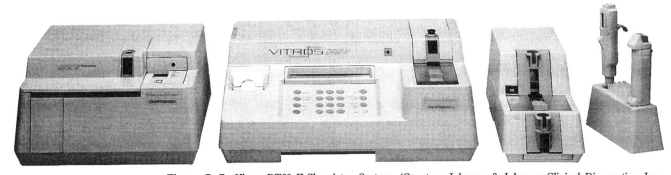

Figure 5–5 Vitros DT60 II Chemistry System. (Courtesy Johnson & Johnson Clinical Diagnostics, Inc., Rochester, NY.)

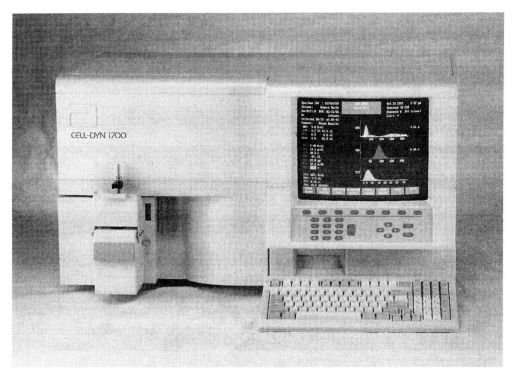

Figure 5-6 Cell-Dyn 1700. (Courtesy Abbott Diagnostics, Abbott Park, Ill.)

In light-scattering cell counting, the concept of cell counting is based on a laser beam or a tungsten-halogen light beam directed at a single stream of blood cells in a narrow channel. The light beam scatters when it strikes a cell at an angle that allows sensors to detect the amount of light scattered and how much of the beam is absorbed by the cell. Each type of cell creates a different angle of scatter. This angle depends on the volume, shape, and the **refractive index** of the blood cell. This type of analyzer is not usually found in a POL.

The QBC Autoread from Becton Dickinson is an automated hematology instrument that uses an undiluted blood sample. The QBC *(quantitative buffy coat)* has its own special centrifuge that separates the blood into layers. The sample is inserted into the instrument, which reads, displays, and prints the results (Fig. 5-7).

Refractive index: *the angle at which light is bent as it passes from a medium of one density to a medium of another density*

QUALITY CONTROL

Perform quality control procedures on laboratory instruments by calibrating according to the manufacturer's directions. Calibration checks the accuracy and precision of the testing instrument. The accuracy of the instruments can also be checked by using control samples. Run control samples daily and compare them to the known values provided by the manufacturer of the controls. If the controls match the known values, the instrument is working properly, the reagents are working properly, and the procedure was performed accurately.

Quality control includes using normal and abnormal controls daily and for each analyte tested. Controls are available in three levels: abnormally low values, abnormally high values, and normal values. Record the controls in the daily log book. Because of their convenience, built-in procedural controls in test kits have been approved as meeting the QC requirements for moderate-complexity testing.

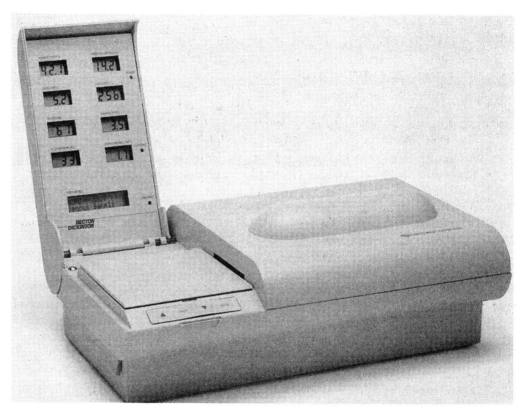

Figure 5–7 QBC Autoread. (Courtesy Becton Dickinson Primary Care Diagnostics, Sparks, Md.)

Clinical Comment: CLIA '88

CLIA '88 requires that two levels of control sample testing for each analyte be performed and recorded each day that a patient's sample is tested for that substance. Control samples should include a normal value and an abnormal value.

EQUIPMENT CARE

Cover all chemistry and hematology instruments when not in use to protect them from dust and spilled reagents. Do not jar or move the instruments. The reagent strips, slides, or electrodes should never be exchanged among the different analyzers. Use only the material designated for a particular instrument and follow manufacturer's instructions regarding each instrument. Follow the maintenance procedures that are provided in the operating manuals for the different instruments and call a representative of the manufacturer when a problem develops that cannot be solved by the laboratorian.

CENTRIFUGES

Centrifugal force: *the force that impels a thing, or parts of it, outward from the center of rotation*

One of the most commonly used laboratory instruments is the *centrifuge.* A centrifuge is an instrument that spins test tubes at high speeds. It separates the liquid contents of the test tube from the solid contents, creating layers according to the weight of the material. It does this by **centrifugal force.** The liquid portion of a centrifuged specimen is known as the *supernatant,* and the solid material is the *sediment.*

When you centrifuge urine specimens, the supernatant is the liquid portion of the urine specimen. The sediment contains all the solid matter found in urine. The microscopic examination of urine is performed on this sediment. See Chapter 13 for more information on microscopic examination of urine.

When a blood specimen is centrifuged, the blood separates into several layers with the red blood cells as the sediment and the plasma or serum as the supernatant. See Chapters 8 and 16 for more detailed descriptions of centrifuged blood specimens.

Some important rules to follow when using a centrifuge are:

- Always make sure the lid is secured before operating a centrifuge.
- Always balance a centrifuge. For example, if only one specimen is centrifuged, it must be balanced with a similar tube of water.
- Always wait until the rotor stops before opening the lid.
- Whenever possible, spin the specimens with caps secured to prevent aerosol contamination.
- Use only tubes specific for the centrifuge.

MICROSCOPES

The microscope is one of the most important pieces of equipment used in the POL. This instrument magnifies objects too small to be seen with the naked eye. It is used in hematology, urinalysis, and bacteriology.

The type of microscope most commonly used in clinical medicine is the *compound microscope*. As the name suggests, the compound microscope uses two different lens systems to produce an image. One lens system compounds, or increases, the magnification produced by the other. The first set of lenses includes the *objective lenses* (objectives). They produce a magnified image of the specimen called the **real image.** The second set of lenses, called the *ocular lenses* (oculars, eyepieces), magnifies the real image to produce a **retinal image.**

> **Real image:** *an inverted magnified image produced by the objective lens*

> **Retinal image:** *the image produced by the ocular lenses and seen by the eye*

COMPONENTS OF THE MICROSCOPE

Framework

All microscopes consist of a framework that includes an *arm* and a *base* (Fig. 5–8). All other components of the microscope are attached to these two structures. In most high-quality microscopes the base houses a *light source*. The light source, usually an incandescent or tungsten bulb, illuminates the specimen. Many microscopes also have a *rheostat*, a device that varies the amount of light produced by the bulb.

Stage

The *stage,* a platform on which the slide is placed for observation, extends from the arm of the microscope. A small **aperture** located in the center of the stage allows light rays from the light source to reach the specimen. The slide is placed on the stage so that the area to be examined is directly over the aperture. A movable clamplike device secures the slide on the *mechanical stage.* Control knobs for the mechanical stage allow the operator to move the slide in a horizontal or vertical direction when it is positioned in the clamp (Fig. 5–9).

> **Aperture:** *a small opening or slit*

Lens System

The lens system consists of the condenser, the ocular lenses, and the objective lenses.

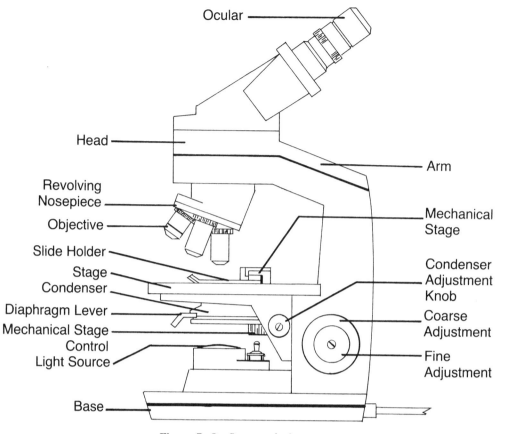

Figure 5–8   Compound microscope.

CONDENSER

The *condenser* is a movable lens located beneath the stage. It can be elevated or lowered using the *condenser control knob.* To the condenser is attached the *iris diaphragm.* The iris diaphragm resembles the shutter of a camera in structure and function. Both the condenser and diaphragm regulate light from the light source. The condenser focuses light on the specimen and fills the lens with light. The iris diaphragm controls the amount of light passing through the stage aperture to the specimen. The condenser and diaphragm assist in achieving the optimum contrast, depth of field, and **resolution.**

Resolution: *the ability to detect the separation of two points or objects*

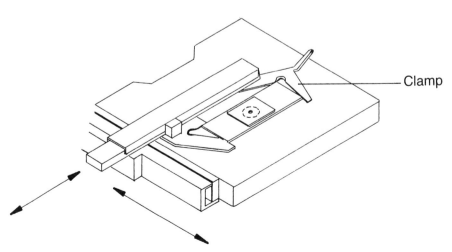

Figure 5–9   Mechanical stage and clamp.

When the condenser is elevated, that is, when positioned nearest the stage, the greatest amount of light is directed toward the specimen. When lowered, less light falls on the specimen. Heavily stained slides, that is, blood smears or dense tissue, require more light for observation than low-contrast or unstained specimens. The use of the oil-immersion *objective* (see discussion that follows) usually necessitates placing the condenser as close to the specimen as possible and fully opening the diaphragm in order to provide the greatest amount of light.

OCULAR LENSES

The ocular lenses are the lenses located closest to the eye when viewing a specimen with the microscope. The microscope typically used in a physician's office laboratory has two ocular lenses that provide *binocular* viewing of the specimen. The magnification of the ocular lenses is generally 10×; that is, the real image produced by the objective lens is further magnified 10 times by the ocular lenses before the operator sees the image. The magnification is etched directly on the side of the ocular.

One ocular is independently adjustable to compensate for differences between the observer's right and left eyes. To determine whether correction is needed, view the specimen with only the right eye, and then, only with the left eye. If a disparity is noted, correction is required. Bring the specimen into sharp focus with the stationary ocular (usually the right ocular) using the fine adjustment knob, and correct the focus by turning the movable ocular (usually the left ocular).

The oculars are movable to accommodate differences in eye span. The distance between oculars can be increased or decreased. They are correctly positioned when a single circle representing the **visual field** is observed. If two circles appear, or if overlapping circles appear, adjust the span of the oculars.

Visual field: *the circular area seen through the oculars*

OBJECTIVE LENSES

There are usually three objective lenses located on a rotating nosepiece. They include the *low-power objective* (10×), *the high-power objective* (40–50×), and the *oil-immersion objective* (95–100×). Variations in magnification strength occur depending upon manufacturer. Check your microscope for the magnification of each objective. The magnification is etched directly on the side of the objective. Note that the oil-immersion lens is characterized by a band that encircles the objective. This highlights that *only* this objective may be used with oil.

The low-power objective is used to focus the microscope initially for all types of specimens. It allows rapid location of the specimen. It is the only objective that will not touch the slide when the microscope's stage is all the way down. The high-power objective, sometimes called the *high-dry objective* or *high dry,* is typically used to observe certain urinary sediment components and to locate and focus bacterial smears before observing them with the oil-immersion objective. The oil-immersion objective is the highest magnification lens on a compound microscope. When using this objective, raise the condenser and open the iris diaphragm to enhance viewing of the specimen.

Light rays *refract* or bend as they pass through media of different densities. As the light rays exit from the glass slide holding the specimen (a dense medium) and pass into the air (a less dense medium) on their journey to the objective, some of them are refracted and scattered away from the objective. The use of a drop of immersion oil eliminates this problem. Since oil has about the same refractive index as the glass slide, the light rays do not scatter but are directed in a straight path as they travel from the slide to the oil-immersion objective (Fig. 5–10). To use the oil-immersion lens properly, cock the nosepiece off to the side, and place a drop of oil directly on the portion of the slide that is to be examined (Fig. 5–11). Rotate the oil-immersion objective directly into the drop of oil. Make sure that the high-power objective does not pass into the oil when the oil-immersion objective is moved into position.

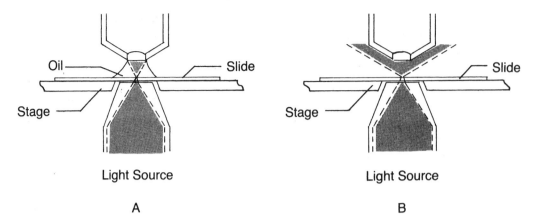

Figure 5-10 *(A)* The drop of oil causes the light rays from the slide to be directed into the oil-immersion lens. *(B)* Without oil, some light rays are scattered as they emerge from the slide and do not pass into the oil-immersion lens.

The compound microscope provides *parfocal* viewing; that is, once the specimen is in focus with the low-power objective, it will almost be in focus when changing to high-power or oil-immersion. In other words, it will require less than one full turn of the fine adjustment to bring the specimen into sharp focus.

USING THE MICROSCOPE

Focusing Adjustment Knobs

Focus the microscope by varying the distance between the specimen and the objective. Use the *coarse adjustment knob* for rapid movement over a large distance to locate the specimen. Use the *fine adjustment knob* for discrete movement over a short distance to sharpen the image.

In early microscopes the draw tube or objectives were raised or lowered to adjust the focus, but in most modern microscopes the focusing mechanism moves the stage rather than the objectives. In either case, the distance is regulated by turning either the coarse adjustment knob or fine adjustment knob.

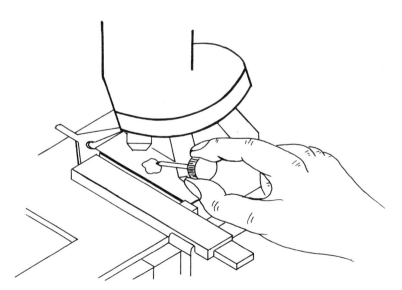

Figure 5-11 Placing oil on a slide.

The coarse adjustment knob is used for initial focusing of the specimen, when the low-power objective is in place. Once the specimen is brought into view, the fine adjustment knob sharpens the image. You can now observe the specimen with either the high-power objective or the oil-immersion objective by rotating the nosepiece. Use only the fine adjustment knob when the high-power objective and the oil-immersion objective are in place. Use the diaphragm and condenser to reach the best resolution or clarity possible.

Working Distance

The *working distance* is the distance between the specimen and the bottom of the objective. The greater the magnifying power of the objective, the shorter its working distance. This fact must be kept in mind when you focus the microscope. Any large movement of the coarse adjustment knob while focusing could cause the oil-immersion objective or the high-power objective to grind against the slide, causing damage to the slide or the lens. Therefore, *only* small focus corrections using the fine adjustment knob should be attempted when using the high-power or oil-immersion objectives. Figure 5–12 shows the magnification, working distance, and required iris diaphragm aperture for proper illumination for each of the objectives.

Total Magnification

The ocular lenses and the objective lenses contribute to the *total magnification* of the specimen. Total magnification is obtained by multiplying the ocular magnification by the magnification of the objective that is used for observing the specimen.

Ocular lens	×	objective magnification	=	total magnification
10×	×	10× (low power)	=	100×
10×	×	40–50× (high power)	=	400–500×
10×	×	95–100× (oil immersion)	=	950–1000×

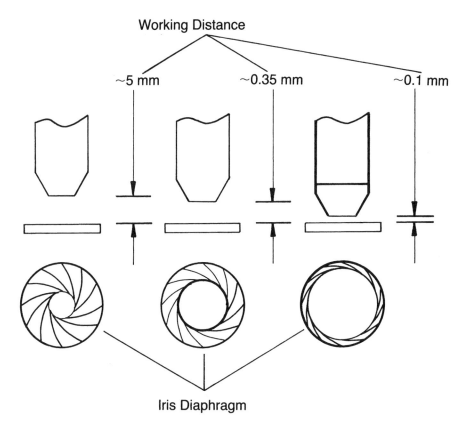

Figure 5–12   Working distance decreases with higher magnification, while the need for light increases.

CARE OF THE MICROSCOPE

The microscope requires very little care with the exception of the stage and the lenses. All nonglass surfaces can be cleaned using a soft cloth, gauze, or commercial products such as Kim-Wipes. Clean lenses *only* with lens paper or lens tissue. Wipe the ocular lenses first, then all the objective lenses, leaving the oil-immersion objective until last. Clean the oil-immersion lens last to avoid carrying oil to other lenses. Occasionally a small amount of lens cleaner may be used to remove excess residual immersion oil. Moisten a lens tissue with a small quantity of commercially available lens cleaner and gently wipe away any oil. Avoid using too much lens cleaner because this may weaken the seal surrounding the lens.

Maintain a supply of light bulbs so that your work schedule will not be interrupted by a burned-out bulb. In POLs, the microscope may be placed in a permanent position on a sturdy laboratory bench, where activity is at a minimum, or kept in a cabinet until it is needed. Transport the microscope by holding it in an upright position, using two hands. Firmly hold the arm of the microscope with one hand, while stabilizing the base with the other hand. Keep the microscope covered when not in use. Disconnect the power by pulling the plug, not the cord.

SUMMARY

Beer-Lambert's law states that the color intensity that results from adding reagents to analytes is directly proportional to the concentration of the analyte. All colorimetric instruments use this law as a basis for operation. Therefore, the intensity of the light passing through the different colors of solutions or the light reflected from a dry-reagent pad determines the quantity of the analyte. Using normal and abnormal controls provides a daily check on the instrument used, the reagents and procedure used, and the technical skill of the person performing the procedure.

The microscope requires minimal but important care in order to function properly. The microscope must be transported carefully, using two hands, and it must be cleaned at the end of the day. With appropriate care, the microscope will require little or no professional servicing.

PROCEDURE FOR FOCUSING THE MICROSCOPE

Focusing the microscope is a relatively simple task once the technique is properly learned. By following these simple guidelines, the beginning student should have little difficulty in mastering this technique:

Turn on the light and adjust the ocular lenses to accommodate your eye span.

Rotate the nosepiece to the low-power (10×) objective. Initial focusing always begins with the low-power objective.

While viewing the microscope *from the side,* increase the working distance as far as possible.

Place a prepared slide on the stage, secure it with the slide clamp, and center it using the horizontal and vertical adjustment knobs.

While still observing the microscope from the side, decrease the working distance as far as possible.

Place your eyes over the oculars and begin the initial focusing of the specimen by slowly increasing the working distance using the coarse adjustment.

After the specimen is in focus, adjust the amount of light using the rheostat, condenser, and iris diaphragm.

Using the fine adjustment knob, focus to the sharpest possible image. With parfocality, when a sharp image is obtained using the low-power objective, you may view the specimen with the high-power objective or the oil-immersion objective, with little or no additional focusing.

- When changing from the low-power objective to high-power objective, view the microscope from the side as you rotate the nosepiece.
- When changing from the low-power objective to the oil-immersion objective, cock the nosepiece off to the side and place one or two drops of immersion oil directly on the slide over the area to be observed. Gently rotate the oil-immersion objective into the drop of oil. Make sure that the high-dry objective does not come in contact with the oil.

Place your eyes over the oculars. Readjust the amount of light using the rheostat, condenser, and diaphragm. More light is required when using high-dry or oil-immersion lens. This will necessitate turning the rheostat to full or near full power, elevating the condenser and opening the iris diaphragm.

Using *only* the fine adjustment, refocus the specimen to produce a sharp image.

Remove the slide and clean the microscope by wiping the lenses. Remember, clean the oil-immersion objective last.

Return the low-power objective to the viewing position, and fully decrease the working distance.

Cover the microscope and place it in the storage cabinet.

Questions

Name _____ Date _____

1. Briefly state Beer-Lambert's law.

2. Describe reflectance photometry and name two types of instruments using this technique.

3. Describe the principle of discrete analysis used in automated chemistry analyzers.

4. Name two types of hematology analyzers and give a brief description of them.

5. Explain how quality control is achieved in instrumentation.

6. What is the purpose of the condenser and iris diaphragm?

7. Give the name of each objective and its magnifying power.

8. Calculate the total magnification when the ocular lens is $10\times$ and the objective lenses are $10\times$, 40–$50\times$, and 95–$100\times$.

9. What is meant by parfocality?

10. Why does initial focusing always begin by using the low-power objective?

11. Briefly explain the care, cleaning, and carrying of the microscope.

SPECIMEN COLLECTION

Introduction to Specimen Collection and Transport

6

Learning Objectives
Cognitive Objectives

The Test Request

Documentation
Directory of Services Manual
Procedure Manual
- ○ Name of test
- ○ Specimen type and quantity
- ○ Method of collection
- ○ Patient preparation
- ○ Labeling information
- ○ Special handling

- ○ Criteria for rejection
- ○ Stability and time constraints
Quality Control Manual

Chain-of-Custody Collections
Testing Programs
Mandatory Testing

Transport

Confidentiality

Summary

Questions

LEARNING OBJECTIVES

On completing this chapter, you will be able to:

COGNITIVE OBJECTIVES
- State the purpose of a Test Request Form and tell what information it provides.
- Name three manuals that are normally available in physicians' offices that contain information on specimen collection.
- State, in general terms, the type of information found in a Directory of Services manual.
- List the types of information found in the physicians' office Procedure Manual.
- List the information that should be included on specimen labels and test request slips.
- Explain the purpose of a chain-of-custody sample.
- State important considerations regarding the transport of clinical specimens.
- State why confidentiality is important in specimen collection.

The accuracy of any laboratory result begins at the beginning—with proper laboratory specimen collection. The foundation of reliable and valid laboratory test results starts with the specimen and the way in which it was obtained. The saying "garbage in, garbage out" applies as accurately to laboratory test results as it does to computer-generated data. Proper collection, handling, and processing are essential for accurate and reliable test results.

The nature of the test dictates the manner in which the specimen is collected. Some specimen collections are complicated and require specially trained technical personnel and elaborate patient preparation. However, most specimen collections, especially those undertaken in the POL, are uncomplicated.

In many instances proper collection depends on giving clear and concise instructions to the patient. Even the simplest urine specimen collection requires some patient education. Patient instruction is the responsibility of clinical laboratorians.

THE TEST REQUEST

Specimen testing is initiated by a physician who requests that certain tests be performed on a patient. This is normally done by means of a *Test Request (Requisition) Form* (Fig. 6–1). The request form contains all relevant information regarding the patient (name, age, sex, sometimes social security number). It identifies the test requested by the physician and provides space for the initials of the laboratorian who obtains the sample. It also contains billing information for test payment. When test requests are made orally by the physician, the laboratorian must follow up with a written test requisition. The test specimen, whether collected by the laboratorian or received by the laboratorian, must be correctly labeled (with the patient's name, age, sex, etc.). The information on the label must match the test request form. Unlabeled or incorrectly labeled specimens must be rejected for testing.

DOCUMENTATION

The variety of biologic specimens, the multitude of analytes, and the various methods of specimen collection and transport all provide opportunities where inaccuracies and errors may be introduced into the test procedure. Because of this, the laboratorian must exercise the highest degree of care and attention from the moment he or she begins undertaking collection of any biologic specimen and meticulously follow all guidelines relating to specimen collection.

The Clinical Laboratory Improvement Amendment (CLIA) requires that documentation of specimen collection procedures be available to all personnel who participate in any aspect of laboratory testing. For this purpose most physician's offices use three manuals:

- Directory of Services manual
- Procedure Manual
- Quality Control Manual

Directory of Services Manual

Referral (reference) laboratories: *laboratories that accept specimens from other sources, including POLs; these laboratories usually have an extensive menu of clinical laboratory tests that they perform*

Most physicians' offices have a limited menu of tests that are performed on-site. Consequently, most specimen collection in the POL is quite routine. When specimens are sent to **referral (reference) laboratories** for more comprehensive testing, the laboratorian must follow the collection procedures required by the referral laboratory. Referral laboratories provide the physician's office with a *Directory of Services* manual, which lists the tests performed by that laboratory, the method of specimen collection for each test, reference ranges, and other information of interest to the physician. This directory must be consulted, and all requirements for specimen collection and handling must be carefully and accurately followed.

Procedure Manual

Physicians' offices must keep a *Procedure Manual* that clearly identifies and details the following information regarding each test performed in the POL:

- Name of the test
- Specimen type and quantity
- Method of collection
- Patient preparation
- Labeling information
- Special handling
- Criteria for rejection
- Stability and time constraints

Lab Test INC. ‖‖‖‖‖‖‖‖	**TEST REQUSITION FORM**	**PATIENT INFORMATION - PLEASE PRINT**

REFERRED BY

Andrew A. Kurtz, M.D.
1234 Playfield Rd
Anywhere, OH 45321

Complete the Shaded Box for Patient and Third Party Billing

PATIENT NAME (LAST)   (FIRST)   (M.I.)

REGISTRATION #

BIRTH DATE (AGE)   SEX   PATIENT I.D.#

ROOM #   LAB REFERENCE #

CHECK CHOICE OF BILLING

( ) Medicare # _____

( ) Medicaid # _____ State _____

( ) Patient Billing

Insurance
Company _____
            ID#   GROUP#   EMPLOYER#
Employer Name
RELATIONSHIP: ( ) SELF ( ) SPOUSE ( ) DEPENDENT
DX #1 _____ CODE _____
DX #2 _____ CODE _____
PATIENT TELEPHONE # (   )

ADDRESS OF RESPONSIBILE PARTY MUST BE PROVIDED

NAME (last) _____ (first) _____

ADDRESS _____

CITY _____ STATE _____ ZIP _____

Collection Date _____ Time _____ By _____
☐ Fasting (Hours) _____
☐ Serum   ☐ Plasma
☐ Urine   Volume _____   Hours _____
☐ Other _____

U.P.I.N. REFFERING PHYSICIAN(S)

( ) B34567 Dr. One   ( ) S15697 Dr. Four
( ) C34907 Dr. Two   ( ) S38887 Dr. Five
( ) D22567 Dr. Three   ( ) L36667 Dr. Six

☐ STAT   ☐ STAT PICK UP
☐ CALL RESULTS TO: (___) _____
☐ SEND DUPLICATE RESULTS TO:

NAME (last) _____ (first) _____

ADDRESS _____

CITY _____ STATE _____ ZIP _____

PROFILES AND TESTS

( ) 223 Albumin
( ) 249 Antinuclear Ab
( ) 303 Calcium
( ) 4643 C-Peptide (U)

( ) 231 Alk Phos Isoenzymes
( ) 285 Bilirubin, Direct
( ) 7943 Creatinine Clearance
( ) 7573 Iron, Total & IBC

( ) 234 Alk Phos, Total
( ) 294 Urea Nitrogen
( ) 5637 Glucose, PP/2 Hour
( ) 4555 Microalbumin (U)

ADDITIONAL TESTS (PLEASE PRINT)

TOTAL NUMBER
OF TESTS ORDERED

REMARKS

Figure 6-1 Test request form.

NAME OF TEST

The Procedure Manual lists the name of the test and also the various synonyms commonly used for that test. For example, the manual may list *Erythrocyte Sedimentation Rate, Sedimentation Rate, Sed Rate,* or *ESR,* all synonyms for the same test.

SPECIMEN TYPE AND QUANTITY

The types of laboratory tests performed in physicians' offices and the types of specimens collected for referral laboratory testing tend to be routine and generally uncomplicated. Usually they include blood, urine, and some microbial cultures. The Procedure Manual gives the quantity for each type of specimen. When more elaborate tests are required, and specimens other than blood, urine, or bacterial cultures are needed, the patient is sent directly to the referral laboratory or hospital, where trained individuals collect the needed specimen.

METHOD OF COLLECTION

The Procedure Manual and the Directory of Services provided by the referral laboratory specify the method of collection. For example, the submission requirements for a urine zinc determination may read as follows:

> 25 mL urine—plastic container. **Aliquot** of well-mixed 24-hour collection. Add 20 mL 6N HCl to container at start of collection. Record total volume on both the specimen container and the test request form.

Aliquot: *a small representative sample; a portion of the whole*

In this example, the submission requirements list the type and quantity of preservative, the quantity of urine required for testing, and the method of collection. It also specifies that the total volume of urine be recorded on both the specimen container and the test request form.

PATIENT PREPARATION

The patient preparation section of the Procedure Manual specifies what has to be done before obtaining a specimen. The most common preparation is the requirement that the patient fast. For example, the submission requirements for a Lipid Panel may state:

> 2 mL serum—plastic vial. *Fasting specimen required.* Patient should fast 12–16 hours prior to test. State patient's age and sex on the test request form.

If fasting is a requirement for a specific test, be sure to check with the patient before drawing blood. Verify that fasting requirements have been met. Gum chewing and smoking are not allowed when fasting samples are required. It is usually a better technique to ask the patient whether he or she had anything to eat or drink over the last 12 to 16 hours, rather than asking whether he or she has fasted during that period. Many people think they have fasted if they have only had a cup or two of coffee and a glass of orange juice!

LABELING INFORMATION

Laboratory reference number (log number): *any number assigned to a particular specimen by a laboratory*

Proper labeling is absolutely essential for all specimen collections. Labeling information must include the patient's name, age, and sex because some test reference ranges may vary accordingly. If additional identification is required, that is, **laboratory reference numbers (log numbers),** be sure that they are properly recorded on the request slip and specimen. The specimen should be identified as to whether it is serum, plasma, urine, throat swab, or bacterial culture. Include the name or initials of the laboratorian who collects the sample. For some urine tests, the total amount of urine collected is necessary for the proper interpretation of the test results. The time of collection (use military time) may also be required on the label and request form. For microbial collections, the site of collection, the **tentative** diagnosis, and whether the patient has taken antibiotics prior to collection are important for testing personnel and must be written on the Test Request Form.

Be sure to complete all billing information on the request slips when specimens are sent to referral laboratories.

SPECIAL HANDLING

Special handling includes any information that is necessary to preserve the integrity of the specimen prior to testing. Handling requirements may include how long a specimen may be kept before it is tested, whether the specimen must be kept frozen, or whether it must be kept out of direct light. For example, a blood specimen collection for an HLA Rheumatology Panel may give the following submission requirements:

> 10 mL heparinized whole blood—1 full green-top tube. Sodium heparin tubes are stable for 48 hours. Do NOT refrigerate or freeze. Send immediately by courier or overnight mail.

CRITERIA FOR REJECTION

The section on criteria for rejection in the Procedure Manual lists criteria that cause a specimen to be rejected for testing. The most common criteria for rejection of a blood specimen are **hemolytic** or **lipemic** appearance. Other criteria for rejection include incomplete filling of vacuum tubes, unlabeled specimens, inappropriate preservative, and incorrect vacuum tubes.

STABILITY AND TIME CONSTRAINTS

Some tests have strict requirements regarding specimen collection, handling, and processing. Time of testing following the collection of the specimen, temperature, and drying of samples are important in some tests, especially those for microbial studies. Follow all special requirements when analytes are unstable or require special attention.

Quality Control Manual

A *Quality Control* (QC) *Manual* defines the limits of acceptable performance for the tests performed in the laboratory. It provides a permanent record of all control sample testing and of any necessary corrective action. It also contains information on specimen collection. General venipuncture, urine collection, and microbial culture collection protocols are frequently referenced in the QC Manual. They need not be repeated for each laboratory assay (test) listed in the Procedure Manual or Directory of Services. When questions arise as to specimen collection, refer to the detailed instructions regarding specimen collection in the QC Manual or Directory of Services.

CHAIN-OF-CUSTODY COLLECTIONS

Some test results have legal ramifications. Physicians' offices are frequently involved in collecting specimens for drug and substance abuse testing. Collection of these specimens must meet rigorous guidelines to ensure that the test results are indeed for the specimen from the particular individual on whom the test was ordered. The collection procedure must ensure that there was no chance for **adulteration** of or tampering with the specimen at any time. The rigorous guidelines and procedures are referred to as a *chain-of-custody collection*.

Tentative: *provisional; not confirmed*

Hemolytic: *pertaining to the breakdown of erythrocytes with the subsequent release of hemoglobin*

Lipemic: *pertaining to an abnormal amount of fat or fatty products in the blood*

Adulteration: *the addition of unwanted substances that make the sample impure*

Testing Programs

The five types of testing programs that may require a chain-of-custody collection include:

- Preemployment physicals
- For **cause**
- Postaccident
- Periodic
- Random

A chain-of-custody procedure is designed to withstand legal scrutiny. It establishes that:

- No adulteration or tampering has taken place
- All personnel who handled the specimen are documented
- No unauthorized access to the specimen was possible
- Specimens were handled in a secure manner
- Specimens belong to the individual identified on the label of the specimen container

Specimens are collected according to rigid guidelines in specimen containers that have tamper-evident tape for sealing. The specimen containers are placed in tamper-evident bags for transport to the testing facility.

Clinical Comment: Preventing Adulteration

Adding water to a urine specimen can dilute it to such an extent that drugs cannot be detected. To protect against adulteration of a specimen by the donor in a chain-of-custody sample, the laboratorian should tape the water faucet in the bathroom used for collection with tamper-proof tape. Blue food dye or a toilet bowl cleaner that contains dye should be put into the toilet bowl or tank. Soap dispensers should also be taped so that the donor does not have access to any substances that can alter or adulterate the specimen.

The temperature of urine specimens must be taken within 2 minutes after voiding. Freshly voided urine will be at normal body temperature (98.6°F). This fact can be used to ensure that the specimen is "freshly voided," and not a specimen collected from another individual and secretly carried into the bathroom. Some specimen cups have a thermometer directly attached so that the temperature can be immediately recorded. The acceptable range is 90.5°F to 99.8°F. Temperatures not in this range may cause the specimen to be rejected. The supervisor or coordinator of the drug-testing program for the company should be notified if a freshly voided sample does not fall within this range.

The custody and control forms (paperwork) for chain-of-custody samples identify the purpose of the specimen collection, the individual who collected the specimen, and the integrity of the specimen when it arrives at the testing facility. Each individual who receives the specimen, from time of collection to the issuing of results, is identified on the custody-and-control requisition form. All who have had custody of the specimen must be in a position to testify that the specimen was not altered or adulterated in any way while in their possession.

Mandatory Testing

Some governmental agencies, including the Department of Transportation and the Department of Defense, have mandatory drug-testing requirements for some of their employees. Any governmental mandatory drug testing must be undertaken by laboratories that are certified to perform these tests. Specimens must be submitted to a National Institute on Drug Abuse (NIDA) certified agency. Not all referral laboratories are NIDA certified.

TRANSPORT

Log the specimen in a log notebook, including date, time, patient's name, and test requested. Follow all special requirements necessary to preserve the specimen. The effects of heat, cold, drying, **agitation,** and time delay are concerns that must be taken into consideration when transporting specimens for testing. When testing is done within the POL, these problems usually do not arise. However, for specimens that will be tested at a referral laboratory, the fastest and most convenient method of transport is pickup service by the referral laboratory's courier. These couriers are trained in the proper handling of specimens. They have the proper equipment (refrigerated containers, ice chests, or other containers) in which to transport specimens. Unless **"Stat"** pick-ups are available, the courier generally makes only one pickup daily. When prompt delivery is essential, the patient appointment should be made immediately prior to the pickup time. Do not collect samples that require immediate transport *after* the time of courier pickup or when holidays or weekends delay delivery.

Postal service is generally inadequate for most specimen transport because delivery time and temperature requirements are of concern. Specimens sent through the U.S. postal service must meet all postal regulations. Generally three containers are used for mailing. A primary container holds the specimen. Sufficient absorbent packing material should surround the primary container. The primary container fits inside a secondary waterproof container. Next, the secondary container is placed in a shipping carton. *A biohazard label must be prominently displayed on the shipping carton* (Fig. 6–2).

Agitation: *turbulence*

Stat: *immediate, immediately*

CONFIDENTIALITY

Some specimen collections involve tests that are very personal and highly confidential. Included in these collections are HIV testing (the organism that causes AIDS), pregnancy testing, and testing for sexually transmitted diseases (STDs). Completed test request slips must never be placed in areas where curious eyes may identify the patient and the test ordered.

Mailing Container

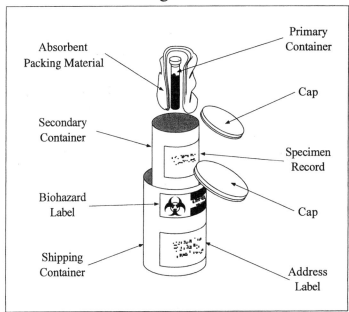

Figure 6–2 Packaging and labeling of etiologic (disease-causing) agents.

SUMMARY

Proper specimen collection is a vital aspect of quality control. It is important that all specimens be collected, processed, and tested so as to represent a clinical picture of the patient. Improper collecting, processing, or testing produces false data. Analytes must be preserved from the time of collection to the time of testing. If preservatives are used in collecting, they must not interfere with the test.

Specimen collection guidelines for chain-of-custody samples must be meticulously followed so as to withstand legal scrutiny. Remember that not only must test results remain confidential, but the ordering of certain tests, especially those involving HIV testing, must also be kept confidential.

Information on specimen collection is available in the Procedure Manual, Directory of Services, and Quality Control Manual. Laboratorians should familiarize themselves with these technical sources and should consult them when questions arise regarding the correct collecting, handling, or processing of any specimen.

Questions

Name _____ Date _____

1. What is a test request form? What information does it provide?

2. What manuals are available in most physicians' offices that describe specimen collecting? What is the purpose of each?

3. What information is given in a Procedure Manual regarding each test that is performed in the physician's office?

4. Give some examples of "special handling" that may apply to specimen collection.

5. What is a chain-of-custody specimen?

6. Why is it necessary to follow rigidly all guidelines regarding specimen collection for a chain-of-custody specimen?

7. What is meant by mandatory testing?

8. What is a courier service? What advantages does courier service have over the U.S. postal service when transporting specimens?

9. Why is maintaining patient confidentiality important in all aspects of specimen collection?

Collection of Urine Specimens

7

LEARNING OBJECTIVES

On completing this chapter, you will be able to:

COGNITIVE OBJECTIVES
- Briefly state the general directions for collection of all types of urine specimens.
- Identify the proper method of urine collection for routine urinalysis, quantitative analysis, and bacterial studies.
- List the responsibilities of the clinical laboratorian for urine specimen collection in the office and for specimen delivered by the patient to the physician's office laboratory.

PSYCHOMOTOR OBJECTIVES
- Consult a Procedure Manual or other sources to determine the type of urine collection for various tests.
- Comply with all safety guidelines for the proper handling and disposal of specimens.
- Instruct patients on the method of collecting a midstream clean-catch specimen.

AFFECTIVE OBJECTIVES
- Identify and assist patients who need special help in collecting the specimens described in this chapter.
- Properly respond to patient inquiries as to the proper method of specimen collection, as described in this chapter.

Urine specimens are used to diagnose and manage urinary tract disorders. They are also used to evaluate **metabolic** and **systemic** function. The type of test that will be performed dictates the manner in which the urine specimen is collected. Some urine samples are collected in the medical office; others are collected at home by the patient. The time and manner of collecting and processing specimens influence the accuracy of urine testing.

Metabolic: *pertaining to the sum of all physical and chemical changes that take place within an organism*

Systemic: *pertaining to the entire body*

GENERAL DIRECTIONS

Proper labeling is essential to all specimen collection. Labels should be placed on the container, not the lid. Since many specimens are kept under refrigeration, use labels that adhere at low temperatures or label the container with a permanent marker.

Preservatives may be required when testing is delayed or when the analyte is unstable. Check the Procedure Manual or Directory of Services to determine the proper preservative for each test. The preservative must not interfere with test procedures or results.

Special pediatric urine collectors made of pliable ethylene are available. These are taped directly to the infant and remain in place until the sample is collected.

SPECIMEN COLLECTION

First Morning Specimen

The *first morning specimen,* collected upon arising, is the specimen of choice for the routine urinalysis. Because it represents the urine formed over approximately an 8-hour period, it is the most concentrated sample of the day. Its high concentration increases the chances of detecting abnormalities. In addition, the microscopic elements tend to remain intact for longer periods of time in a concentrated sample.

It is not practical to collect the first morning specimen at the medical office. The patient collects this sample at home and brings it to the office. Because of the physical and chemical changes that occur as urine ages, the patient must either refrigerate the sample until it is delivered to the office or add a preservative to the container. The clinical laboratory should supply the patient with a suitable container. It must be clean and have a tight-fitting lid. Old pickle jars, jelly jars, and other makeshift containers found at home are not acceptable, especially if they are not thoroughly cleaned and rinsed. Never use prescription bottles, bleach, or cleaning agent containers.

In menstruating women, blood cells may appear in such great quantities as to obscure other structures, so a clean tampon should be used before the collection. If the test is for a routine urinalysis, waiting a few days for specimen collection is advisable.

When the patient delivers a urine specimen to the POL, check that it is properly labeled and note the collection time and details of handling and storage. Test the specimen at once or refrigerate. The urine sample must be fresh and tested not more than 1 hour after voiding or, if refrigerated, not more than 6 hours after collection.

Timed Specimen

Challenge dose: *a measured amount of glucose given to the patient to evaluate how it is used by the body*

Postprandial: *after a meal*

In a *timed urine collection* the sample is obtained at a specified time. This type of sample is required in conjunction with other tests, especially those that assess metabolic activity or renal function. A glucose tolerance test is an example of a metabolic test that requires timed urine samples. In this test the patient drinks a **challenge dose** of glucose. Every hour, for 3 to 6 hours after the ingestion of the glucose, a blood sample and urine sample are collected and tested to determine the quantity of glucose.

Another timed specimen is a 2-hour **postprandial.** The patient is instructed to void, and then consume a routine meal. A specimen is collected 2 hours following the meal and tested for glucose. This test is used to evaluate insulin therapy. With controlled diabetes, the urine should not test positive for glucose.

Renal clearance tests evaluate the body's ability to remove urea and other nitrogenous wastes from the body. Some renal clearance tests incorporate timed urine samples. In one such clearance test, dye is injected into the bloodstream of the patient. The ability of the kidneys to remove the dye is assessed by determining the amount of dye found in urine samples collected at intervals after the dye is administered.

Laboratorians must carefully follow instructions for collection of timed samples. It is vital that the clinical laboratorian have the proper reagents and containers on hand before beginning any timed tests. Because time is critical to an accurate diagnosis, this collection takes priority over all other tasks except emergencies. As with all tests, fully label all samples. In timed tests, the time that the sample is collected is critical and must appear on the specimen container. Finally, immediately test the sample, refrigerate it for later testing, or send it to a referral laboratory following the directions provided by the testing laboratory.

The 24-Hour Urine Specimen

The *24-hour urine specimen* is a pooling of all urine excreted by the patient over a 24-hour period. Some tests require a pooled collection over a 3-, 6-, or 12-hour period. For all such tests the theory behind the collection and the method of collection are the same. The only variable is the length of time that the urine sample is collected.

The 24-hour sample is required to determine the quantity of an analyte in the specimen. As noted previously, urine concentration varies considerably during the day. To test a dilute sample, or a concentrated one, may give results that do not represent the true clinical picture. To test all urine samples excreted by the patient for the entire 24-hour period and then take their average is highly impractical and costly. To achieve the same results, you need to collect only samples excreted by the patient over the 24-hour period, pool these into one large container, and test a well-mixed representative sample from the 24-hour pool.

Since the urine will not be tested until the completion of the specimen collection time, it is necessary to use a preservative and to refrigerate the urine to avoid decomposition. (See Table 7–1 for information on urine preservatives.) The preservative must not

Table 7–1   **Urine Preservatives**

Preservative	Advantages	Disadvantages	Additional Information
Refrigeration	No interference with chemicals	Raises specific gravity by hydrometer; precipitates amorphous phosphates and urates	Shown to prevent bacterial growth for at least 24 hours
Thymol	Preserves glucose and sediments well	Interferes with acid precipitation tests for protein; large amounts will interfere with o-toluidine glucose tests	
Boric acid	Preserves protein and formed elements well; no interference with routine analysis other than pH	Large amounts are needed to inhibit bacterial growth; large amounts may cause crystal precipitation	Keeps pH at about 6.0; interferes with drug and hormone analyses
Formalin (formaldehyde)	Excellent sediment preservative	Interferes with copper reduction tests for glucose; causes clumping of sediment	Containers for collection of specimens for cell counts can be rinsed with formalin for better preservation of cells and casts
Toluene	Does not interfere with routine chemical tests	Floats on the surface of specimens and clings to pipettes and testing materials	
Hydrochloric acid	Bactericidal	Destroys formed elements and precipitates solutes; unacceptable for routine analysis	May be dangerous to the patient (splashing, etc.)
Freezing	Preserves bilirubin and urobilinogen	Destroys formed elements; turbidity occurs upon thawing	Useful for nonroutine chemical analysis

Adapted from Strasinger, SK: Urinalysis and Body Fluids, ed 3. FA Davis, Philadelphia, 1994, pp 4–5.

interfere with the analyte. Most 24-hour specimen containers are brown. This helps to screen out ultraviolet light, which can further decompose urine. Consult the Procedure Manual for the proper preservative and any special patient instructions, such as diet or medicine restrictions.

The 24-hour urine collection can begin at any time of the day. In practice, however, the collection usually begins upon arising. The first morning sample *is not collected for testing;* it is discarded, and the patient notes the time of this voiding. The test then begins with an empty bladder. The patient collects each urine discharge for the next 24 hours in a small urine cup and pours each sample into a large 24-hour container. The patient collects the last sample 24 hours after the time noted when the first voiding was discarded. For example, if the patient begins the 24-hour collection at 8:30 A.M., this first sample is discarded and the time is noted. At 8:30 A.M. the following day, the patient empties his or her bladder as the final sample and adds this to the 24-hour sample.

Physicians' offices rarely perform the analysis on 24-hour urine samples. They are sent to referral laboratories or hospitals. After the specimen has been logged, the 24-hour specimen is measured and this measurement is recorded on the request slip. A small aliquot is removed from the pooled 24-hour specimen after it has been thoroughly mixed, and this sample is placed in a labeled transport container. Always follow the recommended method of transport required by the referral laboratory.

Midstream Specimen

A *midstream urine specimen* is the middle portion of a single urination. The patient collects the specimen after an initial one-third of the urine is passed into the toilet. The first one-third of urine passed into the toilet "flushes" the lower urinary structures of normal contaminants. It is not part of the specimen. The patient then collects the second one-third portion. This second portion should contain at least 20 mL of urine. The midstream urine more closely represents the environment of the contents of the bladder because it is free of most contaminants found in the urethra or around the urinary meatus. After collecting the middle quantity of urine, the patient completes urination into the toilet.

The midstream method is becoming the accepted way to obtain many urine specimens, especially for routine urinalysis. Obviously this technique is *not* used for 24-hour specimen collection because those specimens require all voided urine to be saved and the total quantity measured.

Midstream Clean-Catch Specimen

Extraneous organisms: *organisms that may be present in a location and may enter a test procedure as a contaminant*

Aseptic technique: *a method used to prevent contamination in procedures where a sterile field is required*

Sterile: *free of living microorganisms, including spores*

The *midstream clean-catch* procedure involves collecting urine in a way that greatly minimizes the chance that it will be contaminated by **extraneous organisms.** Urine specimens for bacterial studies such as cultures for identification of bacterial organisms and antibiotic sensitivity testing must be free of contaminating organisms. The midstream clean-catch specimen collection requires special cleaning of the external genitalia. Most patients are not familiar with **aseptic technique;** therefore, you must carefully instruct them on the procedure for collection. Elderly, young, or disabled patients may require assistance. Some patients experience embarrassment when personal matters are discussed. Be sensitive and try to anticipate any special needs. Assure them that their privacy will be respected when they enter the bathroom. Be helpful, courteous, and professional when you interact with patients. To determine whether patients understand the procedure, you may have them restate the steps of the procedure.

Several companies sell kits that contain all the equipment required for a clean-catch midstream specimen, including illustrated directions for patients, towelettes premoistened with cleaning solution, and a disposable **sterile** urine container (Fig. 7–1).

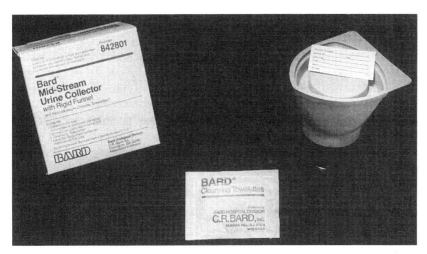

Figure 7–1 Midstream clean-catch kit.

Instruct all patients to wash and dry their hands. Tell male patients to clean the urinary opening with a towelette in a single stroke from the tip of the penis toward the ring of the glans. They should repeat the procedure with a fresh towelette. Uncircumcised males must first retract the foreskin, exposing the urinary opening.

Female patients are instructed to clean the external genitalia by having them sit on the toilet with one leg placed to the side as far as comfortably possible. Next, spread the labia with the nondominant hand and with a fresh towelette in the other hand, clean the labia on one side of the urinary opening in one stroke from front to back. Clean the labia on the other side in the same way using a fresh towelette. Finally, with another fresh towelette, clean the urinary opening itself, in one stroke from front to back. After cleaning, keep the labia spread until the sample is collected using the midstream collection technique, which flushes away any organisms or contaminants that are in the lower part of the urethra.

Patients collect the midstream clean-catch specimen at the physician's office. For the convenience of the patient many offices post illustrations and directions for the clean-catch technique at eye level in the bathroom where urine collections are obtained. When the patient delivers the specimen, wipe the outside of the urine cup with a tissue that has been moistened in a **disinfectant,** dry the container, and apply a label containing all necessary information. After completion of the specimen collection, clean the work area (Table 7–2).

Disinfectant: *substance used to kill microorganisms on inanimate objects, such as equipment, surfaces, and clothing*

Table 7–2 *Types of Urine Specimens Usually Collected in a POL*

Type of Specimen	Purpose
Random	Routine screening
First morning	Routine screening
	Pregnancy tests
	Orthostatic protein
Fasting	Diabetic monitoring
2-hour postprandial	Diabetic monitoring
	Glucose testing
Glucose tolerance test (GTT)	Accompanies blood samples in glucose tolerance tests
Midstream clean-catch	Routine screening
	Bacterial culture

SUMMARY

The nature of the tests to be performed on any specimen determines its method of collection. Refer to the POL Procedure Manual for instructions on the manner of collection, the quantity of specimen needed for the test, whether preservatives are required, and any other relevant information. You must instruct the patient regarding dietary and medicine restrictions. Clearly instruct the patient on the proper method of collection. Be sure all containers and reagents are on hand before the specimen is collected. The clinical laboratorian is responsible for patient instruction, specimen labeling, and specimen testing or preparation for transport.

PATIENT EDUCATION

- Evaluate understanding of the proper procedures for a urine specimen collection by having the patient repeat the steps of the procedure back to you after your instructions.
- When patients show undue concern or embarrassment, be reassuring. Anticipate their needs and be responsive.

TECHNICAL CONSIDERATIONS

- Fully label all specimens.
- Include time of collection on the label for all timed specimens.
- For 24-hour specimens, include the total quantity of urine collected, and prepare a well-mixed aliquot for transport.
- Follow all collection requirements in the Procedure Manual or Directory of Services.

SOURCES OF ERROR

- Test only fresh urines or those that have been properly preserved. "Stale" urines will give erroneous results.
- Makeshift jars supplied by the patient are often unacceptable for transport of specimens to the office. They often contain soap or residual materials that interfere with testing.

Procedure with Rationale

Clean-Catch Specimen Collection

EQUIPMENT AND SUPPLIES

Handsoap	Paper towel moistened with disinfectant
Towelettes with an antiseptic solution	solution
Clean paper towel	Permanent marker
Sterile urine container with lid	Latex gloves
Label	Biohazard container

Assemble equipment.

Wash hands with soap and water. Observe the OSHA Standard for this procedure.

Greet the patient and briefly explain the midstream clean-catch technique. Do not use technical terms.

Assist the elderly, disabled, or young patient.

Have the patient wash and dry his or her hands. ***Handwashing minimizes contamination.***

Instruct the patient to remove the lid of the sterile container and place it so that the inner portion faces upward. ***This minimizes transfer of bacteria to the sample when the lid is replaced on the container after the collection of the sample.***

Tell the patient not to touch the inside of the container or lid anytime during the procedure. ***This minimizes the transfer of extraneous bacteria to the sample.***

Instruct the patient to clean the external genitalia using fresh towelettes.

INSTRUCTIONS FOR MALE PATIENTS

If uncircumcised, retract the foreskin using a sterile towelette. Hold it back throughout the entire procedure. ***This exposes the urinary opening for proper cleaning.***

Using a fresh towelette, clean the urinary opening with a single stroke directed from the tip of the penis to the ring of the glans. ***This avoids carrying bacteria back to the urinary opening.***

Discard towelette. ***The towelette is now contaminated and must not be used again.***

Repeat the cleaning procedure with a fresh towelette. ***Additional cleaning removes bacteria that may still be present.***

INSTRUCTIONS FOR FEMALE PATIENTS

Sit on the toilet and position one leg to the side as far as comfortably possible. ***This position allows the patient room to manipulate the towelettes and container during the procedure.***

Spread the labia with the fingers of the nondominant hand and maintain this position until the specimen is collected. ***This exposes the urinary opening for proper cleaning.***

In a single front-to-back stroke, wipe the labia on one side of the urinary opening with a fresh towelette. ***The single front to back stroke removes bacteria from the urinary opening and avoids recontamination from the rectal or vaginal opening.***

Using a fresh towelette, repeat the procedure on the opposite side of the urinary opening. *(Same rationale as in previous step.)*

Using a third towelette, wipe the urinary opening with a single front-to-back stroke. Keep the labia spread until the specimen is collected. *(Same rationale.)*

INSTRUCTIONS FOR MALE AND FEMALE PATIENTS

Begin urination into the toilet, voiding approximately one-third of the urine. *This initial voiding washes away bacteria that are part of the normal contaminants of the lower portion of the urethra and meatus.*

After passing approximately one-third of the urine into the toilet, interrupt the stream and collect approximately 20 mL of urine in the sterile container. *The midstream collection is part of the clean-catch technique. This urine most closely represents the state of the urine in the bladder.*

After collecting about 20 mL of urine, complete urination into the toilet. *Only the urine that represents the "midstream" is collected.*

Put the lid on the container without touching the inside of it.

Obtain the specimen from the patient. Wipe the outside of the container with a paper towel moistened with disinfectant. *Urine may be on the outside of the cup. Others who handle the container should not be exposed to urine.*

Dry the container and apply a label that has been properly completed using a permanent marker. *A permanent marker ensures that the information will not be eradicated if the label becomes wet during transport of the specimen to the laboratory.*

Clean work area following laboratory protocol.

Remove gloves and wash hands with soap and water.

Questions

Name _____ Date _____

1. When is a urine preservative used? What are the requirements for a urine preservative?

2. What is the specimen of choice for a routine urinalysis? Why?

3. What is a timed urine specimen, and when is this type of specimen required?

4. What is a 24-hour urine specimen? When is it required?

5. Briefly explain the procedure for a midstream collection.

6. When is a midstream clean-catch sample required?

7. What general precautions must be followed when obtaining a midstream collection?

8. Why is the midstream collection part of a clean-catch specimen collection?

9. How can a laboratorian tell whether patients understand the various urine collection procedures?

Terminal Performance Objective

Clean-Catch Specimen Collection

You will assemble the required equipment, instruct a male and a female patient on the proper method for a midstream clean-catch urine specimen, and process the specimen within 5 minutes. For this competency, role-play a situation with one student as the patient and the other as a clinical laboratorian. The clinical laboratorian must respond to any questions or needs of the patient. Your instructions must include all steps to an accuracy level as determined by your instructor. Your instructor will evaluate whether you assembled the proper equipment, whether your role-playing instructions were complete, and whether you properly processed the specimen.

INSTRUCTOR'S EVALUATION FORM

Name _____ Date _____

+ = SATISFACTORY   ✓ = UNSATISFACTORY

_____ Assemble equipment.

_____ Wash hands with soap and water. Observe the OSHA Standard for this procedure.

_____ Greet the patient and briefly explain the midstream clean-catch technique. Do not use technical terms.

_____ Assist the elderly, disabled, or young patient.

_____ Have the patient wash and dry his or her hands.

_____ Instruct the patient to remove the lid of the sterile container and place it so that the inner portion faces upward.

_____ Tell the patient not to touch the inside of the container or lid anytime during the procedure.

_____ Instruct the patient to clean the external genitalia using fresh towelettes.

Instructions for Male Patients

_____ If uncircumcised, retract the foreskin using a sterile towelette. Hold it back throughout the entire procedure.

_____ Using a fresh towelette, clean the urinary opening with a single stroke directed from the tip of the penis to the ring of the glans.

_____ Discard towelette.

_____ Repeat the cleaning procedure with a fresh towelette.

Instructions for Female Patients

_____ Sit on the toilet and position one leg to the side as far as comfortably possible.

_____ Spread the labia with the fingers of the nondominant hand and maintain this position until the specimen is collected.

_____ In a single front-to-back stroke, wipe the labia on one side of the urinary opening with a fresh towelette.

_____ Using a fresh towelette, repeat the procedure on the opposite side of the urinary opening.

_____ Using a third towelette, wipe the urinary opening with a single front-to-back stroke. Keep the labia spread until the specimen is collected.

Instructions for Male and Female Patients

_____ Begin urination into the toilet, voiding approximately one-third of the urine.

_____ After passing approximately one-third of the urine into the toilet, interrupt the stream and collect approximately 20 mL of urine in the sterile container.

_____ After collecting about 20 mL of urine, complete urination into the toilet.

_____ Put the lid on the container without touching the inside of it.

_____ Obtain the specimen from the patient. Wipe the outside of the container with a paper towel moistened with disinfectant.

_____ Dry the container and apply a label that has been properly completed using a permanent marker.

_____ Clean work area following laboratory protocol.

_____ Remove gloves and wash hands with soap and water.

_____ The procedure was completed within 5 minutes.

_____ The results obtained were accurate to the level specified by your instructor.

Final Competency Evaluation

_____ SATISFACTORY   _____ UNSATISFACTORY

Comments:

Instructor _____ Date _____

Collection of Blood Specimens

8

LEARNING OBJECTIVES

On completing this chapter, you will be able to:

COGNITIVE OBJECTIVES

- Identify the sites for capillary puncture and explain why these sites are selected.
- Explain how the capillary puncture is performed using a sterile lancet.
- Name the parts of the vacuum tube system and explain their function.
- List the order of draw for a multiple-draw venipuncture.
- Describe the technique of venipuncture using a syringe and hypodermic needle.

PSYCHOMOTOR OBJECTIVES

- Perform a capillary puncture following the Terminal Performance Objective presented in the chapter.
- Perform a venipuncture following the Terminal Performance Objective presented in the chapter.

AFFECTIVE OBJECTIVES

- Assume responsibility for a clean and safe work environment.
- Maintain laboratory safety for yourself and your coworkers by disposing of the blood and sharps according to laboratory protocol.

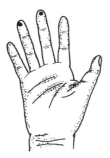 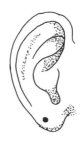 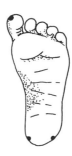

Figure 8-1   Recommended sites for a capillary puncture.

Many laboratory tests require only a few drops of blood. The *capillary puncture,* also known as the *finger stick,* is a safe and efficient method for obtaining smaller quantities of blood for testing. This method of blood collection may eliminate the need for **phlebotomy.** Phlebotomy is sometimes a difficult procedure, especially on infants and children whose veins are too small for venipuncture. Phlebotomy may also be undesirable and difficult for geriatric, cancer, and burn patients.

Phlebotomy: *surgical opening of a vein to withdraw blood*

CAPILLARY PUNCTURE

Commonly Used Sites

Capillaries are microscopic blood vessels that pass through virtually all tissues of the body. Although any surface of the body will yield a small quantity of blood when punctured with a **lancet,** the most common sites are shown in Figure 8-1. They include:

Lancet: *metal device ending in a pointed blade sharpened on both sides*

Plantar: *pertaining to the sole of the foot*

- The ring finger or middle finger on adults
- The earlobe on adults and children
- The great toe on infants
- The medial and lateral **plantar** surface of the foot of newborns

These sites are preferred because of their *vascularity* and "fleshiness." Vascularity is the density of capillaries within tissues. The lancet must puncture sufficient capillaries so that enough blood is available to perform all requested tests. The site must also be fleshy enough to ensure that the lancet does not penetrate underlying bone or dense connective tissue.

Because a puncture on the plantar surface of the foot on a newborn baby may cause injury to the underlying bone, use only the fleshy area of the heel. For infants, the great toe is often the best site. With children and adults, the middle finger or ring finger is the site of choice.

Sterile Lancets

Many devices are used in the medical office for the capillary puncture. Disposable sterile lancets (Fig. 8-2) are used for microcollection of blood from the heel of an infant or fin-

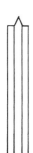

Figure 8-2   Blood lancet.

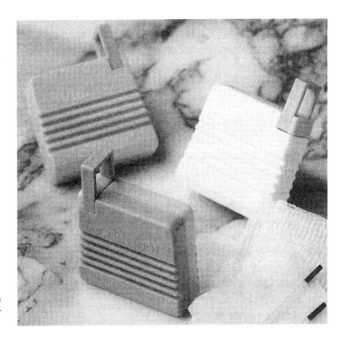

Figure 8-3 Tenderfoot heel incision device. (Courtesy International Technidyne Corporation, Edison, NJ.)

ger of a child or adult. Capillary puncture is performed on adults when there are no accessible veins. It is used for bedside, point of care testing (POCT), and for glucose monitoring at home.

Lancets come in sterile packages. Follow package directions for opening to maintain sterility. The blade size used depends on the size of the puncture required. Blade sizes also vary according to manufacturer. The Tenderfoot (Fig. 8-3) is a disposable device available for heel incision. Use this device to make an incision 1.0 mm in depth and 2.5 mm in length, not a puncture wound. The Tenderlett is a disposable spring-loaded device for fingertip puncture. Both are available from International Technidyne Corporation.

Monolet blood lancets are a product of Sherwood-Davis & Geck. The tribeveled point of the Monolet is used for easy penetration with minimum pain. Depth of penetration is controlled to provide an adequate capillary blood sample with minimum dilution by tissue fluids. The Monojector is a compact, spring-loaded, fingertip puncture tool specifically designed for use with the Monolet. The Monolettor Safety Lancet, which retracts and locks the lancet within the case after puncturing the skin (Fig. 8-4), is also available.

The Microtainer Safety Flow Lancet by Becton Dickinson is similar to other spring-loaded devices, but the entire mechanism is discarded (Fig. 8-5). Three puncture depths are available, 1.4, 1.9, and 2.2 mm, and they are color-coded.

Method for Capillary Puncture

When you perform a fingertip puncture, make the puncture slightly to the side of the fingertip, holding the blade so that the cut is perpendicular to the **whorls** on the fingerprint (Fig. 8-6). This causes the blood to form as a drop on the end of the finger instead of running down the grooves of the fingerprint ridges.

The entire lancet tip must penetrate the skin. The penetration is controlled by the design of the lancets. If the penetration is not complete, another puncture might be necessary. If this happens, *always use a new lancet. Never* use any blood-collecting device more than once, even on the same patient. Once used, the lancet is no longer sterile and must be disposed of in a **sharps** container.

Seat the patient in a blood-drawing chair. These decklike chairs are designed with arms that protect the patient from falling in case of fainting. Do not allow the patient to

Whorls: *swirls of the fingerprint*

Sharps: *medical articles that may cause punctures or cuts to those handling them, including syringes, needles, lancets, scalpel blades, suture needles, razors, and broken medical glassware*

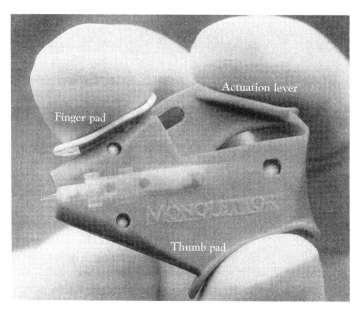

Figure 8–4 Monolettor blood lancet. (Courtesy Sherwood-Davis & Geck, St. Louis, Mo.)

Edematous: *having an excessive amount of tissue fluid; swollen*

Cyanotic: *having slightly bluish discoloration of the skin due to abnormal amounts of reduced hemoglobin in the blood*

Interstitial fluid: *fluid that surrounds cells*

Tissue thromboplastin: *a blood coagulation factor (factor III) found in tissues, platelets, and leukocytes*

stand or sit on a stool during any blood-collecting procedure. After the patient is seated, select the site for puncture. Avoid any area that is red, **edematous,** calloused, wounded, or **cyanotic** or that exhibits a rash.

If the site is unusually cold, or appears pale, place the finger in warm water for 2 to 3 minutes or gently massage the finger to increase circulation. Cleanse the area with a 70 percent isopropyl alcohol pad, allow it to air-dry, or wipe the area with a sterile gauze pad. Prepare all equipment required to perform the tests requested by the physician. Securely hold the patient's finger and puncture the site with a swift stabbing motion of the lancet. After the puncture has been made, use a sterile 2 × 2 inch gauze pad to wipe away the first drop of blood. This drop may be diluted by **interstitial fluid** and **tissue thromboplastin,** which could activate clotting of the specimen.

All blood collected must be *free-flowing.* Blood is free-flowing if a slight amount of pressure near the site of the puncture causes a drop of blood to be present immediately.

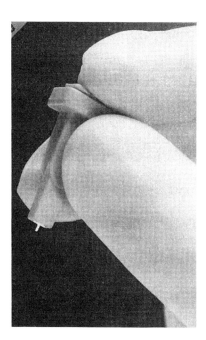

Figure 8–5 Microtainer safety flow lancet. (Courtesy Becton Dickinson, Franklin Lakes, NJ.)

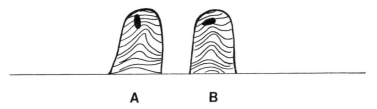

A   **B**

Figure 8–6 Lancet should penetrate slightly to the side of the fingertip so that the cut is perpendicular to the whorls of the fingerprint as shown in *(A)*. It should not penetrate as shown in *(B)*.

If you must squeeze the finger to get blood, you will be diluting the sample with tissue fluid. Adding tissue fluid to the sample will cause inaccuracies in test results.

Excessive squeezing of the finger may also cause **hemolysis** of the red blood cells. The specimen will no longer be usable for testing. If blood is not free-flowing, make another puncture using a *new sterile* lancet. At the end of the collection, give the patient a sterile gauze pad to press against the puncture site to stop the bleeding. This prevents *extravasation,* that is, the leaking of blood into the surrounding tissues.

Hemolysis: *destruction of the red blood cells*

Check to see that the bleeding has stopped. You may apply a small adhesive bandage if necessary. Exercise caution when using adhesive bandages. Some patients are allergic to adhesive tape, and young children may pull off bandages, put them in their mouths, and choke.

Place all sharps into a puncture-resistant, leakproof sharps biohazard container (see Chapter 2).

CAPILLARY BLOOD COLLECTION

The capillary puncture allows for the collection of blood for many different tests. The nature of the test and instrumentation used determine the manner in which blood is collected. Specimens are collected for hematology studies, such as complete blood counts (CBCs), red blood cell (RBC) counts, white blood cell (WBC) counts, and hematocrits.

Several micro-blood-collecting tubes are available for capillary blood collection for chemistry analysis. Small glass or plastic specimen tubes fitted with a wide-mouth blood collector and color-coded plug are used to collect a single-tube skin puncture on infants, children, and geriatric, cancer, and burn patients with whom venipuncture may be difficult. The Microtainer with Microgard closure by Becton Dickinson (Fig. 8–7) is one type of micro-blood-collecting tube. It is available with or without additives. The blood sample is ready for transport or centrifugation right in the collection tube.

Samplette (Fig. 8–8) capillary blood separator by Sherwood-Davis & Geck contains a barrier gel that provides one-step processing to separate **serum** from cells during centrifugation. Follow the manufacturer's instructions for the proper use of these micro-blood-collecting tubes.

Serum: *the liquid portion of coagulated blood*

VENIPUNCTURE

When more than a few drops of blood are required for hematology and clinical chemistry analysis, a *venipuncture* is necessary. Clinical laboratories usually perform blood studies on venous blood samples collected by phlebotomy.

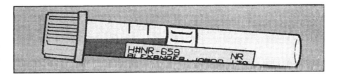

Figure 8–7 Microtainer blood collector tube. (Courtesy Becton Dickinson, Franklin Lakes, NJ.)

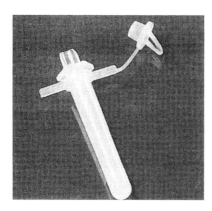

Figure 8–8 Samplette capillary blood separator. (Courtesy Sherwood-Davis & Geck, St. Louis, Mo.)

To collect a venous blood sample, the phlebotomist either pierces the vein with a **hypodermic needle** and draws blood into a syringe or uses commercially available apparatus specifically designed for collecting venous blood, such as the Vacutainer, Veniject, or Monoject systems. Using a hypodermic needle and syringe requires more skill and gives the phlebotomist more control for drawing blood from small or difficult veins.

BLOOD SAMPLE COLLECTION SYSTEMS

Vacuum Tube System

The vacuum tube system is the most popular method for collecting blood samples by venipuncture. It consists of a double-pointed needle, a plastic holder, and a series of vacuum tubes with rubber stoppers (Fig. 8–9).

Vacuum Needle

The vacuum needle (Fig. 8–10) is pointed at both ends, with one end shorter than the other. The shorter end goes through the rubber stopper of the vacuum tube, and the longer end is for insertion into the vein. Needles are available in several sizes, determined by the length and gauge of the needle that goes into the vein. Vacuum needles range from 1 to 1.5 inches in length. The *gauge* of a needle is a number that indicates the diameter of its *lumen* (also called the bore), which is the circular hollow space inside the needle. The higher the gauge number, the smaller the lumen. The most frequently used gauges for phlebotomy are 20, 21, and 22.

The *bevel* is the slanted opening at the end of the needle. The phlebotomist performs a venipuncture so that the bevel of the needle is facing upward when the needle is inserted into the vein. When the slanted opening of the needle faces upward, the needle will cause less pain and enter the vein more smoothly. Vacuum tube needles come in sterile packages, either peel-apart envelopes or plastic cases.

Vacuum system needles are available with single-draw or multiple-draw capabilities. The multidraw needles have a rubber sheath on the end of the needle that penetrates the rubber stopper. The sheath prevents the leaking of blood when switching tubes.

Vacuum Needle Holder

The vacuum needle holder is a plastic sleeve into which the phlebotomist screws the double-pointed needle. The vacuum tubes are pushed onto the needle inside the holder, but not past the line shown on the holder. After entry into the vein the tube is pushed into the holder all the way. This causes the vacuum to draw the blood from the vein. If the tube is pushed onto the needle past the line, the vacuum will be exhausted and the tube will be unusable. Holders are available in two sizes, one for adult venipuncture and one for pediatric procedures.

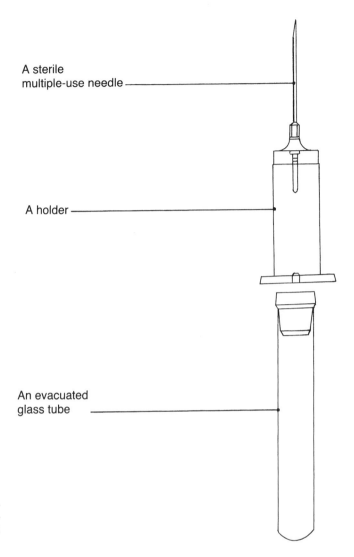

A sterile
multiple-use needle

A holder

An evacuated
glass tube

Figure 8–9 The vacuum tube system consists of a double-pointed needle, a plastic holder, and a vacuum tube with rubber stopper.

Vacuum Tubes

Vacuum tubes are glass or plastic tubes, sealed by color-coded rubber stoppers, that contain a partial vacuum. The air pressure inside the tube is negative, less than the normal environment. After inserting the longer needle into the vein, the phlebotomist pushes the tube into the holder, so that the shorter needle pierces the stopper. The difference in pressure between the inside of the tube and the vein causes blood to fill the tube. The tubes are available in various sizes for adult and pediatric phlebotomies. Adult tube sizes are 5, 7, 10, and 15 mL and pediatric tube sizes are 2, 3, and 4 mL.

Different blood tests require a variety of tubes with additives. For instance, some specimens require the addition of an **anticoagulant** in the tube. In the vacuum collection tube system, the additives are already in the tubes in the precise amount needed to mix with the amount of blood that will fill the tube. The color of the stopper on each vacuum tube indicates what, if any, anticoagulants the tube contains. Table 8–1 identifies the con-

Anticoagulant: *a substance that prevents or delays coagulation of the blood*

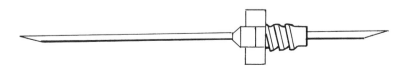

Figure 8–10 Vacuum tube needle, pointed at both ends with one end shorter than the other

Table 8-1 *Vacuum Tube Stopper Color Code in Order of Draw*

Stopper Color	Additive	Specimen Use
Red	No additive; no anticoagulant	Serum determinations in chemistry, serology, and blood banking
Red and black mottled top	Clot activator and gel for serum separation	SST brand tube for serum determinations in chemistry (Tube inversion ensures mixing of clot activator with blood and clotting within 30 minutes.)
Red Monoject Corvac	Silicone coated tube; gel barrier	Tests using serum for general chemistry, serology, and toxicology procedures
Blue	Sodium citrate	Coagulation determinations on plasma specimens (Tube inversion prevents clotting.)
Green	Sodium heparin; lithium heparin; ammonium heparin	Plasma determinations in chemistry (Tube inversion prevents clotting.)
Lavender	EDTA (ethylenediaminetetraacetic acid)	Whole blood hematology determinations (Tube inversion prevents clotting.)
Gray	Potassium oxalate; sodium fluoride; lithium iodoacetate or lithium heparin	Glucose determinations (Glycotic inhibitors stabilize glucose values for 24 hours at room temperature with iodoacetate and for at least 3 days with fluoride.)

Note: Certain tests require chilled specimens. Follow recommended procedures for collection and transport of specimens.

tents of the vacuum tubes and their corresponding stopper colors. Remember, it is important to fill each tube completely, so that the proportion of blood to chemical additive is correct; otherwise, the test results may not be accurate. Failure to obtain the correct amount of blood in proportion to the anticoagulant is called a "short draw." .

When drawing blood for a blood profile, or panel (see Chapter 20 for an explanation of "profiles"), the phlebotomist fills several vacuum tubes, each with a different color stopper, in what is called a multiple draw, or *multidraw*. The phlebotomist must fill these tubes in a certain order. This is necessary to avoid contaminating the blood in one tube with traces of chemicals from a previous tube, which might interfere with the test results. For this reason, red-stoppered tubes—with no anticoagulants—are filled first.

Blood for **coagulation studies** is never drawn first, because the first blood taken from a punctured vein may contain the body's naturally occurring coagulant, *tissue thromboplastin,* which would affect the accuracy of coagulation time. Always draw a red-stoppered tube before the blue-stoppered tube, which is for coagulation studies. Table 8-1 indicates the order of draw according to stopper color. Draw specimens for **blood culture** first, followed by the tubes without anticoagulants, and finally, draw the tubes that contain anticoagulants in the order shown. If a blood culture is not ordered, the first tubes collected are the red-stoppered tubes.

Coagulation studies:
analysis of the ability of the blood to clot

Blood culture:
collection of blood into vacuum tubes with special media to grow pathogenic organisms

Needle and Syringe

Use the needle and syringe method of venipuncture to obtain specimens from fragile, thready veins that might collapse from the vacuum of collection tubes and from the veins in the hands and feet. The hypodermic needle consists of the bevel (opening), the shaft, and the *hub* (Fig. 8-11). The hub attaches the needle to the syringe. The recommended length for the hypodermic needle is 1 to 1.5 inches. Use a gauge of 20, 21, or 22 for venipuncture. The 22-gauge needle is preferred for pediatric phlebotomy or very small veins of the hands or feet.

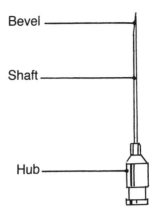

Figure 8–11   The hypodermic needle consists of the bevel, the shaft, and the hub.

The syringe consists of a barrel and a plunger. The barrel is graduated into milliliters (mL) or cubic centimeters (cc) (Fig. 8–12). Sizes vary from 2 to 20 mL or larger. Loosen the plunger of the barrel to break the seal created in the manufacturing process and force out all the air before inserting the needle into the vein. After inserting the needle into the vein, the phlebotomist retracts the plunger slowly. Withdrawing blood with a syringe causes a pressure (back pressure) in the vein. Pulling the plunger slowly prevents the collapse of the vein because of this back pressure. The larger the barrel, the greater the back pressure.

Winged Infusion Set (Butterfly)

The winged infusion set (butterfly) is an intravenous device that phlebotomists sometimes use for collecting blood from pediatric patients and patients with difficult or small veins. The butterfly set consists of a needle with plastic wings for gripping, plastic tubing, and an adapter to attach the tubing to the holder of the vacuum collection system (Fig. 8–13). The length of the needle is a half inch, which limits its use to surface veins. The gauge ranges between 22 and 25. No adapter is necessary for using the butterfly-winged infusion set with the needle and syringe method.

PATIENT PREPARATION

Before beginning a venipuncture, the laboratorian must wash his or her hands and follow the OSHA Standard. To help prevent patient anxiety, explain the procedure to the patient. For phlebotomy, choose the appropriate vacuum tubes for the tests requested and label the tubes after collecting the specimen. Have many additional tubes available within reach in case the vacuum of the tubes has been destroyed. Laboratories identify the number and color of the stoppered vacuum tubes needed for all the tests that they perform.

It is important that the phlebotomist correctly identify the patient. Verify the patient's identity by having the patient spell his or her own name. Record the name of the

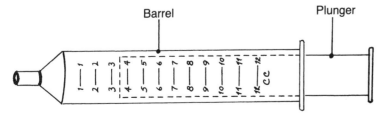

Figure 8–12   Syringe consisting of a barrel and plunger.

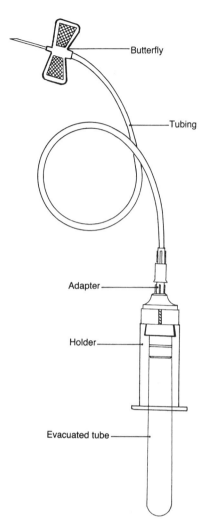

Figure 8-13 Butterfly-winged infusion set with adapter, holder, and evacuated tube.

patient, the date, the time, and the phlebotomist's initials on all the vacuum tubes collected during the venipuncture. The patient's ID or social security number, the test ordered, billing information, and the name of the physician may also be required.

Position the patient in a phlebotomy chair with a tray for support of the arm and body. The arm must be positioned downward to prevent **reflux.** Drawing blood from the patient who feels faint is accomplished more easily with the patient in a reclined position. Know where first aid kits are located before you begin the procedure. If the patient appears pale or complains of feeling faint, terminate the phlebotomy and have the patient breathe deeply. Apply cold compresses to the back of the neck. Have the patient lower his or her head below the knees; use an ammonia capsule if the patient loses consciousness. If this treatment is not effective, call for assistance immediately. Remain with the patient until he or she is fully recovered. Instruct the patient to remain in the area and not to drive for at least 30 minutes. Document this instruction in the patient's chart, in case of future litigation.

Reflux: *a return or backward flow*

SITE PREPARATION

Tourniquet: *any constrictor used to distend veins to facilitate venipuncture*

Apply a **tourniquet** above the elbow to impede blood flow and make the veins more prominent. Tie the tourniquet in a way that it may be removed with one hand (Fig.

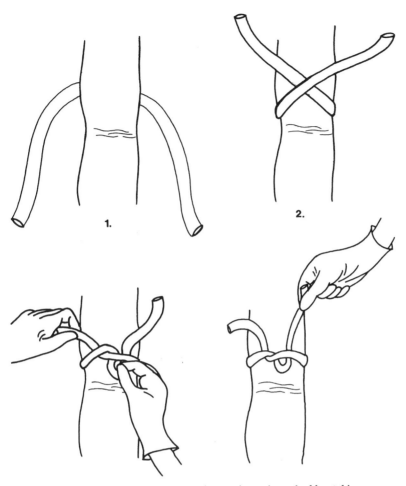

Figure 8–14 Application of tourniquet using a piece of rubber tubing.

8–14). Do not apply the tourniquet so tightly as to prevent flow of blood in the arteries, but make it tight enough to stop the flow of blood in the veins. A flat piece of rubber tubing functions best as a tourniquet and is more comfortable for the patient than the small tubular tourniquet. Velcro tourniquets are also available. After applying the tourniquet to the arm, choose the puncture site. The arm has many veins from which to choose a venipuncture site. Use the large *median cubital, cephalic,* or *basilic* veins (Fig. 8–15) for venipuncture. The median cubital, cephalic, and basilic are veins of the forearm. The basilic vein veers toward the anterior surface of the forearm and is joined to the cephalic vein by the median cubital vein. Use of the basilic is more painful. The cubital area is the obvious choice. The blue superficial veins of the forearm are not adequate for a venipuncture.

Using the fingertips, **palpate** the veins to determine their direction, depth, and size. Choose veins that are large and accessible. Large veins frequently roll, so if you choose one, be sure to anchor it with the thumb of your nondominant hand when you penetrate it with the needle. Do not choose veins that feel hard (sclerosed). Blood is not easily collected from veins that are scarred and hardened from repeated use. They are difficult to enter, and if obstructed or occluded, will not permit blood to flow through them. Veins sometimes collapse from the vacuum pressure of vacuum tubes or the back pressure of a syringe.

After selecting a vein, remove the tourniquet to clean the site. Clean the puncture site with 70 percent isopropyl alcohol and allow it to air-dry. Rub the alcohol gauze in one smooth circular pass of the venipuncture site with enough pressure to remove all perspi-

Palpate: *to examine by touch; to feel*

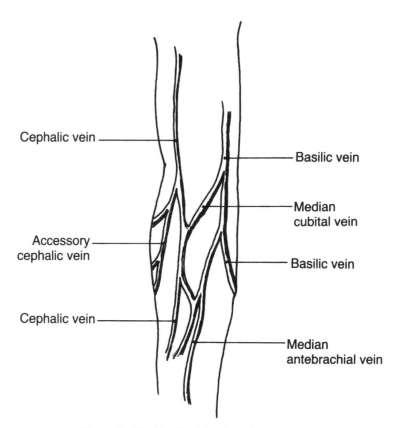

Figure 8–15 The blood-drawing veins of the arm.

ration and dirt from the puncture site. Use a second alcohol gauze at your discretion if the site is extremely dirty. Touching the site after cleaning with alcohol requires cleaning the area *again* with a new alcohol preparation.

Reapply the tourniquet after cleaning the puncture site. Hold the prepared vacuum tubes or needle and syringe in your dominant hand. Place the thumb of the non-dominant hand below the puncture site to anchor the vein and pull the skin taut. The needle entering the site should not touch the thumb of the phlebotomist. Position the needle in the same direction as the vein with the bevel of the needle facing upward. Enter the skin and penetrate the vein at a 15° angle in a swift but smooth motion to decrease the patient's discomfort. The bevel of the needle should enter and remain in the center of the vein (Fig. 8–16). Remove the tourniquet as soon as the blood begins to flow.

When switching vacuum tubes in a multidraw, it is very important to steady the holder to prevent the needle from accidentally pulling from the vein. Use a multiple-draw needle for the vacuum tube system when filling more than one tube. This prevents the blood from escaping into the holder when switching tubes. Release the tourniquet as soon as the blood begins to flow. When all tubes of blood have been collected, place a sterile gauze pad over the site and withdraw the needle in a smooth and cautious manner (Fig. 8–17).

After withdrawing the needle fully, press the gauze over the puncture site to prevent a **hematoma** and ask the patient to apply pressure with the arm elevated and straight for at least 3 to 5 minutes until bleeding stops. Apply an adhesive pressure bandage after 3 to 5 minutes only if bleeding has ceased and the patient is not allergic to the adhesive. Warn the patient not to lift or carry any heavy items in the arm of the venipuncture for at least an hour. Document patient instructions.

Hematoma: *a swelling or mass of blood confined to an organ, tissue, or space caused by a break in a blood vessel*

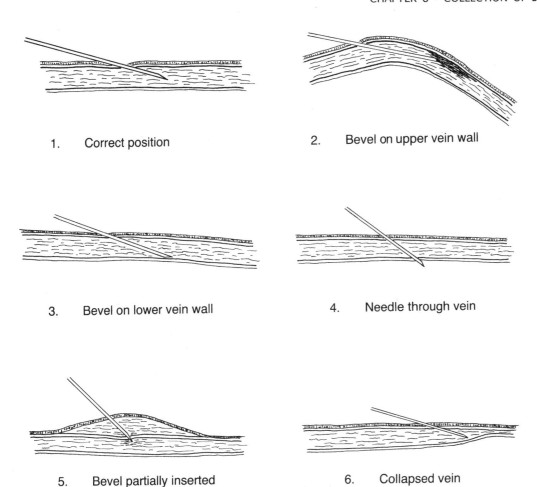

1.   Correct position

2.   Bevel on upper vein wall

3.   Bevel on lower vein wall

4.   Needle through vein

5.   Bevel partially inserted

6.   Collapsed vein

Figure 8–16   Correct and incorrect positions of the needle in the vein.

Clinical Comment: Vasovagal Syncope (Fainting)

Vasovagal syncope or sudden fainting is due to hypotension induced by the response of the nervous system to abrupt emotional stress, pain, or trauma. It is accompanied by pallor, sweating, hyperventilation, and **bradycardia.** Have the patient lie flat and make sure of a clear airway; treat the cause of the condition, if possible. In the case of venipuncture, stop the procedure and treat the symptoms. Vomiting does not usually occur, but if it does, position patient to prevent aspiration of vomitus.

Bradycardia: *a slow heartbeat usually with a pulse rate that is under 60 beats per minute*

Discard the needle of the syringe or vacuum tube into a biohazard sharps container *without recapping* the needle. Invert gently any tube containing an anticoagulant at least 8 to 10 times or until the anticoagulant is thoroughly mixed with the blood. Label the collection tubes and also observe the patient for any signs of fainting.

If the needle and syringe method of collection is used, gently retract the plunger of the syringe, making sure the needle and syringe do not move or pull from the vein during the procedure. After collecting the blood, place a dry, sterile gauze pad over the puncture site, remove the tourniquet, and carefully withdraw the needle. Ask the patient to apply pressure for 3 to 5 minutes.

Insert the needle into the stoppered tube and allow the vacuum to pull the blood slowly into the tube. Invert gently at least eight times any tube containing an anticoagu-

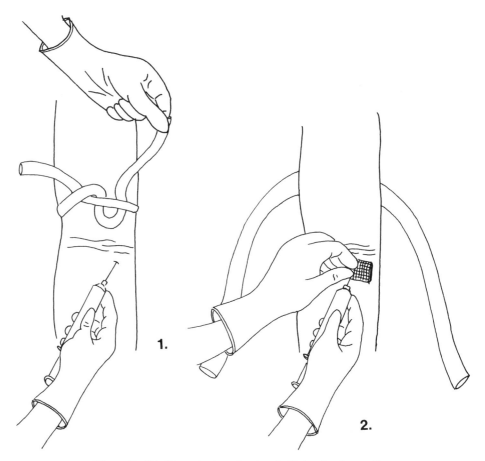

Figure 8–17   Removing tourniquet and withdrawing the needle.

lant to mix the anticoagulant with the blood. Do not shake the tubes because this may cause hemolysis. Many laboratory studies cannot be performed on hemolyzed blood.

HANDLING AND PROCESSING BLOOD SAMPLES

Handle blood specimens with extreme care and, if necessary, centrifuge within 1 hour after collection. Blood collected in vacuum tubes without anticoagulants must remain in a vertical position for 20 to 30 minutes before centrifuging. Coagulation of the blood occurs within this time. If the specimen has to be placed in ice, let it stand for 30 to 60 minutes before refrigerating.

When collecting the specimen in a Serum Separator Tube (SST) by Vacutainer or the Corvac by Sherwood-Davis & Geck, the silicone gel separates the serum from the red cells during centrifuging. The silica glass beads speed clot formation and retraction. Once centrifuged, store the serum on the gel barrier up to 48 hours with the tube stoppered and refrigerate at 2°C to 8°C. If the blood specimen must be kept longer than 48 hours, remove the serum and freeze.

Perform hematology studies on well-mixed EDTA anticoagulated whole blood. Otherwise, anticoagulated blood may be centrifuged immediately after collecting. When this blood is centrifuged, remove the **plasma** from the remaining blood cells as soon as possible. Using a transfer Pasteur pipette, transfer the plasma to a dry, clean test tube and label. Some laboratory tests are performed on plasma.

When centrifuging, keep stoppers on all tubes of blood. Certain test results may be altered or inaccurate if the stopper is removed too soon. Keeping the tube stoppered during centrifugation prevents aerosol contamination and evaporation of the specimen.

Plasma: *liquid portion of uncoagulated blood*

Some analytes such as bilirubin will be destroyed when exposed to light. Vacuum tubes with special coating are available to prevent exposure of the specimen to light.

The recommended time for centrifugation of blood is 10 to 15 minutes at 3000 rpm; however, follow the recommendations of the manufacturer for the different tube types and centrifuges. (See Chapter 5 for information on centrifuging, including balancing the vacuum tubes.) Serum or plasma specimens sent to a referral laboratory must be submitted in accordance with that laboratory's instructions.

SUMMARY

A capillary puncture is a method for obtaining a blood specimen when you need only a small amount of blood or when a venipuncture may be difficult. The area selected for the puncture must be vascular and fleshy. Sites commonly selected are the ring finger or the middle finger on adults, the great toe on infants, and the medial and lateral plantar heel surfaces of the foot on newborns.

Phlebotomy is the technique of entering a vein for the removal of a blood specimen for hematology and chemical analysis. Whole blood, serum, or plasma is used for testing. The hypodermic needle and syringe, the vacuum tube system, and the winged infusion system are the three collection methods available for phlebotomy. When drawing multiple samples, follow guidelines on the order of draw. In addition to blood drawing, the phlebotomist must prepare each sample for testing or transport to a reference laboratory. Proper specimen collection and preparation are essential to accurate test results.

PATIENT EDUCATION

- Advise patients not to lift or carry heavy objects with the arm used for venipuncture for an hour.

TECHNICAL CONSIDERATIONS

Capillary Puncture

- Avoid any puncture site that appears to show pathology (cyanosis, puffiness, rashes, redness, etc.).
- If the finger site is unusually cold or appears pale, place the finger in warm water for 2 to 3 minutes to increase circulation.
- If the patient is allergic to adhesive bandages, do not use.

Venipuncture

- If the needle passes through the vein and a hematoma results, immediately remove the tourniquet, retract the needle, and apply pressure.
- Patients taking a blood anticoagulant medication, for example, warfarin sodium (Coumadin), require *more* than 5 minutes of pressure to stop bleeding.
- If the patient has had a mastectomy, choose the opposite arm for venipuncture.

SOURCES OF ERROR

Capillary Puncture

- Penetrate the skin to the depth of the lancet or blood flow may be scanty, necessitating another puncture.
- Never use any lancet more than once.

Box continues on following page

- Never "squeeze" a capillary puncture site to obtain blood since this may dilute the sample with excessive tissue fluid or cause hemolysis.

Venipuncture

- Not using the correct order of draw in a venipuncture may interfere with testing or cause the results of the test to be inaccurate.
- Not removing the tourniquet as soon as blood begins to flow may create the possibility of backflow when performing a venipuncture.
- Release the tourniquet within 1 to 2 minutes of application.
- Take caution to label the tubes immediately after drawing the blood.
- Do *not* recap needles or bend them before discarding them into a biohazard sharps container. Recapping needles increases the risk of needle-stick injury.
- Always centrifuge blood specimen tubes with the rubber stoppers in place to prevent aerosol contamination and spillage.
- Submit serum or plasma specimens to a referral laboratory in accordance with the laboratory's instructions.
- Do not centrifuge blood specimens more than once.
- Never use vacuum tubes after the expiration date.
- When using vacuum tubes with an anticoagulant, always fill the tubes with blood until the vacuum is exhausted.

Procedure with Rationale

Capillary Puncture
EQUIPMENT AND SUPPLIES

Hand soap
Latex gloves
70 percent isopropyl alcohol
Sterile 2 × 2 inch gauze
Sterile lancet

Blood collection container (Microtainer, etc.)
Biohazard container
Sharps container
Surface disinfectant

Assemble equipment.

Wash hands with soap and water. Observe the OSHA Standard for this procedure.

Identify the patient by having the patient spell his or her name.

Identify the site that will be used for the capillary puncture.

Cleanse the area with 70 percent isopropyl alcohol and allow the site to air dry or wipe the site with sterile gauze. *If alcohol remains on the finger when it is punctured, it will dilute the specimen and cause an error in test results.*

While the puncture site is drying, prepare a sterile lancet.

Remove the lancet cap immediately prior to the capillary puncture.

Secure the finger and hold the lancet firmly, then puncture the site with a quick stabbing motion.

Gently squeeze the finger below the puncture site and wipe away the first drop of blood using a sterile gauze. *The first drop of blood contains tissue fluid and tissue thromboplastin, which dilutes the specimen and may cause clotting.*

Collect a blood specimen suitable for diagnostic testing.

At the completion of blood collection, have the patient apply a sterile 2 × 2 inch gauze pad to the puncture site. *The pressure stops the flow of blood and prevents extravasation.*

Observe the puncture site to make sure bleeding has stopped and determine whether an adhesive bandage should be applied.

Label the specimen with all required information.

Dispose of the lancet in a sharps container.

Clean the work area following laboratory protocol.

Remove gloves and wash hands with soap and water.

Procedure with Rationale

Venipuncture

EQUIPMENT AND SUPPLIES

Hand soap	Vacuum needle and holder
Tourniquet	Vacuum tubes
Sterile gauze or cotton ball	Adhesive bandage
70 percent isopropyl alcohol	Latex gloves
Sterile needle: 20 to 22 gauge, 1.5-inch	Biohazard container
length	Biohazard sharps container
Syringe and collection tubes	Surface disinfectant

Assemble equipment.

Wash hands with soap and water. Observe the OSHA Standard for this procedure.

Prepare needle and syringe or vacuum tube collection system.

Identify the patient. Verify identity by having the patient spell his or her name.

Explain the procedure to the patient. *Frequently, anxiety is reduced when the patient understands the procedure.*

Apply the tourniquet. Make sure the tourniquet is tight enough to distend the vein but not so tight as to interfere with arterial circulation.

Examine arms for suitable veins. Use median cubital and cephalic veins as first choice, then basilic. Never use the small superficial veins. *These veins might be destroyed by the vacuum of the vacuum tubes or the back pressure of a syringe.*

Palpate the vein and remove tourniquet. *Palpating the vein gives information on size, direction, and depth of the vein.*

Clean the puncture site. Use one smooth circular pass with the alcohol prep and rub briskly. Let the site air dry. *If you touch the area after cleaning the puncture site, the site will be contaminated and you must clean it again.*

Apply the tourniquet and with the nondominant hand anchor the vein. Perform the venipuncture at a 15° angle with the bevel facing up using a swift but smooth continuous movement. Use the thumb of the nondominant hand to secure the vein and pull the skin taut. *Entering the skin swiftly reduces discomfort to the patient.*

Remove the tourniquet when the blood begins to enter the tube. *Removing the needle before the tourniquet is released will cause bleeding from the puncture site, producing a hematoma and possibly aerosol contamination.*

When the tube has filled, cover the puncture site with a sterile gauze and remove the needle from the arm in a swift movement. Immediately apply pressure to the puncture site with a sterile gauze. *Bleeding occurs if pressure is not applied immediately, resulting in a hematoma.*

Ask the patient to continue applying pressure to the puncture site, keeping the arm extended. *Pressure should be applied at least 3 to 5 minutes so that a hematoma does not occur. For patients on blood anticoagulant medication, the time should be extended.*

Discard the needle into a sharps biohazard container without recapping the needle.

Gently invert the additive tubes of blood at least eight times as they are removed from the holder and again at the completion of the collection. *Specimens collected with an additive must be thoroughly mixed or coagulation of the specimen may occur.*

Label all tubes. *Correct labeling of the specimen is extremely important, because improper identification of specimens may result in erroneous laboratory reports.*

Remain with the patient until bleeding has stopped. *If an adhesive bandage is applied before the bleeding has stopped, a hematoma may occur.*

  Clean work area following laboratory protocol.

Remove gloves and wash hands with soap and water.

Questions

Name _____ Date _____

1. List the sites for a capillary puncture and tell why these are selected.

2. List several devices for a capillary puncture.

3. What may occur to the blood sample if the puncture site is squeezed in order to obtain the specimen?

4. List four instances when a capillary puncture may be the preferred method of blood collection.

5. Why are the stoppers of the vacuum tubes color-coded? What do the tubes contain? For what purpose is each tube used?

6. Explain the term "multidraw" and give the order of draw.

7. Blood drawn for coagulation studies must never be the first tube collected. Why not?

8. When do you use a syringe and needle for phlebotomy?

9. Explain how hemolysis may occur during a venipuncture.

10. How do you properly identify a patient?

11. What instructions must be given to a patient who faints?

Terminal Performance Objective

Capillary Puncture

Given the necessary equipment, you will be able to collect a capillary blood specimen suitable for diagnostic testing. This procedure must be performed within 5 minutes with a level of accuracy specified by your instructor.

INSTRUCTOR'S EVALUATION FORM

Name _____ Date _____

+ = SATISFACTORY   ✓ = UNSATISFACTORY

_____ Assemble equipment.

_____ Wash hands with soap and water. Observe the OSHA Standard for this procedure.

_____ Identify the patient by having the patient spell his or her name.

_____ Identify the site that will be used for the capillary puncture.

_____ Cleanse the area with 70 percent isopropyl alcohol and allow the site to air-dry or wipe it with a sterile gauze pad.

_____ While the puncture site is drying, prepare a sterile lancet.

_____ Remove the lancet cap immediately prior to the capillary puncture.

_____ Secure the finger and hold the lancet firmly, then puncture the site with a quick stabbing motion.

_____ Gently squeeze the finger below the puncture site and wipe away the first drop of blood using sterile gauze.

_____ Collect a blood specimen suitable for diagnostic testing.

_____ At the completion of the blood collection, have the patient apply a sterile 2 × 2 inch gauze pad on the puncture site.

_____ Observe the puncture site to make sure bleeding has stopped and determine whether an adhesive bandage should be applied.

_____ Label the specimen with all required information.

_____ Dispose of the lancet in a sharps container.

_____ Clean the work area following laboratory protocol.

_____ Remove gloves and wash hands with soap and water.

_____ The procedure was completed within 5 minutes.

_____ The procedure was performed with the accuracy determined by your instructor, and the blood sample was suitable for diagnostic testing.

Final Competency Evaluation

____ SATISFACTORY   ____ UNSATISFACTORY

Comments:

Instructor _____ Date _____

Terminal Performance Objective

Venipuncture

Given the necessary equipment, you will be able to perform a venipuncture. This procedure must be performed within 15 minutes to a level of accuracy specified by your instructor.

INSTRUCTOR'S EVALUATION FORM

Name _____ Date _____

+ = SATISFACTORY   ✓ = UNSATISFACTORY

_____ Assemble equipment.

_____ Wash hands with soap and water. Observe the OSHA Standard for this procedure.

_____ Prepare needle and syringe, or vacuum-tube collection system.

_____ Identify the patient by asking the patient to spell his or her name.

_____ Explain the procedure to the patient.

_____ Apply the tourniquet.

_____ Examine the patient's arms for suitable veins.

_____ Palpate the vein and remove the tourniquet.

_____ Clean the puncture site.

_____ Apply the tourniquet and with the nondominant hand anchor the vein. Perform a venipuncture at a 15° angle with bevel facing up using a swift but smooth continuous movement.

_____ Remove the tourniquet when the blood begins to enter the tube.

_____ When the tube has filled, cover the puncture site with a sterile gauze pad and remove the needle in a swift movement. Immediately apply pressure to the puncture site with a sterile gauze.

_____ Ask the patient to continue applying pressure to puncture site, keeping the arm extended.

_____ Discard the needle in a sharps biohazard container without recapping the needle.

_____ Gently invert the additive tubes of blood at least eight times as they are removed from the holder and again at the completion of the collection.

_____ Label all tubes.

_____ Remain with the patient until bleeding has stopped.

_____ Clean work area following laboratory protocol.

_____ Remove gloves and wash hands with soap and water.

_____ The procedure was completed within 15 minutes.

_____ The results were to the level of accuracy specified by your instructor.

Final Competency Evaluation

_____ SATISFACTORY   _____ UNSATISFACTORY

Comments:

Instructor _____ Date _____

Collection of Microbial Specimens

9

LEARNING OBJECTIVES

On completing this chapter, you will be able to:

COGNITIVE OBJECTIVES
- Briefly state the general requirements for collecting microbial specimens.
- Define aseptic technique and explain why it is necessary in collecting specimens for bacterial studies.
- List the specimen sites generally used for microbial testing.
- Differentiate the two types of wet mounts and tell when each is used.

PSYCHOMOTOR OBJECTIVES
- Explain the procedure for home collection of specimens for pinworm examination.
- Collect and process a throat specimen in accordance with the Terminal Performance Objective presented in this chapter.

AFFECTIVE OBJECTIVES
- Show concern for others by wiping the outside of specimen containers with disinfectant after specimens for microbial studies are obtained from the patient.
- Understand the importance of referring technical questions regarding the collection of microbial specimens to skilled microbiologists.

Microbiology is the scientific study of all organisms (living things) too small to be seen with the naked eye. These microorganisms or microbes include bacteria, viruses, protozoa, and fungi. Most microorganisms live in a harmonious relationship with humans. When they maintain a neutral role, not harming or helping their host, they are called *commensals.* When we rely on them, and they rely on us to provide certain benefits, they are called *mutualists.* Most of the bacteria that populate our body and mucous membranes, and those that reside in our gastrointestinal tract, are mutualists or commensals. We provide them "free room and board" and they keep unwanted bacteria from "taking up residence." They also synthesize vitamins that we need and help digest food. The mutualists and commensals that populate our bodies are called *normal flora.*

The microorganisms that cause disease or are harmful to humans are called *pathogens.* They are identified by testing various body specimens. As in all other laboratory testing, correct and valid results depend on a properly collected microbial specimen.

GENERAL REQUIREMENTS FOR COLLECTION OF MICROBIAL SPECIMENS

Aseptic Technique

Sterile: *totally free of all living organisms, including spores*

Aseptic technique is a method used to control, exclude, or eliminate unwanted microorganisms (contaminants) from a test procedure. **Sterile** instruments and specimen containers are required when specimens are collected aseptically. Commercial sterile collection systems are available (Fig. 9–1) and can be used for most specimen collections.

Because suspected pathogens are often found in nonsterile sites where normal flora abound, the laboratorian must make every effort to use proper aseptic technique to remove, exclude, or control normal flora. If the specimen is not collected properly, normal flora often obscure the suspected pathogen, making the pathogenic organism difficult to isolate and identify properly.

Also some pathogenic organisms are immediately infective and pose a threat to others. Using aseptic technique helps control or minimize the spread of pathogens from the specimen to others or to the surrounding environment.

Collector Transport System

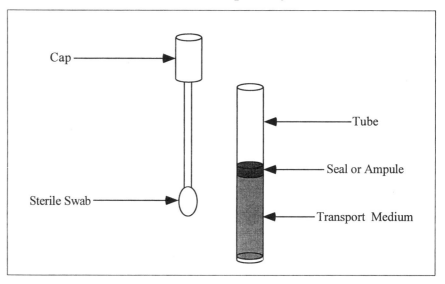

Figure 9–1   Collector transport system.

Proper Handling and Processing

Many pathogens do not survive well outside of the host. Special handling and processing may be required to keep them **viable** until the laboratory receives the specimen. Extended exposure to drying, adverse temperature, environmental stresses, and overgrowth by contaminating bacteria and fungi may kill a suspected pathogen.

Specimens must be **inoculated** immediately after collection or sent in **transport media** to referral laboratories before relevant organisms either die or multiply to levels that distort the clinical picture. Care must be taken to preserve them during transit. Avoid sending a microbial specimen to a referral laboratory when a long weekend or holiday may delay delivery. Check with the laboratory when specific situations arise.

Diagnostic Relevance

The type of test selected for a microbial study depends on the physician's **tentative diagnosis.** Testing personnel use this tentative diagnosis to select media and to make other decisions associated with handling and processing. For example, if a tentative diagnosis suggests **septic sore throat,** the type of bacterial testing will focus on identifying group A beta-hemolytic streptococcus, the organism responsible for "strep throat."

The exact anatomic location and description of the specimen must accompany all request slips for microbial testing. This helps to limit the type of testing for the pathogen and gives information on the possible flora that may appear in the specimen.

Clinical Comment: Self-Medicating

Always check with patients to determine whether they have taken any medications. Even though the physician may not have prescribed antibiotics, the patient may have some "leftovers" at home and have taken them prior to the office visit. This information must be included when submitting a specimen. Additional steps are required by the laboratorian to counteract the effects of the antibiotic, and growth of the pathogen is often delayed.

Adequate Quantity

Often it is difficult to obtain an adequate sample size for testing. For example, the organism responsible for gonorrhea is not evenly distributed in the patient; it is frequently **focally distributed.** The collection of an appropriate sample depends on vigorously and completely swabbing all sites (cervix, urethra, rectum, and vagina) to ensure collecting a sufficient sample of the pathogen.

In **abscesses** and wounds, the infecting organism is usually located deep within the lesion. Pus and other debris make it difficult to obtain a specimen with sufficient pathogens for testing. Interfering material must be removed before the specimen can be collected. Ideally, the sample should be aspirated using a sterile syringe to ensure an adequate sample. This procedure is performed by the physician.

SPECIMEN SITES FOR MICROBIAL TESTING

In POLs, specimens for microbial studies are normally collected from the upper respiratory tract (throat and nasopharynx), lower respiratory tract (sputum), urine, and stool and from wounds and abscesses. Table 9–1 summarizes the source of specimens, method of collection, and the pathogen usually found.

Viable: *capable of living*

Inoculated: *placed in or on a bacterial culture medium*

Transport media: *containers that hold nutrients and other materials that provide an environment that supports microbial viability while in transit from one location to another*

Tentative diagnosis: *provisional "best guess" diagnosis*

Septic sore throat: *an inflammatory sore throat caused by hemolytic streptococci; also called "strep throat"*

Focally distributed: *distributed or located in patches; not evenly distributed*

Abscesses: *localized areas of pus resulting in tissue injury*

Table 9–1 *Commonly Cultured Bacteria*

Source	Method	Organism
Throat and Nasopharynx	Culturette swab touched to the site of inflammation and/or pus at the back of the throat	Streptococcus (Group A), Staphylococcus, Pneumococcus, Candida, Bordetella, Haemophilus
Sputum	Sterile sputum collection container (The patient must obtain a sputum specimen by coughing deeply when getting up in the morning.)	Diplococcus pneumoniae, Streptococcus, Staphylococcus, Mycobacterium, Haemophilus, Klebsiella, Neisseria
Wounds and Abscesses	Culture swab collected from wound or lesion and placed in both aerobic and anaerobic environments	Staphylococcus, Clostridium, Bacteroides, Pseudomonas, Proteus, E. coli
Urine	First morning, midstream clean catch (Refrigerate if transport is delayed.)	E. coli, Klebsiella, Enterobacter, Serratia, Proteus, Pseudomonas, Streptococcus, Staphylococcus, Candida, Neisseria
Stool	Stool specimen collected in a sterile container or with sterile swab	Salmonella, Shigella, Proteus, Pseudomonas

Upper Respiratory Tract (Throat and Nasopharynx)

For a throat specimen, use sterile Dacron or polyester-tipped swabs. Cotton-tipped swabs contain substances that often interfere with the growth of the bacteria. Seat the patient and make sure that if the patient wears dentures they are removed before you begin the procedure. Use a tongue depressor to hold the tongue down and expose the back of the throat. Instruct the patient to say "ahh." Rotate a sterile swab across the back of the throat and over the tonsils. Gray or white patchy areas and **tonsillar crypts** are very productive for streptococcal isolation; be sure to include them in the specimen. Do not touch the swab to the tongue, uvula, teeth, or cheeks during the procedure since these structures have large quantities of flora. Place the swab in a transport system or immediately inoculate a blood agar plate (see Chapter 25).

Tonsillar crypts: *small sacs or cavities located in the tonsils*

The nasopharynx specimen is usually obtained using a Dacron or polyester-tipped swab on a bent wire. The swab is passed through the nose, or by way of the mouth to the *nasopharynx,* the area lying above the soft palate. Avoid touching the tongue or the back of the throat below the soft palate. Place the swab in a transport system or inoculate a blood agar plate.

Lower Respiratory Tract (Sputum)

When attempting to obtain lower respiratory tract specimens, the laboratorian must be sure that the patient knows the difference between sputum and saliva. Saliva is a product of the mouth; sputum is produced in the bronchial tree and lungs. Sputum must be deliberately coughed up from the lungs and lower bronchial structures. It is produced only when pathology is present. Have the patient gargle prior to collection. This decreases the resident flora. Give patients plenty of tissues so that they may use them to cover their mouth when they cough. Keep the lid on the container until the patient has produced a sputum sample. Once the specimen is in the container, wipe the outside of the container with a disinfectant. Inoculate the culture medium at once or send the specimen sample directly to the laboratory. Do not delay.

Debilitated: *weakened*

Very young children, **debilitated** patients, and comatose patients require a transtracheal aspiration. This procedure is performed by a physician in the hospital.

Clinical Comment: Tuberculosis

Tuberculosis (TB) is the leading infectious killer of adults worldwide. One-third of the world's population is already infected with the TB organism. The symptoms of TB include:

- Productive cough
- Coughing up blood
- Weight loss
- Loss of appetite
- Lethargy and weakness
- Night sweat or fever

Collecting a sputum sample from a patient infected with TB can place the health-care worker and others at risk. Coughing to produce a sputum sample places infectious droplets in the air (*airborne droplet nuclei*) that may infect others. Patients suspected of having TB should be sent to facilities that have isolation rooms with properly ventilated systems to control the spread of infection when sputum samples are required.

Urinary Tract Specimens

Most bladder infections are caused by the organisms that are part of the normal flora of the gastrointestinal tract. These bacteria leave the colon and find their way to the urinary bladder. A urethral catheter provides a method of collecting a urine sample for culturing and diagnosis with minimal contamination by adjacent structures. However, this procedure also carries a risk of introducing unwanted bacteria into the bladder, thereby causing new infection. Unless otherwise indicated, the midstream clean-catch urine collection (see Chapter 7) is preferred over the catheterization method. Make sure the patient is familiar with the procedure prior to the specimen collection.

Wound and Abscess Specimens

Most wounds and abscesses contain **anaerobic organisms.** They are generally located deep within the lesion. Remove debris using sterile saline or sterile water. Collect a specimen with a sterile Dacron swab, or sterile aspiration syringe, from the area that appears visibly active. As noted previously, aspiration is performed by a physician. Be sure to identify the site from which the sample was obtained. It is insufficient to identify "wound" when submitting a specimen. The exact location must be identified, for example, "Wound—left foot, plantar surface." Provide the referral laboratory with a tentative diagnosis (i.e., **mycotic** abscess) if possible. Ask the physician for this tentative diagnosis.

Collect a minimum of three swabs to increase the chance of collecting viable organisms. One specimen should be placed in an aerobic medium, and one specimen should be placed in an anaerobic medium.

Anaerobic organisms: *organisms that thrive in an atmosphere low in or absent of oxygen*

Mycotic: *pertaining or relating to fungus*

Clinical Comment: Exudates

Although not considered diagnostic, skilled medical microbiologists sometimes get "hints" as to the cause of a wound exudate from its appearance. Frequently the pus from a streptococcal wound is thin and watery; from a staphylococcal wound it often appears gelatinous. Pus from a wound infected with *Pseudomonas aeruginosa* is characteristically blue-green. Actinomycosis infections are associated with "sulfur" granules.

Stool Specimens

Ova: *eggs*

Parasites: *organisms that live in, on, or at the expense of other organisms*

Stool specimens are used to identify **ova** and **parasites** (O & P), pathogenic viruses, and pathogenic bacteria found in the intestinal tract. Some bacteria are always considered pathogenic in stool specimens, including *Salmonella* and *Shigella.*

Stool specimens should be collected in a sterile, wide-mouth container or bed pan, free of urine contamination. Do not allow toilet paper to contaminate the sample since toilet paper contains bismuth, a substance that interferes with laboratory testing. Although a walnut-size sample is sufficient for testing, the entire sample should be submitted to the laboratory.

A single negative report for O & P is inconclusive; the test should be repeated if clinical symptoms persist.

In POLs, rectal swabs are often collected in place of a stool specimen. Care must be taken to ensure that the rectal area is tested, and not merely the anus.

Insert the sterile swab approximately 3 cm, and rotate it to collect a fecal sample. Immediately place the swab in a clean container provided by the referral laboratory and prepare it for transport.

PINWORM COLLECTION

Pinworms (enterobiasis) frequently occur in pediatric patients. The female pinworm migrates from the cecum to the anus to deposit her ova, generally during the night. Therefore, the specimen should be collected in the morning before bathing or defecating. Ova are rarely found in the feces, but can be detected near the anus. To collect a specimen, place cellophane tape, sticky side out, on the end of a tongue depressor. Press the tape against the anus and the perianal area. Apply the tape, sticky side down, to a microscope slide and examine for ova. Since the test is most reliable in the early morning, parents may be requested to obtain the specimen. Give clear and accurate directions for the procedure. Be ready to answer any questions regarding the collection and how the specimen is to be returned to the office. Commercially made paddles are also available for collecting pinworm specimens. The pinworm specimen is examined by a physician or medical technologist.

WET-MOUNT PREPARATIONS

Wet-mount preparations are used to identify fungi that may infect hair, nails, or skin. They are also used to identify genital tract infections caused by *Trichomonas vaginalis* ("Trich"), *Candida* (yeast), or *Gardnerella vaginalis.*

Two types of wet-mount preparations are currently performed in POLs, the saline prep and the KOH (potassium hydroxide) prep. Medical assistants aid in setting up wet-mount preps; however, skilled laboratorians or physicians perform the actual microscopic examination.

Saline Wet Mount

The saline wet-mount prep is useful in identifying "clue cells" from the genital tract of female patients. Clue cells are vaginal epithelial cells covered with tiny bacteria called *Gardnerella vaginalis.* These tiny organisms cause vaginal epithelial cells to show a speckled appearance with an indistinct cell margin. The organism cannot be identified using only the microscope, but the finding of clue cells is presumptive of *Gardnerella* infection. The wet preparation is made by touching the tip of a vaginal swab to a sterile drop of saline placed on a clean glass slide. A coverslip is placed over the drop. The slide is examined first under low-power magnification to locate any cellular material, and then under high-power magnification to identify the presence or absence of clue cells.

Adding a drop of 10 percent solution of KOH to the discharge from an infected female produces a characteristic "fishy odor." This test is frequently performed in conjunction with the saline wet-mount preparation for *Gardnerella*.

The saline wet-mount prep is also useful in diagnosing *T. vaginalis*. This organism is a protozoan with four anterior hairlike structures called *flagella*. Trichomoniasis is a fairly common condition in women, especially during pregnancy or following vaginal surgery. The presence of the "Trich" organism causes a frothy discharge with burning and itching of the vulvar tissue. It may be transmitted to the male during sexual intercourse.

Collect a vaginal swab and place it in a tube containing sterile saline. Using the cotton-tipped applicator, transfer one drop of the saline suspension to a slide and cover it with a coverslip. The physician examines the slide, first with low power and then with high power to determine the presence or absence of *T. vaginalis*. The organism moves in a characteristic jerky, undulating motion.

KOH Wet Mount

KOH is an alkaline solution that dissolves proteinaceous material. It is frequently used to identify fungal elements.

For hair, skin, or nails, cleanse the suspected site with 70 percent alcohol. Collect a specimen by scraping the area with a scalpel or small wooden spatula. Place the scrapings in a drop or two of KOH on a glass slide and cover with a cover slip. A physician or trained laboratorian examines the slide using a microscope to check for yeast or fungal elements.

Candida is a genus of yeastlike fungi that normally inhabit the mouth, skin, intestinal tract, and vagina. Occasionally, an overgrowth occurs in the vagina, causing "yeast infection" or candidiasis. An overgrowth in the mouth is called *thrush*. Fungal elements, especially budding yeast, can be observed in a KOH wet mount. Place the specimen (either vaginal or mouth) directly in a drop of KOH that has been applied to a slide. The physician observes the slide under low-power magnification and then under high-power magnification to identify the organism.

SAFETY CONCERNS

Exercise extreme caution when collecting specimens for microbial studies. They frequently contain pathogens that may be *immediately infective*. Always wear latex gloves. Keep specimen containers tightly closed to prevent spillage. Wipe soiled containers with a disinfectant solution to protect others. Disinfect any surface that comes in contact with the specimen. Commercial products are available for this purpose. They vary in concentration and effectiveness. The most common error made in disinfection is failure to allow the required time for the disinfectant to remain in contact with the organism. Read and follow directions and product inserts to ensure that all organisms are destroyed.

SPECIMEN TRANSPORT

Because of the complexity of medical microbiology, many of the specimens obtained in a medical office are sent to referral laboratories for isolation, culturing, and identification. Medical assistants or other laboratorians are often assigned the responsibility of logging specimens and preparing them for transport. Any delays or errors in processing or transporting the specimen may invalidate test results. Follow all requirements for specimen transport. The Directory of Services of the referral laboratory gives all requirements for collecting, handling, and transporting specimens (see Chapter 6).

Transport Systems

Many referral laboratories provide collection and transport systems for use by the POL. These systems can also be purchased commercially. Culturette, manufactured by Marion Scientific Corporation; Precision Culture CATS, manufactured by Precision Dynamics Corporation; Vacutainer Brand Anaerobic Specimen Collector, manufactured by Becton Dickinson; and Difco Culture Swab Transport System, manufactured by Difco Laboratories, are some of the culture collection and transport systems for POL use. All transport systems contain sterile swabs for specimen collection and a medium to preserve the viability of the organisms during transit. Each of these systems comes with directions for proper use. Most systems must be delivered to the laboratory for culturing within 72 hours.

MEDIA

Transport media are used for preserving and transporting a specimen to a referral laboratory for testing. They may be liquid, semisolid, or solid. *Nonselective media* support the growth of most bacteria. Blood agar is an example of a nonselective medium. The presence of blood encourages some **fastidious** pathogens to remain viable while in transit. A general nonselective liquid medium is tryptic soy broth (TSB).

Selective media support the growth of certain bacteria while preventing the growth of others. An example of a selective medium is the Jembec plate, a modified Thayer-Martin agar that supports the growth of bacteria responsible for gonorrhea. The organism that causes gonorrhea must be cultured in an atmosphere containing approximately 10 percent carbon dioxide. The Jembec plate contains an ampule that releases carbon dioxide when it is crushed. MacConkey's medium is also a selective medium; it supports the growth of a large group of bacteria called *gram-negative organisms,* but it inhibits the growth of another large group of bacteria, the *gram-positive organisms* (see Chapter 23).

> **Fastidious:** *in microbiology, an organism that has precise nutritional and environmental requirements for growth and survival*

LABELING AND TRANSPORT GUIDELINES

Follow these guidelines when collecting a specimen for microbial studies:

- Carefully label all specimens with the patient's name, date and time of collection, and site from which the specimen was obtained.
- List the date of birth and sex of the patient on the request slip.
- Note any tentative diagnosis provided by the physician on the request slip to facilitate media selection and staining.
- Indicate whether the patient is taking any chemotherapeutic drugs (antibiotics, etc.). This frequently delays the growth of the organism.
- Use only sterile containers, swabs, and transport systems when collecting specimens for bacteriologic studies.
- Use aseptic technique for collecting and processing clinical specimens.
- Carefully follow safety guidelines regarding collecting, handling, processing, and transporting of clinical specimens.

Remember, specimens for microbial studies may carry infectious organisms. Be careful. Follow all safety procedures found in the procedural manual.

SUMMARY

The accuracy of the test results in medical microbiology depends not only on the skills of the microbiologist performing the tests but also on the skills and attention of the laboratorian who collects the specimen and prepares it for transport to the laboratory.

Although most microbial testing is performed by physicians and medical technologists, routine collections and setting up and assisting at more complex collections may be part of your employment duties. Medical assistants routinely log specimens and prepare them for transport.

Because of the diversity of specimens, and the special requirements of various microorganisms, always check the Directory of Services manual or the Procedure Manual for important information regarding microbial testing. When questions arise, call the referral laboratory for specific details.

PATIENT EDUCATION

- Explain specimen collection procedures to the patient.
- Respond to questions and reassure the patient if necessary.
- Have patient remove dentures, if necessary, for throat and nasopharynx specimen collection.

TECHNICAL CONSIDERATIONS

- Make sure all equipment and media are available before the actual collection begins.
- Follow all labeling requirements.
- Check with the referral laboratory when questions arise.
- Immediately process or transport specimens.

SOURCES OF ERROR

- Failure to use aseptic technique.
- Inappropriate technique in specimen collection or processing.
- Inappropriate selection of media for inoculation of the specimen.

Procedure with Rationale

Throat Specimen Collection

EQUIPMENT AND SUPPLIES

Hand soap	Tongue depressor
Latex gloves	Surface disinfectant
Culturette or Culturette II collection package	Lab absorbent towel for counter top
	Biohazard container

Assemble equipment.

Wash hands with soap and water. Observe the OSHA Standard for this procedure.

Greet patient. Seat the patient and remove dentures, if necessary.

Explain the procedure to the patient and request his or her cooperation.

Place the tongue depressor on the back of the tongue. Ask the patient to say "ahh." Observe the oropharynx and tonsillar area for white patches and crypts. *White patches and crypts are productive for the strep organism and must be included in the throat swab for culturing.*

Using a rotating motion, swab the back of the throat and the tonsillar area. Include white patchy areas and tonsillar crypts. Do not touch the tongue, uvula, teeth, or cheeks with the swab.

Insert the swab into the plastic tube and replace the cap.

Crush the ampule of holding medium. *The ampule contains 0.5 mL of modified Stuart's transport medium to prevent drying or deterioration of the specimen.*

Place the plastic tube in the envelope and staple the ends securely.

Complete the laboratory request slip and log the specimen.

Remove gloves and wash hands with soap and water.

Clean work area following laboratory protocol.

Arrange for immediate transport of the specimen to the referral laboratory.

Questions

Name _____ Date _____

1. What are commensals, mutualists, normal flora, and pathogens?

2. What is aseptic technique?

3. What external influences negatively affect the viability of a microbial specimen?

4. List the various types of microbial specimen collections.

5. Briefly describe the pin worm specimen collection.

6. What is a wet mount preparation? What are the two types of wet mount preps?

7. List some safety procedures that will decrease the chance of spreading infection when handling and processing specimens.

8. Describe three types of media used in a transport system and the purpose of each.

9. What information must be included on a label for a microbial specimen?

Terminal Performance Objective

Throat Specimen Collection

You will assemble the required equipment, perform a throat specimen collection, and process the specimen, following the manufacturer's directions. You will complete the laboratory request slip and arrange for immediate transport of the specimen. This procedure must be completed within 5 minutes to a level of accuracy specified by your instructor.

INSTRUCTOR'S EVALUATION FORM

Name _____ Date _____

+ = SATISFACTORY   ✓ = UNSATISFACTORY

_____ Assemble equipment.

_____ Wash hands with soap and water. Observe the OSHA Standard for this procedure.

_____ Greet patient. Seat the patient and remove dentures, if necessary.

_____ Explain the procedure to the patient and request his or her cooperation.

_____ Place the tongue depressor on the back of the tongue. Ask the patient to say "ahh." Observe the oropharynx and tonsillar area for white patches and crypts.

_____ Using a rotating motion, swab the back of the throat and the tonsillar area. Include white patchy areas and tonsillar crypts. Do not touch the tongue, uvula, teeth, or cheeks with the swab.

_____ Insert the swab into the plastic tube and replace the cap.

_____ Crush the ampule of holding medium.

_____ Place the plastic tube in the envelope and staple the ends securely.

_____ Complete the laboratory request slip and log the specimen.

_____ Remove gloves and wash hands with soap and water.

_____ Clean work area following laboratory protocol.

_____ Arrange for immediate transport of the specimen to the referral laboratory.

_____ The procedure was completed within 5 minutes.

_____ The level of accuracy determined by the instructor was attained.

Final Competency Evaluation

_____ SATISFACTORY   _____ UNSATISFACTORY

Comments:

Instructor _____ Date _____

URINALYSIS

Introduction to Urinalysis Procedures

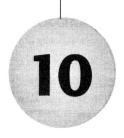

10

Learning Objectives
Cognitive Objectives

Structures of the Urinary System
Kidneys
○ Nephrons
Ureters
Bladder
Urethra

Function of the Urinary System
Urine Formation
○ Filtration
○ Reabsorption
○ Secretion

Urinalysis
Quality Control

Summary

Questions

LEARNING OBJECTIVES

On completing this chapter, you will be able to:

COGNITIVE OBJECTIVES
- Describe the four main structures of the urinary system and briefly state their function.
- Describe the structure of the nephron.
- List the steps in urine formation and briefly define each.
- Explain renal threshold.
- Define the terms *oliguria, polyuria, anuria,* and *nocturia.*
- Name the three major diagnostic methodologies of the urinalysis.

The urinary system consists of two kidneys, two ureters, a bladder, and a urethra. These structures remove waste material from blood and temporarily store it in the form of urine until it is finally expelled from the body.

Approximately one-fourth of the total cardiac output is directed to the kidneys. This means that about 1200 mL of blood enters the renal arteries each minute. In the kidneys, microscopic filtering units called *nephrons* continually regulate the composition and quantity of blood. They remove unwanted substances while preserving those that are needed by the body. In some disease states, abnormal products appear in blood, and finally "spill over" into the urine. By examining the composition of urine, physicians can sometimes identify abnormal substances, often before signs and symptoms of disease appear.

Urine formation is a complex process that includes several physiological processes including filtration, reabsorption, and secretion.

STRUCTURES OF THE URINARY SYSTEM

Kidneys

The kidneys are dark red, bean-shaped structures about 4 to 5 inches long. They lie within the posterior wall of the abdominal cavity, slightly above the waistline, behind the

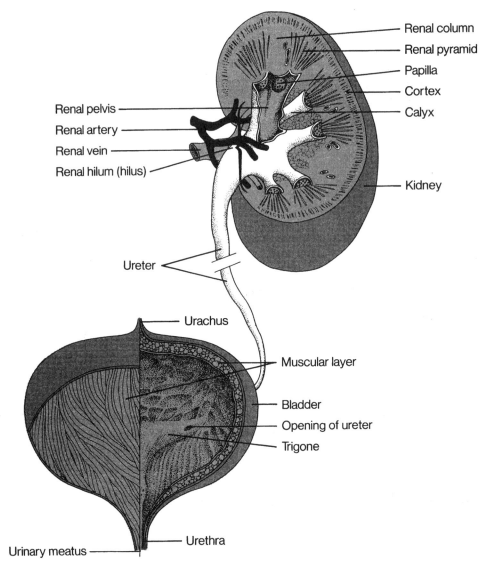

Figure 10–1 Structures of the urinary system. (From Gylys, B, and Wedding, ME: Medical Terminology: A Systems Approach, ed 3, FA Davis, Philadelphia, 1995, p 240, with permission.)

Peritoneum: *a double-folded serous membrane located in the abdominopelvic cavity.*

peritoneum. This membrane covers but does not surround the kidneys. The concave medial border of the kidney has a notch called the *hilum* that leads to a cavity in the kidney called the *renal pelvis.* Nerves, blood vessels (renal artery and renal veins), lymphatic vessels, and ureter pass through the hilum. The outer portion of the kidney, the *cortex,* encloses the inner portion, the *medulla.* Sinuses or *calyces* (sing. calyx) within the kidney converge to form the renal pelvis. Urine formed in the cortex drains through the calyces and enters the renal pelvis (Fig. 10–1).

Clinical Comment: Dialysis

Dialysis machines are able to remove waste products from blood when renal function is temporarily lost or permanently impaired. Two methods are currently used: *hemodialysis* and *peritoneal dialysis.* In both methods, the process relies on the principle of *osmosis,* that is, the passing of substances from a region of high concentration to a region of low concentration
Box continues on following page

through a semipermeable membrane. In hemodialysis, the membrane is cellophane; in peritoneal dialysis, the membrane is the peritoneum. With hemodialysis, blood from the patient is shunted through a machine to remove waste products. Once the blood is filtered of its toxic products, it is returned to the patient. In peritoneal dialysis, a dialyzing solution is introduced into the peritoneal cavity. Waste products transfer across the peritoneal membrane and enter the dialyzing solution. The dialyzing fluid is then removed.

NEPHRONS

There are about 1 million microscopic filtering units, called *nephrons,* in each kidney. They function in the production of urine. Each nephron consists of a *renal corpuscle* and a *renal tubule.* The renal corpuscle is composed of the *glomerulus* and *Bowman's capsule.* The renal artery divides to form the renal arterioles, which further divide into microscopic tufts of capillaries called the glomerulus. The glomerulus is nestled within Bowman's capsule. Bowman's capsule is a thin-walled saclike structure that surrounds the glomerulus. It is the expanded end of the renal tubule.

There are four sections of the renal tubule: (1) the proximal tubule, (2) the loop of Henle, (3) the distal tubule, and (4) the collecting tubule or duct (Fig. 10–2).

Ureters

The *ureters* are slender muscular tubes approximately 10 to 12 inches long that carry urine from the kidneys to the bladder. At the hilum, the ureters funnel outward to form a hollow chamber called the *renal pelvis.* Urine produced in the kidneys passes to the renal pelvis and begins the descent through the ureters to the bladder.

Bladder

The *urinary bladder* is a hollow muscular sac that holds urine until it is ready to be expelled from the body. It is relatively small when empty but expands as it fills with urine. Urine passes from the body by an act called *micturition* (voiding, urination), which is a combination of voluntary and involuntary nerve responses.

Like the kidneys, the bladder lies outside the peritoneal cavity. It is positioned behind the *symphysis pubis,* the junction of the pubic bones, near the floor of the pelvis.

Urethra

The *urethra* is the tube that carries urine from the bladder to the outside of the body. The female urethra is approximately 1.5 inches in length; the male, approximately 8 inches. In males the urethra carries reproductive products as well as urine. The external opening of the body where urine is expelled is called the *urinary meatus.*

FUNCTION OF THE URINARY SYSTEM

When blood passes through the millions of capillary beds found throughout the body, it collects a variety of substances from the billions of cells found in these capillary beds. Some of the substances collected by blood include:

- **Nitrogenous wastes** (urea, uric acid, creatine, creatinine, and ammonia)
- Hormones from glands (i.e., thyroid, pancreas, gonads)
- Products from the digestive system (amino acids, sugars, fats, and vitamins)

Nitrogenous wastes: *products of cellular metabolism that contain nitrogen*

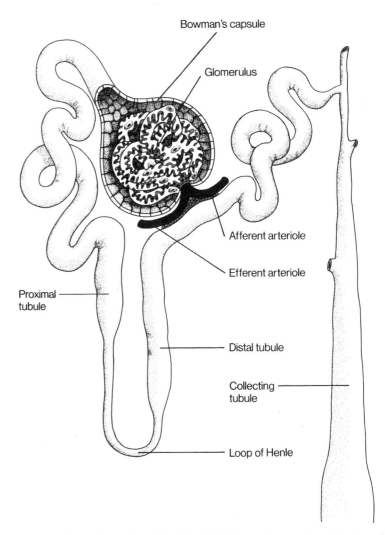

Figure 10–2   A nephron. (From Gylys, B, and Wedding, ME: Medical Terminology: A Systems Approach, ed 3, FA Davis, Philadelphia, 1995, p 241, with permission.)

Electrolytes: *substances in blood, tissue fluid, and cells that conduct an electric current*

Homeostasis: *a state of equilibrium of the internal environment of the body*

Extracellular fluids: *chiefly plasma, tissue fluid, and lymph*

- **Electrolytes** (sodium [Na], potassium [K], calcium [Ca], magnesium [Mg], chloride [Cl], phosphate [PO$_4$], sulfate [SO$_4$], and carbonate [CO$_3$]).

Ladened with these substances, blood is pumped to the kidneys. Unwanted products are removed from the blood as the kidneys produce urine. Urine is then expelled from the body. The kidneys also stabilize blood volume, acidity, and electrolytes. The adjustments made by the urinary system are designed to maintain or reestablish **homeostasis.**

The kidneys play a vital role in monitoring and regulating the **extracellular fluids** of the body. They also secrete a hormone called *erythropoietin* when blood oxygen level is low. Erythropoietin acts on bone marrow, causing the production of red blood cells. Finally, the kidneys assist in vitamin D metabolism.

Urine formation begins in early fetal life. As urine is produced, it passes into the amniotic fluid for disposal through maternal circulation. Throughout life the formation of urine is a constant process and continues until death. When kidney function ceases, death results within a few days.

Urine Formation

The formation of urine involves three distinct processes, all of which occur in the nephrons of the kidneys:

- *Filtration* of substances from the blood in the glomerulus into Bowman's capsule
- *Reabsorption* of some of the filtered substances back into the bloodstream
- *Secretion* of products from the peritubular capillaries to tubules, a process similar to reabsorption, but in the opposite direction

FILTRATION

Urine formation begins when blood pressure causes fluids and dissolved substances found in blood plasma to pass from the glomerulus into Bowman's capsule (Fig. 10–3). The resulting fluid is called *glomerular filtrate*. In a healthy person, the glomerular filtrate consists of all the materials present in the blood except for blood cells and most proteins, since these elements are too large to pass through the glomerular membrane. Except for the size of the substances that pass through the glomerulus, this process is nonselective. In other words, many substances pass through the glomerulus to become glomerular filtrate, even those that are needed by the body.

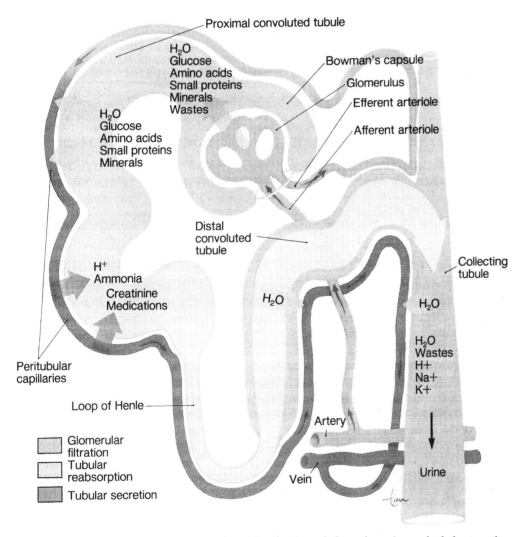

Figure 10–3   Schematic representation of glomerular filtration, tubular reabsorption, and tubular secretion. The renal tubule has been uncoiled, and the peritubular capillaries are shown adjacent to the tubule. (From Scanlon, VC, and Sanders, T: Essentials of Anatomy and Physiology, ed 2, FA Davis, Philadelphia, 1995, p 423, with permission.)

REABSORPTION

As glomerular filtrate journeys through the proximal tubule some substances partially or completely pass back into the peritubular capillaries. Some of these substances include glucose, water, and amino acids. Also, some electrolytes may reenter the peritubular capillaries. The return of these substances to the blood from the glomerular filtrate is called *reabsorption*. Many of these substances have a *threshold level* or *renal threshold*. This means that when blood levels of these substances are high, no more of that particular substance will be reabsorbed by the blood. Therefore that particular substance will remain in the filtrate to become part of the urine. Blood glucose has a renal threshold of 160 to 180 mg/dL. Once this level is reached, no more sugar will be reabsorbed by the peritubular capillaries, and the excess glucose will remain in the filtrate to be passed in the urine. This condition is called *glycosuria*. It is often found in diabetes.

SECRETION

While filtrate is in the distal tubule, more water returns to the vascular system. At the same time potassium and hydrogen ions are secreted; that is, they pass from the blood into the tubule. This is especially important in maintaining a stable blood **pH.**

pH: *the symbol used to express acidity and alkalinity: pH less than 7 is acidic; pH greater than 7 is alkaline (basic)*

When the journey through the tubules is completed, the resulting fluid is called urine. Urine passes from the collecting tubules to the renal pelvis. From there it descends through the ureters to the bladder. Urine is stored in the bladder until urination.

The approximate daily output of urine ranges from 1200 to 1500 mL, but may vary considerably depending on the state of hydration, fluid intake, fluid loss, and other factors. A decrease in urine volume, *oliguria,* often occurs with dehydration because of vomiting, diarrhea, or severe burns. An increase in urine flow is called *polyuria.* The complete absence of urine flow is called *anuria.*

Other terms associated with the urination process include *dysuria,* painful urination; *nocturia,* excessive urination during the night; and *diuresis,* the passage of abnormally large amounts of urine.

URINALYSIS

A routine urinalysis (UA) consists of three major diagnostic methodologies:

- Physical assessment
- Chemical analysis
- Microscopic examination

Each of these methodologies will be covered in detail in Chapters 11, 12, and 13.

A urinalysis provides specific data on abnormalities of the urinary system, such as infections, tumors, and stones. In addition, it gives general information on the health of other body systems. A correctly performed urinalysis can give information to confirm a diagnosis or rule out a suspected disease. A change in the chemical composition of urine is often an early indicator of disease states.

Quality Control

Quality control is a vital aspect of urine testing. To ensure quality control, use positive and negative controls when required. Verify that instruments are in proper working order. Collect specimens as indicated in the Procedure Manual and properly label them at the time of collection. Perform each test in exact compliance with the Procedure Manual. Report and record all results (see Chapter 4).

The laboratorian must perform the urinalysis in a careful and conscientious manner. Fresh urine is required for testing. Stale urine is unacceptable for testing. When urine stands for over an hour without refrigeration or preservatives, bacteria multiply and urine constituents decompose. The laboratorian must perform the urinalysis promptly or take precautions to preserve the specimen (see Chapter 7).

As in all laboratory testing, specimens must be properly labeled with the patient's name, date, and time of collection. Collection containers should have a capacity of 50 to 100 mL with an opening of about 2 inches in diameter. Pediatric collection cups are slightly smaller. Specimens going to a referral laboratory need a screw-on lid. Label the specimen as soon as it is collected. Discard any unlabeled specimens and obtain a new sample for testing.

SUMMARY

Urine is a complex excretory product of the body. Its composition gives valuable clues as to the well-being of the urinary system and all other body systems.

The routine urinalysis includes three diagnostic methodologies: the physical assessment, the chemical analysis, and the microscopic examination. Quality control ensures that the results obtained are valid and accurate.

Questions

Name _____ Date _____

1. List the four main structures of the urinary system and briefly describe their function.

2. Describe the nephron.

3. What are nitrogenous wastes and where do they originate?

4. What are electrolytes? List some of the body electrolytes.

5. List three processes in the formation of urine and briefly describe them.

6. What is meant by renal threshold? Explain glycosuria in terms of renal threshold.

7. What is the normal urinary output for 24 hours? What terms are used to express a marked decrease and a marked increase in urinary output?

8. List the three diagnostic methodologies of the routine urinalysis.

Physical Assessment of Urine

11

LEARNING OBJECTIVES

On completing this chapter, you will be able to:

COGNITIVE OBJECTIVES
- Name the tests included in the physical assessment of urine.
- Identify various pathologies associated with abnormal results obtained during the physical assessment of urine.
- Explain the relevance of the specific gravity results and the protein reading.

PSYCHOMOTOR OBJECTIVES
- Standardize a refractometer following the manufacturer's directions.
- Perform a physical assessment of a urine sample that meets the Terminal Performance Objective presented in the chapter.
- Record the results of the physical assessment of urine.

AFFECTIVE OBJECTIVES
- Recognize the importance of following safety guidelines to help minimize the spread of infection when working with a urine specimen.
- Assume responsibility by maintaining a laboratory that meets safety guidelines with respect to the processing and disposal of urine specimens.

One of the oldest and most frequently performed laboratory tests is the routine urinalysis. A carefully performed urinalysis not only provides information on the health status of the urinary system, but also gives important clues to abnormalities in other body systems. Urinalysis is one of the most frequently ordered laboratory tests for the following reasons:

- A urine specimen is easily obtained.
- Little or no specialized equipment is required to perform the test.
- Abnormal results may be early detectors of disease.

THE ROUTINE URINALYSIS

The routine urinalysis consists of a physical assessment, a chemical analysis, and a microscopic examination of the urine specimen. The physical assessment of urine includes observation of the color, odor, and transparency of a urine specimen. The specific gravity of the urine is also measured as part of the physical assessment.

Those who perform the physical assessment of urine must be able to identify the physical properties that constitute normal findings and those that do not. Any abnormalities detected during the physical assessment of the urine sample must be identified during the chemical analysis or the microscopic examination. Although a random sample is acceptable for the routine urinalysis, the first morning void is usually more desirable. In either case, the sample should not be tested more than 1 hour after voiding or 6 hours after voiding if refrigerated (see Chapter 7).

Urine is potentially infectious, and care must be exercised when performing the urinalysis. Be sure to follow all regulations for specimen handling. In physicians' offices, it is generally recommended that urine specimens be flushed down the toilet after testing. Clean and disinfect all work areas after testing is completed. Dispose of equipment properly. Disinfect all equipment that will be reused. A safe work area is the responsibility of all members of the health-care team.

PHYSICAL PROPERTIES OF URINE

Color

Urine derives its yellow color primarily from the presence of a bile pigment called *urochrome.* As red blood cells age, they disintegrate, releasing hemoglobin. Urochrome is one of the products formed when hemoglobin breaks down into simpler compounds. The color of normal urine ranges from light yellow through dark yellow to amber. The intensity of urine color depends on its concentration. When kidneys excrete large quantities of water, urine becomes dilute and appears light colored. When the body is dehydrated, kidneys excrete small quantities of water and urine becomes concentrated and takes on a darker color. Dehydration can result from **diaphoresis,** vomiting, diarrhea, or taking certain medications.

Diaphoresis: *profuse sweating*

Since color perception is subjective, individuals may differ when they describe the color of urine. For example, one laboratorian may call a urine dark yellow, and another may call it amber. Such a distinction is unimportant. What is important is that the person making the assessment know whether the color is normal or not.

Pigments other than urochrome may appear in urine and affect color. Some of these pigments are associated with disease states; others are not. Food dyes (e.g., beets or carrots) and some medications (e.g., sulfa drugs) and vitamins give characteristic colors to urine. Colors associated with food or medications usually are unimportant, and once they are identified, no further testing is required. Some pigments associated with pathology include bile pigments, bilirubin, biliverdin, myoglobin, hemoglobin, and porphyrin.

Clinical Comment: Foam Test

Bile pigments often give urine a greenish yellow or yellow-brown color. When such a urine sample is placed in a small vial and vigorously shaken, the resulting foam will be stained with these bile pigments. Early physicians tested urine in this manner to identify the presence of bile pigments. Today, concerns over biohazards and innovations in chemistry testing have virtually rendered this early test obsolete.

Table 11–1 **Abnormal Urine Colors Associated with Pathology**

Color	Possible Source	Possible Pathological Cause
Yellow-brown	Bilirubin	Excessive destruction of erythrocytes Obstruction of the bile duct Diminished function of liver cells
Orange-yellow	Urobilin, bilirubin	Excessive destruction of erythrocytes Diminished function of liver cells
Dark red	Porphyrin products	Disturbance in porphyrin metabolism (needed for heme synthesis)
	Erythrocytes	Hemorrhage from urinary structures Menstrual contamination
	Hemoglobin	Lysed erythrocytes Excess free hemoglobin in plasma
Red-brown	Myoglobin	Excessive destruction of skeletal or cardiac muscle
	Erythrocytes	Same as above
	Hemoglobin	Same as above
Clear red	Hemoglobin	Same as above
	Porphyrin products	Same as above
Cloudy red	Erythrocytes	Same as above
Green	Biliverdin	Oxidation of bilirubin

Table 11–1 shows some of the abnormal urine colors and gives some possible pathologic causes.

When an abnormal color is present, only the abnormal color is recorded. Often, the cause of the abnormal color is identified during the chemical analysis or the microscopic examination of the specimen.

Odor

Normal urine odor is pungent or aromatic, but not necessarily unpleasant. Other odors can sometimes be detected in urine. Foods, notably garlic and asparagus, give a characteristic odor to urine. These odors are not associated with disease. Some serious diseases, however, produce characteristic odors in the urine. In the past, physicians frequently smelled urine samples to assist in diagnosis. Today, because of concern over biohazardous substances, including urine, and the fact that we have accurate and sophisticated methods of urine testing, the practice of directly smelling urine is no longer a part of the urinalysis procedure.

Skilled laboratorians sometimes detect a specific identifiable odor in a urine sample, which may offer clues to a particular pathological condition. Although odor cannot be used in diagnosing, it may indicate areas that need further investigation. Some odors that may warrant further investigation include ammonia, sweet or fruity, and putrid or foul. In addition, a serious metabolic disease found in newborn infants called **phenylketonuria (PKU)** produces an unpleasant odor often referred to as "mousey." Although newborns are routinely checked for PKU, the increase in home births and the rise in poverty in the United States have allowed some cases to go undetected. Therefore, always investigate further a complaint by a mother who reports her baby's urine "does not smell right." Table 11–2 lists some abnormal urine odors with possible causes.

Phenylketonuria (PKU): *a recessive hereditary disease caused by the body's failure to oxidize an amino acid (phenylalanine) to tyrosine because of a defective enzyme*

Transparency (Appearance or Character)

Transparency, also called appearance or character, refers to the clarity of the specimen. As with urine color, the terms that describe this feature are subjective. Terms that denote transparency in urine or the lack of it include *clear, hazy,* and *cloudy.* The term for excessively cloudy urine is *turbid.*

Table 11–2 **Abnormal Urine Odors**

Odor	Possible Source	Possible Cause
Ammonia	Splitting of urea molecule by bacteria	Urinary tract infection "Stale" urine
Sweet or fruity	Acetone and acetoacetic acid (ketones)	Fat metabolism due to starvation, diabetes mellitus, etc.
Putrid or foul	Decomposition of leukocytes Bacterial growth	Leukocytes associated with urinary tract infections
"Mousey"	PKU (phenylketonuria)	Congenital metabolic disease

Freshly voided urine is usually clear or transparent but becomes cloudy upon standing. As urine cools, dissolved substances crystallize. In alkaline urine, these substances include phosphate and carbonate crystals. In acid urine, they include uric acid, calcium oxalates, and urates. As urates precipitate, a pinkish cloud forms. This cloud is called "brick dust." Phosphate, carbonate, uric acid, oxalates, and urate crystals are not associated with pathology.

Other substances that cause urine cloudiness are mucus threads, bacteria, cells, and casts. These substances may be clinically important in diagnosis and can be confirmed during the microscopic examination of urine, or in some cases, during the chemical analysis of urine.

Specific Gravity

Solutes: *substances dissolved in a solution*

The specific gravity (sp. gr.) of urine measures the concentration of **solutes** in a urine sample. Therefore, specific gravity provides information regarding the concentrating ability of the kidneys. The two major solutes found in urine are urea and salt (sodium chloride). A concentrated urine contains more of these two substances than does a dilute sample; therefore, the concentrated sample will have a higher specific gravity.

Specific gravity is the ratio of the weight of a given volume of urine to the weight of the same volume of distilled water at the same temperature:

$$\text{Specific gravity} = \frac{\text{weight of urine}}{\text{weight of water}}$$

The specific gravity of urine can be obtained by weighing a measured amount of the sample or by using a urinometer, a refractometer, or a reagent strip. (The reagent strip method is described in Chapter 12.)

Weighing a measured amount of urine is time consuming and impractical. This method is not used in clinical practice.

The *urinometer* is an instrument with a weighted float that is placed in a sample of urine. The concentration of the urine sample affects its buoyancy. The more concentrated the urine, the higher the urinometer floats in the specimen. A scale on the urinometer records the height at which the urinometer floats in the specimen (Fig. 11–1). The urinometer method of obtaining a specific gravity requires a relatively large quantity of the specimen. This test method cannot be used when small quantities of urine are collected, which often occurs with pediatric patients. Newer and more convenient methods of obtaining a specific gravity have made this method obsolete.

Refractive index: *bending of a ray of light as it passes from one substance (or interface) to another*

REFRACTOMETER METHOD OF DETERMINING SPECIFIC GRAVITY

A common method for determining specific gravity, especially in physicians' offices, incorporates a total solids meter (TS meter), also called a *refractometer* (Fig. 11–2). The refractometer indirectly measures specific gravity by obtaining the **refractive index** of

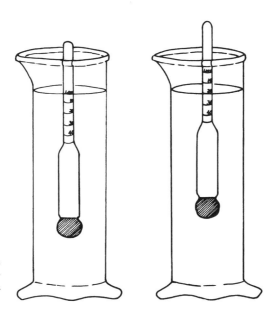

Figure 11–1 Urinometers representing various specific gravity readings. (From Strasinger, SK: Urinalysis and Body Fluids, ed 3, Revised Reprint, FA Davis, Philadelphia, 1994, p 44, with permission.)

urine. The refractive index is the ratio of the velocity of light in air to the velocity of light in solution. Light passes more slowly through a solution than it does through air. It passes even more slowly through a solution that contains a high concentration of dissolved substances. In other words, the more concentrated the solution, the slower the passage of the light through the solution.

The refractive index varies with, but is not identical to, the specific gravity. The refractometer scale is calibrated so that the refractive index is shown in terms of specific gravity. The TS meter is capable of determining specific gravities from 1.000 to 1.035.

To find the specific gravity of a urine sample using the refractometer, wipe the surface of the prism dry and place one drop of urine on the prism using a pipette. Look through the ocular and read the specific gravity from the scale that appears at the boundary line between the light and dark areas (Fig. 11–3). Record the results on the request slip.

A Clinical Refractometer

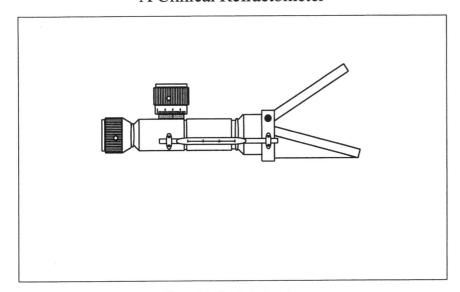

Figure 11–2 Refractometer.

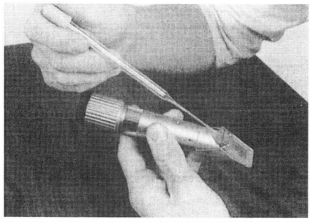

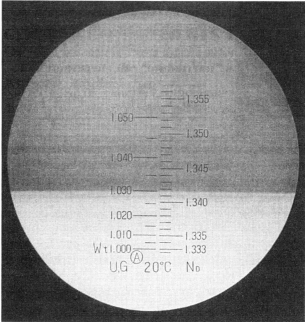

Figure 11–3 *(Top)* Place one drop of urine in the refractometer. Hold the refractometer toward a light source and view the scale through the eyepiece. *(Bottom)* The reading is determined by interpreting the line represented by a light and dark contrast area and reading the scale on the left side. This reading is 1.030. (From Frew, MA, Lane, K, and Frew, DR: Comprehensive Medical Assisting: Competencies for Administrative and Clinical Practice, ed 3, FA Davis, Philadelphia, 1995, p 759, with permission.)

The refractometer method of obtaining a specific gravity reading requires only a single drop of urine. This is a distinct advantage over the urinometer method in which a relatively large quantity of specimen is required. In addition, temperature correction required in the urinometer method is not necessary with the refractometer because this instrument is temperature-compensated between 60°F and 110°F.

The specific gravity often helps the physician to interpret urine test results more accurately. For example, 1 gram of protein in a very dilute sample of urine is more clinically significant than 1 gram of protein in a highly concentrated specimen.

QUALITY CONTROL—CALIBRATION OF THE REFRACTOMETER

The standard used for the calibration of the refractometer is distilled water. To calibrate the refractometer, place a drop of distilled water on the prism and observe the scale. If the scale does not show 1.000, adjust the scale screw with a small screwdriver. Some instruments have a knob screw for adjustments. Run daily control samples representing low, medium, and high concentrations. Document instrument calibration and control results in a daily log book.

INTERFERING SUBSTANCES

Whether the urinometer or refractometer is used to determine specific gravity, the laboratorian needs to make corrections to the reading when large amounts of glucose and/or protein are present. Both glucose and protein elevate the specific gravity reading but have no relationship to the concentrating ability of the kidneys.

For each gram of protein or glucose per deciliter of urine, 0.003 must be subtracted from the specific gravity reading. For example, if a urine specimen contains 1 gram of glucose per deciliter, subtract 0.003 from the specific gravity reading. If the sample also contains 1 gram of protein per deciliter, subtract an additional 0.003 from the specific gravity reading. Corrections are made for interfering substances after the chemical analysis of urine has been performed, since the quantity of both of these analytes is determined at that time.

SPECIFIC GRAVITY REFERENCE RANGE

An individual specific gravity reading ranges from 1.003 to 1.030. If a pooled 24-hour sample of urine is tested for specific gravity, the normal value usually ranges between 1.015 and 1.025. The kidney can only concentrate urine to a specific gravity of 1.040. When readings exceed this value, check for interfering substances, including sugar, protein, and contrast media from x-ray studies. Specific gravity values vary considerably and an isolated reading has little clinical value other than the interpretation of the other analytes in the specimen. Under controlled conditions of fluid intake, however, and with other diagnostic criteria taken into consideration, the specific gravity reading can provide valuable information regarding the ability of the kidneys to reabsorb essential chemicals and water selectively.

SUMMARY

The physical assessment of urine is an important part of the routine urinalysis. The person performing the physical assessment evaluates urine for color, transparency, and specific gravity.

The results obtained during the physical assessment of urine should correlate with information from the chemical analysis and microscopic evaluation. For example, red, cloudy urine is associated with erythrocytes in the urine. Therefore, it is reasonable to anticipate a positive reading for blood during the chemical analysis and to observe erythrocytes during the microscopic examination. An intensely yellow or brownish yellow urine is suggestive of bile pigments. This may be confirmed during the chemical analysis of urine. Cloudy urine is suggestive of microscopic elements including cells, crystals, and bacteria. These can be identified during chemical analysis or microscopic examination.

Many variations from normal in the physical properties of urine have little or no clinical significance, but some can provide the first hint of pathology. Abnormalities observed during the physical assessment of the specimen should be identified either to confirm or to rule out pathology.

PATIENT EDUCATION

• Some foods and medications affect the results of the urinalysis. Check to see whether the patient is taking any medications or vitamins. Document this information on the urine request slip.

Box continues on following page

TECHNICAL CONSIDERATIONS

- Take special care when handling specimens that appear to have excessive bile pigments. These may carry hepatitis B virus (HBV), a disease that can be transmitted through body specimens, including urine.
- If testing cannot be immediately performed, refrigerate the urine specimen.

SOURCES OF ERROR

- If the urine specimen is not collected at the physician's office, determine whether it has been properly refrigerated or was collected within the hour. "Stale" urines give inaccurate results.

Procedure with Rationale

Physical Assessment of Urine
EQUIPMENT AND SUPPLIES

Hand soap	Latex gloves
Urine specimen	Surface disinfectant
Refractometer	Biohazard container
Gauze or soft tissue	

Assemble equipment.

Wash hands with soap and water. Observe the OSHA Standard for this procedure.

Observe and record a urine sample for color. *Be sure you have good lighting to clearly see the color of the specimen.*

If any unusual odor of the sample is noted, record your observation.

Observe and record the transparency of the specimen.

SPECIFIC GRAVITY—REFRACTOMETER METHOD

Calibrate a refractometer following the manufacturer's directions.

Document calibration and controls in a log book.

Using the calibrated refractometer, place one drop of urine on the prism.

Read and record the specific gravity at the boundary line between the light and dark areas.

Dispose of urine following laboratory protocol.

Disinfect and wash all nondisposable equipment.

Clean work area following laboratory protocol.

Remove gloves and wash hands with soap and water.

Questions

Name _____ Date _____

1. Why is the routine urinalysis a test frequently used by physicians?

2. List four abnormal urine colors and give possible source and pathological cause.

3. Which abnormal urine odors are associated with pathology?

4. What is phenylketonuria?

5. What information is provided by the specific gravity of urine?

6. In addition to assessing the concentrating ability of the kidneys, why is it important to determine the specific gravity of a specimen?

7. What substances falsely elevate the specific gravity reading and are not associated with the concentrating ability of the kidneys? How do you correct for this?

8. Give the reference ranges associated with the specific gravity of urine.

Terminal Performance Objective

Physical Assessment of Urine

Given a urine specimen and the necessary equipment, you will perform a physical assessment of urine within 5 minutes and record the results accurately. This procedure must be performed to include all steps to an accuracy level determined by your instructor.

INSTRUCTOR'S EVALUATION FORM

Name _____ Date _____

+ = SATISFACTORY   ✓ = UNSATISFACTORY

_____ Assemble equipment.

_____ Wash hands with soap and water. Observe the OSHA Standard for this procedure.

_____ Observe and record a urine sample for color.
RESULTS _____

_____ If any unusual odor of the sample is noted, record your observation.
RESULTS _____

_____ Observe and record the transparency of the specimen.
RESULTS _____

Specific Gravity—Refractometer Method

_____ Calibrate a refractometer using the manufacturer's directions.

_____ Document calibration and controls in a log book.

_____ Using the calibrated refractometer, place one drop of urine on the prism.

_____ Read and record the specific gravity at the boundary line between the light and dark areas.   RESULTS _____

_____ Dispose of urine following laboratory protocol.

_____ Disinfect and wash all nondisposable equipment.

_____ Clean work area following laboratory protocol.

_____ Remove gloves and wash hands with soap and water.

_____ The procedure was completed in 5 minutes.

_____ The recorded results were within the level of accuracy specified for this procedure.

Final Competency Evaluation

_____ SATISFACTORY   _____ UNSATISFACTORY

Comments:

Instructor _____ Date _____

Chemical Analysis
of Urine

Learning Objectives
Cognitive Objectives
Psychomotor Objectives
Affective Objectives

Analytes of Urine
Glucose
○ Glycosuria
Bilirubin
Ketones
Specific Gravity
Blood
pH
Protein
Urobilinogen
Nitrite
Leukocytes

Specimen Collection

Reagent Strips
Method of Testing

Quality Control
Care of Reagent Strips
Automation

Reporting

Alternate Testing Methods
Clinitest
○ Method of performing a Clinitest

Summary
Patient Education
Technical Considerations
Sources of Error

Procedure with Rationale
Chemical Analysis of Urine

Questions

Terminal Performance Objective
Chemical Analysis of Urine
○ Instructor's evaluation form

LEARNING OBJECTIVES

On completing this chapter, you will be able to:

COGNITIVE OBJECTIVES
- Differentiate between a quantitative and qualitative test.
- Identify the analytes that are generally included in the chemical analysis of a routine urinalysis.
- Give the clinical significance for each of the analytes when abnormalities are noted.
- Name three confirmatory tests performed on urine and explain when they are used.

PSYCHOMOTOR OBJECTIVES
- Store, maintain, and use reagent strips in accordance with the manufacturer's directions to ensure quality control.
- Using a reagent strip, perform a chemical analysis of urine that meets the Terminal Performance Objective presented in this chapter.
- Using Clinitest, perform a test for glycosuria and record the results.

AFFECTIVE OBJECTIVES
- Recognize the importance of logging quality control and test results when performing the chemical analysis of urine.
- Show professional courtesy to other laboratorians by cleaning work areas after testing specimens.

157

The chemical analysis is an important part of a routine urinalysis. It helps to identify substances in the urine that may indicate pathology. A convenient and simple technique for determining many chemical components is the *reagent strip* method. Reagent strips are thin disposable plastic strips that contain small pads impregnated with chemicals that react with **analytes** in the urine. Each pad on the strip contains a reagent specific to one of the urinary components that is the focus of the chemical analysis of urine. The reagent on each pad produces a color change when it reacts with its specific analyte. A test that determines whether an analyte is present is called a *qualitative test.*

Analyte: *the substance or chemical that is analyzed*

The intensity of color change on each of the pads indicates the approximate quantity of the analyte in the urine. When the approximate quantity of an analyte is determined, the test is called a *semiquantitative test.* Accordingly, the reagent strip method used in urinalysis is qualitative and semiquantitative.

Usually the color change that occurs is *time dependent.* This means that time is essential to the accuracy of the test; therefore, the test must be read at a specific time or results may be inaccurate.

Reagent strips are frequently used for *screening tests.* A screening test is any test used on large groups of individuals to separate those who show results within a normal reference range from those who do not. Because they are used on large populations, a screening test should be inexpensive and easy to use. When an abnormality is found, additional tests are used to confirm the accuracy of the original test. Such tests are referred to as confirmatory or alternate tests. These tests are generally more expensive to use and more complicated to perform.

ANALYTES OF URINE

The routine urinalysis usually involves reagent-strip testing for the following analytes: glucose, bilirubin, ketones, specific gravity, blood, pH, protein, urobilinogen, nitrite, and leukocytes. When abnormalities are found, further testing is usually required to verify or further identify the cause of the abnormality. Table 12–1 provides normal urine values using reagent strips.

Glucose

The sugar most commonly found in urine is glucose, but other sugars, including lactose, fructose, galactose, and pentose, may also be present under certain circumstances. Ex-

Table 12–1 **Normal Urine Values Using Reagent Strips**

Analyte	Reference Range and Value
Glucose	Random: Negative 24 hr: 1–15 mg/dL
Bilirubin	Negative to 0.02 mg/dL
Ketones	Negative
Specific gravity	Random: 1.015–1.025 24 hr: 1.003–1.030
Blood	Negative
pH	Range: 4.6–8 24 hr: 6
Protein (albumin)	Random: negative or trace 24 hr: 10–140 mg/L
Urobilinogen	Random: 0.1–1 Ehrlich units/mL; 24 hr: 1–4 mg
Nitrite (bacteria)	Negative
Leukocytes (esterase)	Negative

cessive glucose in the urine is called either *glycosuria* or *glucosuria*. It is often found in patients with diabetes, but it may also occur in acute emotional stress or after vigorous exercise when glucose is liberated from the liver for energy.

GLYCOSURIA

Glycosuria occurs any time blood sugar levels exceed the reabsorption capacity of the renal tubules. Sugar in the blood passes through the glomerulus into the glomerular filtrate during the initial stages of urine formation. Normally, it is reabsorbed back into the blood through the renal tubules. However, when the *renal threshold* is reached, that is, the blood sugar level is so high that complete reabsorption through the renal tubules is impossible, sugar remains in the filtrate and glycosuria results. For most individuals a blood glucose level in excess of 170 mg/dL (normal is about 90 mg/dL) results in glycosuria.

The reactive substance on a reagent strip that identifies the presence of urinary glucose is *glucose oxidase*. This substance is an **enzyme** that reacts specifically with glucose. Consequently, the reagent strip detects only glucose and none of the other sugars that may be present in the urine.

The presence of large quantities of aspirin, ascorbic acid (vitamin C), and levodopa may produce false-positive results. Therefore, glucose results should be correlated with ketone results.

Enzyme: *an organic catalyst that acts only on a certain substance or on a closely related group of substances to cause a chemical change*

Bilirubin

Red blood cells live approximately 120 days. After that, they **lyse** and release hemoglobin. The heme portion of the hemoglobin molecule decomposes to *bilirubin*. Bilirubin is an intensely yellow-colored, pigmented compound. It is not soluble in water and must attach to a protein, primarily albumin, for transportation through the blood. When attached to albumin, it is referred to as *free* or *unconjugated bilirubin*. Free bilirubin cannot pass through the glomerular membrane because of its large size. Instead, it enters the liver where it becomes a water-soluble compound. The water-soluble form of bilirubin is referred to as *bound* or *conjugated bilirubin*. Conjugated bilirubin can be excreted from the body by way of the intestines or the kidneys. Most bilirubin enters the gallbladder and is excreted through the intestines. In the intestines it is converted to a colorless compound called urobilinogen. Whenever the level of bilirubin is elevated because of excessive **hemolysis** and/or the inability of the liver to eliminate bilirubin (liver damage or obstruction of the bile duct), it remains in the body. The yellow color associated with bilirubin, called *jaundice,* appears in the skin, mucous membranes, sclera of the eye, plasma, and urine. Since excess bilirubin can be associated with hepatitis, be very careful when processing any intensely yellow urine specimen and rigorously follow the OSHA Standard.

Lyse: *rupture*

Hemolysis: *rupture of blood cells*

Clinical Comment: Viral Hepatitis

Viral hepatitis is an infection caused by a variety of different viruses that often leads to inflammation of the liver. Two of these important viruses are hepatitis A virus (HAV), sometimes called infectious hepatitis, and hepatitis B virus (HBV), sometimes called serum hepatitis. *HAV* is highly contagious through the fecal-oral routes or **parenterally.** It is usually nonfatal and nonchronic. *HBV* is usually transmitted by way of infectious body fluids including blood, urine, vaginal secretions, and so forth. It is a potentially fatal virus and may increase the risk of cancer of the liver. Health-care workers are at risk for HBV infections. Immunization against this virus is especially important to health-care providers.

Parenterally: *routes other than the gastrointestinal system, that is, vascular, intramuscular, subcutaneous, and so forth*

Bilirubin is an unstable compound. If urine stands, especially in a lighted room or in sunlight, bilirubin oxidizes to a green compound called *biliverdin,* which does not react with the bilirubin reagent on the reagent strip pad.

Ascorbic acid and nitrite in urine may produce false negatives.

Ketones

Cells usually use carbohydrates for energy. When carbohydrates are completely metabolized, they produce water and carbon dioxide. If there is a decreased dietary intake of carbohydrates, such as in starvation, extreme dieting, or certain metabolic disorders, the body uses fats in the form of fatty acids rather than carbohydrates for energy. When excessive fatty acids are used and their metabolism is incomplete, intermediary products are formed. These products, called *ketone bodies,* are composed of acetoacetic acid, acetone, and betahydroxybutyric acid. The ketone reagent on the reagent strip shows positive when acetoacetic acid is present in urine.

Ketones in the urine *(ketonuria)* are most frequently associated with uncontrolled diabetes mellitus. In diabetes, body cells are unable to use glucose effectively as a source of energy because of the lack of insulin. Thus, fatty acids are metabolized to meet energy needs. Ketone bodies are formed as fatty acids are metabolized. Ketone bodies often "spill" into the urine when their level is elevated in the blood. Testing for ketones helps in monitoring diabetes mellitus, because a deficiency in insulin may cause ketonuria. Therefore, ketone and glucose results should be correlated.

Fevers, anorexia, episodes of prolonged diarrhea, vomiting, and any other conditions that accompany restricted carbohydrate intake may lead to ketonuria. Since ketones are acid compounds, ketonuria is correlated with low (acid) urine pH. Levodopa and some dyes produce false positives.

Specific Gravity

The Bayer Multistix 10 SG reagent strip is designed to determine specific gravity. This reagent strip replaces the urinometer and the refractometer method for determining specific gravity. The Multistix 10 SG permits determination of urine specific gravity between 1.000 and 1.030. The results obtained with this reagent strip correlate within 0.005 of values obtained with the refractometer method. A low specific gravity correlates with a dilute, light-colored urine specimen. If this correlation does not exist, high concentrations of sugar, protein, or x-ray dye material may be present. Cells tend to lyse in a urine with a low specific gravity. When urines with low specific gravities are not promptly examined microscopically, the laboratorian may fail to identify cellular elements because they will have disintegrated.

Excessive sugar and protein in urine will produce elevated readings, which are not necessarily associated with the concentrating ability of the kidneys.

Blood

Hematuria, the presence of intact red blood cells in urine, occurs when there are urinary tract disorders associated with bleeding. Bleeding occurs when stones, tumors, or lesions are present anywhere in the urinary tract.

The presence of hemoglobin in the urine is called *hemoglobinuria.* It occurs when there is excessive destruction of red blood cells within the vascular system or when hematuria is present and urine specific gravity is low. When red blood cells are found in a dilute urine, they tend to burst and release hemoglobin into the urine. Hemoglobinuria of vascular origin is found in hemolytic anemias, transfusion reactions, and severe infectious diseases.

When either intact red blood cells or free hemoglobin are present in urine, the blood test reagent pad reacts. Reagent strips show green spots when intact, nonhemolyzed red cells are present, and a homogeneous green to dark blue when free hemoglobin is present. This test is highly sensitive to hemoglobin. A positive test for the presence of blood is complemented by cloudy or clear red urine and the presence of red blood cells in the microscopic examination.

The most frequent cause of hematuria is menstruation, and this should be ruled out or noted on the request slip. Menstruating women should use a clean tampon prior to collecting a specimen for urinalysis.

Although not a product of red blood cells, **myoglobin** also causes a reaction on the blood indicator of the urine reagent strip. The red-brown or black color associated with myoglobin remains in the plasma just a short time and is rapidly excreted by the kidneys. In the absence of erythrocytes or hemoglobin in the urine, a positive blood reaction may be caused by myoglobin in the urine.

> **Myoglobin:** *a substance released from skeletal muscles and cardiac tissue when they are injured*

False negatives may occur with ascorbic acid, nitrite, protein, pH below 5.0 or with high specific gravity.

pH

The abbreviation pH stands for the potential hydrogen ion concentration (H^+). It expresses the acidity or alkalinity of a solution. The pH scale ranges from 0 to 14, with 7 being neutral. A solution with a pH from 0 to 7 is acidic. A solution with a pH from 7 to 14 is basic (alkaline). The further a solution varies from 7, the more acid or alkaline it is. Distilled deionized water has a pH of 7 and is considered neutral; that is, it is neither acidic nor alkaline. The number of acid ions and alkaline ions are equal.

The pH of urine is about 6, slightly acidic, but it may vary from 4.5 to 8.0. This large variation in values for pH is due to the fact that the kidneys, along with the lungs, are responsible for maintaining blood and extracellular fluids at a stable pH. When blood or extracellular fluids change in pH, even slightly, a correction must be made by the lungs and/or kidneys in order to reestablish a normal blood pH (7.35 to 7.45). If this does not occur, the condition of *acidosis* (blood pH less than 7.35) or *alkalosis* (blood pH greater than 7.45) results and may lead to death. The kidneys aid in maintaining a stable pH by removing the substances that are responsible for the abnormal acidic or basic condition. Urine becomes more acidic or more basic in response to excessive acid or alkaline products in the blood.

Patients who are on high-protein diets, who are taking certain medications, or who have uncontrolled diabetes mellitus often excrete urines with a pH lower than 6.0. Renal tuberculosis and fever may cause the urine to become acidic. Alkaline urine can be found in patients who consume diets high in vegetables, citrus fruits, milk, and other dairy products. Other causes of alkaline urine are infection, some metabolic disorders, medications, and respiratory disorders. Stale urines often show high pH because of the growth of bacteria that converts urea to ammonia, an alkaline compound.

Protein

Under normal conditions the kidneys continually excrete very small or trace quantities of protein. This is due to the fact that protein molecules are relatively large and cannot easily pass through the glomerular membrane. When large amounts of protein are present in urine, this is called *proteinuria.* Most of the protein found in urine is albumin. The remaining proteins are microglobulins, **Tamm-Horsfall protein,** and proteins from prostatic, seminal, and vaginal secretions. In practically all instances the protein excreted in pathological conditions is albumin.

> **Tamm-Horsfall:** *a normal mucoprotein found in most urine, produced by the ascending limb of the loop of Henle*

Fever, exposure to heat or cold, excessive exercise, and emotional stress may cause protein to appear in urine. Such findings are usually temporary, and they may not necessarily be associated with pathology.

Excessive and regular excretion of proteins, however, almost always suggests renal disease. Pathological proteinuria may result from damage to the glomerulus or a defect in the reabsorption process of the renal tubules. Some of the causes of proteinuria that is due to a damaged glomerulus include glomerulonephritis, hypertension, amyloidosis, diabetes mellitus, and lupus erythematosus. Proteinuria associated with a defect in the reabsorption process in the renal tubule may be caused by pyelonephritis, tubular acidosis, Wilson's disease, Fanconi's syndrome, and medullary cystic disease.

It is especially important to monitor pregnant women because proteinuria is one of the signs of pre-eclampsia.

Clinical Comment: Acute Glomerulonephritis

Acute glomerulonephritis is an inflammation of the glomerular membrane of the nephron, causing it to become highly permeable. Red blood cells and protein enter the filtrate. Both of these substances appear in the urine.

One of the most common causes of glomerulonephritis is an immunologic inflammatory response in another area of the body, especially the throat and middle ear as a result of strep infections. Antigen-antibody complexes associated with the strep infection become trapped within the network of capillaries that compose the glomerulus and destroy it. Glomerulonephritis is also associated with the autoimmune diseases, including systemic lupus erythematosus, polyarthritis, and scleroderma.

Leukocytes, erythrocytes, epithelial cells, vaginal cells, and bacteria release protein when they rupture, so large quantities of these cells in urine cause the reagent strip to show a positive reading for protein. Urines containing hemoglobin, a protein product, may also show a positive urine protein with reagent strips.

A very dilute urine may give a false negative because the concentration of protein fluctuates with urine flow. A trace or small amount of protein in a very dilute urine sample may indicate significant proteinuria. Therefore, it is important to correlate protein and specific gravity.

Urobilinogen

Like bilirubin, urobilinogen is a bile pigment that results from the degradation of hemoglobin. Bilirubin is broken down in the intestines by bacteria to form urobilinogen. About one half of the urobilinogen is absorbed by the circulatory system and reenters the liver for elimination by the intestines. A very small amount of the urobilinogen escapes liver clearance and remains in the blood to be excreted by the kidneys. This represents about 1 percent of the total urobilinogen of the body. Urobilinogen in the intestine is either eliminated by the body unchanged or is oxidized by **intestinal flora** into urobilin, a pigmented compound that gives feces its color. Urobilinogen is normally found in small amounts in urine. Nitrite and formalin may produce false-negative results. Table 12–2 interprets urobilinogen values in context with bilirubin results.

Intestinal flora: *normal microbial organisms found in the intestinal tract*

Table 12–2 *Urine Bilirubin and Urobilinogen*

Urine Constituent	Reference Value	Hemolytic Disease	Hepatic Disease	Biliary Obstruction
Urine bilirubin	Negative	Negative	Positive or negative	Positive
Urine urobilinogen	Normal	Increased	Increased	Low or absent

Nitrite

Several urinary tract bacterial pathogens produce an enzyme that converts nitrate in urine to nitrite. In order for this to occur, urine must remain in the bladder for a minimum of 4 hours before voiding. This allows time for the bacterial pathogen to convert enough nitrate to nitrite to be detected on the reagent strip. Therefore, the specimen of choice for nitrite detection is the first morning specimen. This test provides early detection of bacteriuria even when the patient does not experience symptoms. A positive result should be confirmed with cultures and smears and with microscopic examination for bacteria and leukocytes. No attempt is made in the routine urinalysis to identify pathogenic organisms associated with urinary tract infections.

Leukocytes

Leukocytes are white blood cells that frequently leave the vascular system and wander throughout the body. They are chiefly responsible for defending and protecting it when harmful substances gain entry. Their level in blood frequently increases in response to infection.

There are two major types of leukocytes, those with granules in the cytoplasm called *granulocytes,* and those without granules in the cytoplasm called *mononuclear leukocytes* or *agranulocytes.* The finding of white blood cells in urine, especially granulocytes, is characteristic of urinary tract infections (UTIs).

A recent development in reagent strip testing is the ability to detect granulocytic leukocytes in urine. Previously, leukocytes could be detected only during the microscopic examination.

The granulocytic cells must lyse to release **esterase** before the test will show positive. If they do not lyse, the test will appear negative. The test is not sensitive to agranulocytic leukocytes, which may also be present in UTIs.

Esterase: *an enzyme found in granulocytic leukocytes, especially neutrophils*

A trace finding is regarded as questionable, and a finding of more than a trace reading is usually clinically significant. When positive readings are found in the leukocyte test and the nitrite test, it is reasonable to assume that there is a UTI. This is confirmed by more elaborate testing methods.

SPECIMEN COLLECTION

Since the chemical analysis is part of a routine urinalysis, the specimen is often a random sample. However, a fresh, first morning midstream specimen is most desirable. If a first morning specimen is not available, the urine should be one that has remained in the bladder at least 4 hours so that the nitrite test results are valid. When testing will be delayed for more than an hour, the specimen must be refrigerated; many urinary compounds are affected by standing at room temperature or by exposure to light.

Ketones, bilirubin, and urobilinogen are unstable at room temperature. Ketones are volatile organic compounds that may escape into the air, producing results that are lower than those that would have resulted had the urine been fresh. In the presence of light, bilirubin is changed into biliverdin, a compound that cannot be detected using the standard chemical testing methods. Finally, a decrease in urobilinogen may occur because of its chemical breakdown to urobilin. In each of these instances the compound is lost to the analysis, and the test results do not reflect the true picture of the urine.

Urine is an excellent medium for bacterial growth. Hence untreated urine left unrefrigerated for over an hour at room temperature may be rendered unsuitable for testing. Bacterial growth causes the urine to become cloudy. Bacteria metabolize urinary glucose for energy, possibly lowering the glucose results. Many bacteria convert nitrate in urine to nitrite, producing an elevated nitrite result. Many bacterial strains decompose urea to form ammonia, resulting in an elevated pH.

Many medications affect test results and give inaccurate readings. The diagnosing physician should be aware of any medications, including vitamins, that are currently being used by the patient. Refer to Chapter 7 for an in-depth discussion of urine specimen collection and transport.

REAGENT STRIPS

Two brands of reagent strips are available for urine chemical testing. They are manufactured under the trade names Multistix (Bayer Corporation, Diagnostics Division, Elkhart, Ind.) and Chemstrip (Bio-Dynamics/BMC, Indianapolis, Ind.). Some of the reagent strips produced by these manufacturers test for only one or two urine constituents, and others test for as many as 10. These reagent strips provide clinical and office practices with a flexible testing method. The order of the reagent pads and reading times vary with each product. They should be timed exactly as required to ensure accuracy.

Method of Testing

There are differences in sensitivity and testing techniques between the two product lines. You should, therefore, read all directions before using these reagent strips. The technique for both products is similar, however.

Immerse the reagent strip in a fresh, uncentrifuged well-mixed urine sample. Make sure that all pads are covered with urine. This may necessitate holding the specimen container at an angle to ensure that the pads closest to the hand are completely immersed in the urine. Immediately remove the reagent strip from the sample and gently wipe the strip, pad side up, against the side of the container to remove excess urine and begin timing. Do not allow the reagent strip to remain in the urine for more than a brief moment, since the chemicals on the pad leach (wash out) into the urine sample. Hold the color chart close to the reagent strip for accurate color comparisons for each of the tests. Make sure that you have adequate lighting for accurate color comparison. Avoid touching the strip against the chart. Hold the strip parallel to the floor to avoid runover of the colors from one pad to another. Remember to read each test at the time specified by the manufacturer (Fig. 12–1).

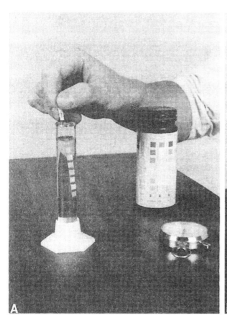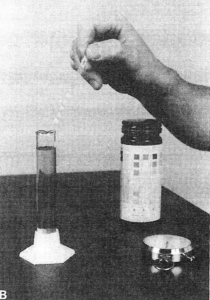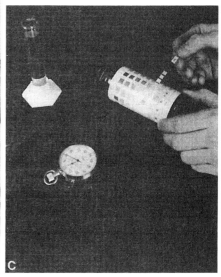

Figure 12–1   Reagent strip procedure. *(A)* Immerse the reagent strip in a fresh, well-mixed urine specimen. *(B)* Drain excess urine by gently wiping the strip on the side of the container. *(C)* Begin timing. Observe the color changes for each constituent by comparing the reagent strip pads with the color chart found on the reagent strip bottle. (From Frew, MA, and Frew, DR: Comprehensive Medical Assisting: Administrative and Clinical Procedures, ed 2, FA Davis, Philadelphia, 1988, Fig. 31–15, with permission.)

Quality Control

Clinical laboratories must have an established quality control system to ensure that test results are accurate. Inaccuracies occur when reagents are faulty or outdated, instruments are not functioning properly, or the laboratorian improperly performs or interprets test results. You should test controls daily and whenever you open a fresh bottle of reagent strips. Bayer Corporation manufactures two control systems that are convenient and easy to use, including Tek-Chek and Chek-Stix. Each of these control systems contains instructions for use and expected values.

When changing reagent strip lots, conduct parallel testing of old and new lots with both controls and patient specimens. Record all control results, lot numbers, and expiration dates in a log book each day and whenever a new bottle of reagent strips is opened (Fig. 12–2).

Care of Reagent Strips

The reagent strip bottle must be tightly closed after you remove the reagent strip. Moisture from the air, light, and aerosol chemicals can react with the reagents on the pads to produce erroneous test results. Do not touch the test pads or lay the strips on any sur-

Figure 12–2 Urine chemistry QC record. (Courtesy Bayer Corporation, Diagnostics Division, Elkhart, Ind.)

faces. Keep reagent strips in a cool, dry place but do *not* refrigerate. Discard any bottles when you see visible changes in the test pads. Before beginning the chemical analysis of urine, read product inserts carefully. Follow all directions in the package insert and on the side of the reagent strip bottle. It is critical to the accuracy of the results that the test is read at the time specified by the manufacturer.

The test bottle displays an expiration date, the date after which the test strips may not be used. Discard any product that has exceeded the expiration date. Any bottle of reagent strips that has been opened for longer than 2 months must likewise be discarded even though the expiration date has not been reached. Repeated exposure to the air may adversely affect the accuracy of the reagents, even though there are no visible changes noted on the reagent strips. Write the date on the label using an indelible marker so that you can discard unused strips after 2 months. Never combine strips from different containers.

Automation

Instruments are available that can detect reagent strip color changes electronically. Using this type of instrument eliminates inaccurate readings associated with individual variations in interpretation. As with all tests, the accuracy of test results depends on following manufacturers' directions. This requires knowing the proper use and limitations of the equipment used for testing. All quality controls applicable to instrumentation must be carefully followed. If necessary, review information in Chapter 5.

REPORTING

Manufacturers provide information on reporting and recording results. The color chart on the side of the reagent strip bottle gives the correct interpretation for each of the colors that can appear during the testing of the urine sample. Match the color obtained on the reagent strip as closely as possible to the color chart, and report the results shown on the bottle. Correlate findings with physical and microscopic findings. For example, a cloudy urine showing high nitrite values probably indicates bacteriuria. This should be confirmed during the microscopic examination.

ALTERNATE TESTING METHODS

When a screening test shows abnormalities, it may be necessary to verify these results. Another testing method may be used to confirm the results of the screening test. If the alternate test is specific for the analyte in the screening test, the test is called a *confirmatory test*. If the test is not specific for the analyte found in the screening test, but verifies results using a different testing technique, the method is referred to as an *alternate test method*.

Three common urine tests that are performed in a physician's office when reagent strip testing shows abnormalities include Acetest, Ictotest, and Clinitest. Acetest is a confirmatory test for ketones; Ictotest is a confirmatory test for bilirubin; Clinitest is an alternate test method for glucose. These tests are manufactured by the Diagnostic Division of Bayer Corporation. Test methods and interpretation of results are provided by the manufacturer.

Clinitest

Clinitest is one of the urine tests most frequently performed when reagent strip results show glucose abnormalities. It not only identifies glucose in the urine, but also reacts when other compounds are present. These compounds are referred to as **reducing substances** because of certain chemical properties that they share. Reducing substances found in urine that react with Clinitest include glucose, galactose, lactose, fructose, pentose, creatinine, uric acid, and ascorbic acid. Galactose in pediatric urine is suggestive of galactosemia, a metabolic disease that may cause nutritional failure and mental retardation. The most significant finding in pediatric urine testing is a negative reagent strip test for glucose and a positive Clinitest for galactose because this is suggestive of galactosemia.

Reducing substances may sometimes appear in the urine of pregnant women. Prior to delivery, the reducing substance is frequently glucose. In postpartum women, the reducing substance is frequently lactose.

> **Reducing substance:** *a substance that loses electrons easily*

Clinical Comment: Galactosemia

Galactosemia is an inborn error of metabolism that results in galactosuria. A child with this disorder lacks an enzyme necessary to convert galactose to glucose and its derivatives. The infant fails to thrive because of anorexia, vomiting, and diarrhea. There may be an enlargement of the liver and spleen, with cirrhosis, cataracts, and mental retardation. In extreme cases, permanent brain damage or even death may result.

The active reagent on reagent strips is glucose oxidase, an enzyme; Clinitest, on the other hand, is based on copper reduction. Table 12–3 compares the interpretations when glucose oxidase and Clinitest are used to test urine.

While reagent strips react only when glucose is present, the Clinitest reacts when any reducing substances are present. Consequently, the reagent strip is said to be a *specific test* and Clinitest is a *nonspecific test*.

METHOD OF PERFORMING A CLINITEST

To use Clinitest, place 5 drops of urine in a glass test tube and add 10 drops of water. Next add a Clinitest tablet to the test tube. Do not touch the tablet since it contains very strong chemicals that will harm the skin. Dispense the tablet into the bottle cap and pour it into the test tube from the cap. In this way the skin does not come in direct contact with the tablet. The contents of the test tube will become hot and begin boiling as the chemicals in the tablet react with the water and urine. When the boiling stops, gently shake the tube and match the color of the solution with a color chart. If no reducing substances are present, the solution will be blue. If reducing substances are present, the color of the solution will range from blue-green to orange, depending on the concentration of the reducing substance. Be sure to watch the entire time the solution begins to boil. When extremely high concentrations of reducing substances are present, the color change occurs very rapidly and returns to the original blue color showing an erroneous negative end result. This is called the *pass-through effect*. Therefore, the clinical laboratorian must observe the sample during the boiling process to be sure that the orange color does not appear.

Table 12–3 **Comparison of Glucose Oxidase Test with Clinitest**

Reagent Strip	Clinitest	Interpretation
Positive	Positive	Glucose present
Negative	Positive	Reducing substances present (galactose, lactose, etc.)

SUMMARY

Reagent strips are thin, disposable plastic strips, with pads impregnated with reagents that test for urine analytes. Reagent strip testing is easy to perform and is a relatively inexpensive method for screening urine samples for possible abnormalities. When abnormalities are found, further testing is frequently undertaken to confirm or rule out pathology.

The accuracy of the results depends on testing only fresh urine samples and following an established quality control program. As part of a quality control program, read all package inserts, record expiration dates, and run positive and negative controls. Record this information in a daily log book. All results obtained during the chemical analysis of urine must correlate with information found during the physical and microscopic examination.

PATIENT EDUCATION

- Some foods and medications interfere with results. Check with the patient and record any medications and/or vitamins on the request slip.
- Instruct menstruating females to use a clean tampon prior to collecting a urine specimen for routine urinalysis.

TECHNICAL CONSIDERATIONS

- Specimens that show an intense yellow color may indicate hepatitis. Exercise caution when handling these specimens.
- Testing must be performed on freshly voided urine or on urine that has been refrigerated for no longer than 8 hours.
- Discard outdated reagent strips or reagent strips open for more than 2 months.
- Do not combine strips from different bottles.
- For Clinitest, observe the entire boiling procedure to determine if the "pass-through effect" has occurred.

SOURCES OF ERROR

- Keep the lid tightly closed on the bottle. Moisture, light, and aerosols affect the reagents.
- Check the manufacturer's directions for correct reading times.
- Avoid prolonged immersion of the reagent strip in the urine, since leaching (washing out) of the reagents may occur.

Procedure with Rationale

Chemical Analysis of Urine
EQUIPMENT AND SUPPLIES

Multistix 10 SG or BMC Chemstrip 9	Distilled water
Color chart	Hand soap
Clock with second hand	Latex gloves
Urine specimen	Disinfectant
Clinitest and color chart	Lab absorbent towel for countertop
Test tube	Biohazard container
Eyedropper	

Assemble equipment.

Wash hands with soap and water. Observe the OSHA Standard for this procedure.

Check the expiration date on the reagent strip bottle and record information. ***Results are not reliable if the expiration date has been exceeded.***

Remove a reagent strip and recap the container. ***The reagent strip bottle must never be left open, since moisture and other substances react with the chemicals on the reagent strip.***

Dip the reagent strip in the urine, making sure to moisten all the pads. Immediately remove the strip from the urine. ***Reagents on the pads may be washed away if excessive wetting of the reagent strip occurs.***

Wipe the reagent strip against the side of the specimen bottle to remove the excess urine.

Hold the strip parallel to the ground, close to the color chart, but avoid touching the strip to the bottle. ***Holding the reagent strip parallel with the ground helps to minimize the runover of colors from one pad to the next.***

At each appropriate time interval, compare the color of the reagent pad against the color chart on the reagent strip bottle. ***Failure to read at the appropriate time interval may result in inaccurate readings. Use a bright light for color comparison. Inaccurate results also occur when the reagent strip is not held close enough to the color chart to discern variations in shade.***

Record the results of the control.

Record your results with correct units.

CLINITEST

Use a disposable dropper to dispense five drops of urine into a glass test tube. Hold the dropper perpendicular to the test tube to ensure uniform drop sizes.

With a clean disposable dropper, dispense 10 drops of distilled water into the test tube. Be sure to hold it perpendicular to ensure uniform drop sizes.

Pour a Clinitest tablet into the cap and then dispense it into the test tube containing the specimen. Recap the Clinitest bottle. ***The tablet contains strong chemicals that can injure the skin. Also, moisture from hands will destroy the tablet.***

Watch the solution until the boiling stops so that the "pass-through effect" can be noted if it occurs. Be careful; the test tube will be hot.

Gently shake the test tube after boiling ceases.

Compare the color of the solution against the color chart.

Record your results with correct units.

Dispose of urine following laboratory protocol.

Clean work area following laboratory protocol.

Remove gloves. Wash hands with soap and water.

Questions

Name _____ Date _____

1. Why is it necessary to read each reagent strip result at the time specified in the directions?

2. The presence of glucose in the urine indicates that the blood glucose level has exceeded the renal threshold. Explain this statement.

3. What causes ketone bodies to appear in urine?

4. What is the relationship of acidosis or alkalosis to urine pH?

5. Name two major renal disorders that lead to proteinuria.

6. What condition is signaled by a positive nitrite test and a positive leukocyte test?

7. For the nitrite test to be valid, urine must remain in the bladder at least 4 hours before voiding. Why?

8. What is the Clinitest? How does this test differ from the glucose oxidase test? What results are noted in Clinitest and glucose oxidase testing method when galactosuria is present?

Terminal Performance Objective

Chemical Analysis of Urine

Given a urine specimen and the necessary equipment, you will be able to perform a chemical analysis of a urine sample using the reagent strip method and test for glycosuria using the Clinitest within 5 minutes. This procedure must be performed to an accuracy level determined by your instructor. Record results.

INSTRUCTOR'S EVALUATION FORM

Name _____ Date _____

+ = SATISFACTORY   ✓ = UNSATISFACTORY

_____ Assemble equipment.

_____ Wash hands with soap and water. Observe the OSHA Standard for this procedure.

_____ Check the expiration date on the reagent strip bottle and record information. Exp.
       date _____.

_____ Remove a reagent strip and recap the container.

_____ Dip the reagent strip in the urine, making sure to moisten all the pads.
       Immediately remove the strip from the urine.

_____ Wipe the reagent strip against the side of the specimen bottle to remove the
       excess urine.

_____ Hold the strip parallel to the ground, close to the color chart, but avoid touching
       the strip to the bottle.

_____ At each appropriate time interval, compare the color of the reagent pad against
       the color chart on the reagent strip bottle.

_____ Record the results of the control. CONTROL _____.

_____ Record your results with correct units. Glucose _____
       Bilirubin _____   Ketones _____
       Specific Gravity _____   Blood _____
       pH _____   Protein _____
       Urobilinogen _____   Nitrite _____
       Leukocytes _____

CLINITEST

_____ Using a disposable dropper, held perpendicular to ensure uniform drop sizes,
       dispense 5 drops of urine into a test tube.

_____ Dispense 10 drops of distilled water into the test tube. Be sure to hold it
       perpendicular to ensure uniform drop sizes.

_____ Pour a Clinitest tablet into the cap and then dispense it into the test tube. Recap the
       Clinitest bottle.

_____ Watch the solution until the boiling stops so that the "pass-through effect" can be
       noted if it occurs. Be careful; the test tube will be hot.

_____ Gently shake the test tube after boiling ceases.

_____ Compare the color of the solution against the color chart.

_____ Record your results with correct units.   RESULTS _____

_____ Dispose of urine following laboratory protocol.

_____ Clean work area following laboratory protocol.

_____ Remove gloves. Wash hands with soap and water.

_____ The procedure was completed within 5 minutes.

_____ The recorded results were within the level of accuracy determined by your instructor.

Final Competency Evaluation

_____ SATISFACTORY   _____ UNSATISFACTORY

Comments:

Instructor _____ Date _____

Microscopic Examination of Urine

13

LEARNING OBJECTIVES

On completing this chapter, you will be able to:

COGNITIVE OBJECTIVES
- Name the two major types of urinary sediment and tell what urinary structures are included in each.
- Tell what actions should be taken when inconsistencies exist among the results obtained in the physical, chemical, and microscopic examination of urine.
- List several pathological states that cause microscopic elements to appear in urine.

PSYCHOMOTOR OBJECTIVES
- Prepare a urine sample for microscopic examination that meets the Terminal Performance Objective presented in the chapter.
- Record microscopic urinary structures using several different accepted methods commonly used by various laboratories.
- Follow all directives for the proper cleanup of laboratory areas used for urinalysis.

AFFECTIVE OBJECTIVES
- Recognize the importance of correlating results obtained in the three testing methodologies used in the routine urinalysis.
- Acknowledge that the identification of microscopic elements in urine requires the expertise of individuals who have received special training in this area of medical laboratory training.

The microscopic examination of urine provides information on the nature of urinary sediment. Urinary sediment consists of all solid particles and formed elements in the urine. The two major types of urinary sediment are the *organized sediment* (also called the biologic sediment) and the *unorganized sediment* (sometimes called the chemical sediment). Organized sediment includes cells, casts, bacteria, parasites, yeast, and fungi. Unorganized sediment includes crystals and **amorphous** material. In general, the organized sediment is clinically more important in diagnosis than the unorganized sediment.

Amorphous: *lacking a definite shape*

Performing the microscopic examination of urine requires more skill and training than the other two parts of the routine urinalysis. Because of this, it is performed by specially trained laboratorians or physicians. The depth of coverage in this chapter depends on your particular academic program of studies. Your instructor will determine the depth of coverage that you need for competency in identifying microscopic urinary sediment. Even if you are not required to identify urinary sediment, you should recognize results that are normal and those that are not so you can render the best care for the patient.

All information obtained during the microscopic examination of urine should be correlated with the information obtained during the physical and chemical assessments of the urinalysis. If there are inconsistencies, the reagents, equipment, specimen, and technique must be evaluated. Retesting may be necessary.

The traditional method for the microscopic examination of urine involves nonstandardized testing techniques. This means that test results may not be precise even when the same individual repeats the test on the same sample of urine. If the test is carefully performed, the urine sample is properly collected (see Chapter 7), and the person performing the test is knowledgeable, valuable information can be obtained from the microscopic examination of a urine specimen.

SPECIMEN PREPARATION

To prepare a sample of urine for microscopic examination, pour a measured quantity of urine into a **centrifuge tube.** A 10- to 15-mL sample from a fresh, well-mixed specimen provides sufficient sediment for observation. Small quantities, that is, 1 to 2 mL, do not contain adequate sediment to assess the sample properly. Set the centrifuge for the length of time and at the speed recommended by the manufacturer (usually 5 minutes at 1500 to 3000 revolutions per minute [rpm]). Place the specimen in the centrifuge. Be sure it is properly balanced (see Chapter 5). When the cycle is completed, remove the sample. The sediment looks like a small "button" of material at the bottom of the centrifuge tube. This is the material that will be examined with a microscope. The clear fluid above the button is the *supernatant.* Using a disposable pipette, syphon off the supernatant leaving behind 1 mL of urine. Resuspend the sediment in the 1 mL of urine by gently tapping the centrifuge tube with the index finger until the entire button disappears. Now the formed elements from the 10- to 15-mL sample are concentrated in only a few drops of urine, thereby increasing the probability that they will be detected when the sample is observed with a microscope. It is important to resuspend the entire button of material.

Centrifuge tube: *a special test tube with a cone-shaped bottom used in centrifuges*

Use a disposable transfer pipette to transfer a drop or two of the resuspended sediment to a microscope slide. Cover the sample with a coverslip by drawing the edge of the coverslip to the drop of urine. Allow the urine to come in contact with the coverslip. Gently lower the coverslip over the drop of urine. This technique avoids trapping bubbles under the coverslip. The volume of urine is standardized by the weight of the coverslip. Be sure not to touch the coverslip once it has been placed over the urine specimen. The specimen is now ready for microscopic examination. Review information on the use of the microscope in Chapter 5.

When examining urine with a microscope, decrease the amount of light on the specimen by lowering the condenser and adjusting the diaphragm. Decreased light enhances the contrast of formed elements, making them easier to see. Urinary sediment stains such as Sedistain are available to aid in visualizing structures. When stain is used, add a drop of stain to the resuspended material in the centrifuge tube. Thoroughly mix the sample with the stain by gentle tapping. Transfer about 2 drops of stained sediment to a glass slide and cover with a coverslip as described above. Whether or not a stain is used, the amount of resuspended sediment placed on the glass slide should be enough so that no dry spots remain under the coverslip but not so much that the coverslip "floats" when placed on the sample. The amount of urine should be approximately the same from sample to sample in order to maintain quality control.

SPECIMEN EXAMINATION

Of the various organized sediments in urine, cells and **casts** have the greatest clinical significance for diagnostic purposes. When other elements such as bacteria, mucous threads, yeast, mold, protozoa, or sperm are observed, note them on the request slip.

> **Casts:** *proteinaceous material that solidifies in the renal tubule and takes the shape of the tubule in which it is formed*

Organized Sediment

CASTS

Renal casts are solidified proteinaceous material formed in the tubules of the kidney. The protein that makes up the matrix of casts is called *Tamm-Horsfall protein.* It originates in the kidneys but does not occur in blood plasma. It is excreted at a relatively constant rate in urine. Even though it is protein in nature, it does not affect the protein pad on reagent strips. Under certain situations Tamm-Horsfall protein solidifies, taking the shape of the tubule in which it is formed. In order for casts to form, there must be a decreased urine flow rate, an acid pH, and an increased urinary protein.

To find casts with the microscope, use low-power (10×) magnification. Decrease the light by adjusting the condenser and diaphragm. Scan 10 fields, especially near the edges of the coverslip. Because of their large size, casts are usually pushed to the edges of the coverslip when it is placed over the urine specimen.

Casts derive their name from their appearance or the materials suspended in their matrix. Hence there are hyaline (glassy or transparent), red-blood-cell, white-blood-cell, epithelial-cell, granular, waxy, fatty, and broad casts. When you find a cast using low-power magnification, examine it with high-power magnification to determine the type of cast. (Table 13–1 lists the types of urinary casts and their possible clinical significance).

Table 13–1 **Summary of Urine Casts**

Type	Origin	Clinical Significance
Hyaline	Tubular secretion of Tamm-Horsfall protein fibrils	Glomerulonephritis; pyelonephritis; chronic renal disease; congestive heart failure; stress/exercise
Erythrocyte	Attachment of RBCs to Tamm-Horsfall matrix	Glomerulonephritis; strenuous exercise
Leukocyte	Attachment of WBCs to Tamm-Horsfall matrix	Pyelonephritis
Epithelial cell	Tubular cells remaining attached to Tamm-Horsfall protein fibrils	Renal tubular damage
Granular	Disintegration of white cell casts, bacteria, urates, tubular cell lysosomes, protein aggregates	**Stasis** of urine flow; urinary tract infection; stress/exercise
Waxy	Hyaline casts	Stasis of urine flow
Fatty	Renal tubular cells	Nephrotic syndrome
Broad	Collecting tubules	Extreme stasis of urine flow

> **Stasis:** *not moving*

Adapted from Strasinger, SK: Urinalysis and Body Fluids, ed 3. FA Davis, Philadelphia, 1994, Table 5–3, with permission.

Normal urines occasionally show one or two hyaline casts per low-power field, with somewhat higher numbers found after extreme exercise. Excessive numbers of hyaline casts or the presence of any other type of cast almost always indicates pathology.

ERYTHROCYTES

It is normal for the microscopic examination of a urine sample to reveal an occasional erythrocyte, or red blood cell (RBC), but more than three per high-power field may indicate pathology. Any abnormal increase in RBCs in urine is called *hematuria*.

Erythrocytes are refractile (shiny) biconcave disks resembling tiny buttons, slightly thinner in the center than around the edge. They do not have nuclei. In concentrated urine, red cells appear "collapsed" (crenated), having lost some of their intracellular fluid. In very dilute urines, the cells "swell" and lose their biconcave appearance. Some of them lyse (rupture), releasing free hemoglobin into the urine.

Hematuria can result from the following conditions:

- Trauma to the kidney
- Passage of stones
- Renal tumors or malignancy
- Inflammation of the renal pelvis, bladder, genitourinary tract, or prostate
- Contamination with menstrual blood
- Vigorous exercise

You should correlate hematuria with a positive blood test in the chemical analysis of urine and a cloudy or clear red urine observed during the physical assessment of the sample. In the absence of erythrocytes, a positive blood result in the chemical analysis may be due to hemoglobin or myoglobin.

LEUKOCYTES

Leukocytes, or white blood cells (WBCs), are normally found in small quantities in most urine samples, especially in female patients. White blood cells are the "scavengers" of the body. They frequently leave blood vessels in search of bacteria and cellular debris. Occasionally they find their way into the bladder and appear in urine samples. However, more than four or five WBCs per high-power field is usually considered abnormal. White blood cells appear "grainy" with dark nuclei often appearing in lobes. If you add 2 percent acetic acid to the concentrated sediment, the nuclei darken, making the lobes more visible. Leukocytes are larger than RBCs.

Pyuria, the abnormal increase of WBCs in urine, is associated with urinary tract infection (UTI) and inflammation of the renal pelvis. A positive leukocyte esterase test and the presence of nitrite in a fresh urine sample, identified by reagent strip, support the diagnosis of UTI.

EPITHELIAL CELLS

Squamous: *resembling a fish scale in appearance*

Microscopic examination of urine can reveal three epithelial cell types: **squamous,** transitional, and renal. Squamous epithelial cells are found in the urethral lining of the male and female and the lining of the vagina in the female. Transitional epithelial cells are found in the lining of the renal pelvis, bladder, and upper urethra. Renal epithelial cells are found in the renal tubules.

Squamous epithelial cells appear flat and contain abundant, irregular cytoplasm and a large central nucleus. They are the least significant of the epithelial cells. Normal urine often shows squamous epithelial cells from the vagina of female patients, especially when the specimen is not a clean-catch sample.

Transitional cells, also called caudal or "tail cells," are smaller than squamous cells. They are pear-shaped with a central nucleus. Their presence usually indicates pathology, especially when many of them have unusual morphology. Pathological conditions, especially nephritis and congestive heart failure, result in urine containing transitional cells. These cells resemble leukocytes but are distinguished from them by the appearance of a single large round nucleus rather than the lobed nucleus of the neutrophil, the cell usually associated with bladder infections.

Renal epithelial cells are the most significant of the epithelial cells and frequently indicate tubular necrosis. They appear round with a central nucleus. Many serious conditions cause an increase in the number of renal epithelial cells.

Unless there is an abundance of squamous cells, or there are transitional or renal epithelial cells, epithelial cells are not routinely recorded.

Other Organized Sediment

Other organized sediment includes bacteria, spermatozoa, protozoa, yeast, and mold. When you observe them, note them on the request slip.

Bacteria are very small organisms. They sometimes appear to "vibrate" as you observe them with the microscope. This type of motility is called *brownian movement.* It is caused by the bombardment of water molecules against the organism. Other bacteria show "purposeful movement" and appear to be "swimming" in a specific direction. These bacteria have *flagella,* whiplike appendages that assist in locomotion.

Always decrease light when you look for bacteria. A finding of a large quantity of bacteria in a fresh midstream clean-catch specimen may indicate UTI, especially if leukocytes are also observed.

Urine from male patients frequently shows sperm after nocturnal emissions or epileptic convulsions. Urine from both male and female patients frequently may show sperm after coitus. Sperm have spherical heads and long thin tails.

Except for *Trichomonas vaginalis,* protozoa are rarely found in fresh urine. When *Trichomonas* is present, it is usually a contaminant from the vagina of females or a result of urethral infection in males. The "Trich" organism is teardrop-shaped with flagella at the smaller end. They are motile and when present can be seen "swimming" in the sample.

Yeast cells are frequently found as a contaminant in the urine of women with *Candida albicans* infection of the vagina. Yeast cells characteristically show budding, the unique feature that helps to differentiate them from RBCs. When in doubt as to whether yeast or RBCs are present, add a small drop of acetic acid to urine sediment. RBCs lyse but yeast cells remain intact.

Mold is rarely found in urine but when present is identified by refractile, jointed, or branched rods (hyphae).

You may occasionally observe contaminants and artifacts including fibers from clothing, talc, and fecal material during the microscopic examination of the urine. These artifacts are not reported.

Unorganized Sediment

Unorganized sediment consists of crystals and amorphous material. These substances are not as clinically important as the cellular components of urine. Most urine samples contain unorganized sediment, especially if the urine has been refrigerated or is not freshly voided. Crystals that normally appear in acid urine include amorphous urates, uric acid, and calcium oxalate. Crystals that normally appear in alkaline urine include triple phosphate, ammonium biurate, calcium phosphate, and calcium carbonate. The presence of cystine, leucine, and tyrosine crystals indicates pathology (Fig. 13–1).

CRYSTALS FOUND IN ACID URINE (X400)

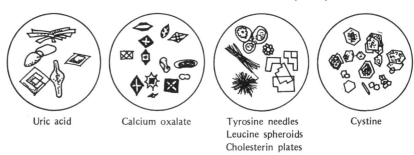

Uric acid   Calcium oxalate   Tyrosine needles   Cystine
                                 Leucine spheroids
                                 Cholesterin plates

CRYSTALS FOUND IN ALKALINE URINE (X400)

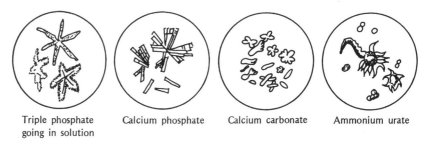

Triple phosphate   Calcium phosphate   Calcium carbonate   Ammonium urate
going in solution

SULFA CRYSTALS

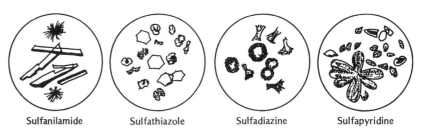

Sulfanilamide   Sulfathiazole   Sulfadiazine   Sulfapyridine

Figure 13-1 Crystals found in urine. (Courtesy Bayer Corporation, Diagnostics Division, Elkhart, Ind. From Frew, MA, and Frew, DR: Comprehensive Medical Assisting: Administrative and Clinical Procedures, ed 2, FA Davis, Philadelphia, 1988, Fig. 31–18, with permission.)

REPORTING

Casts, Erythrocytes, and Leukocytes

When reporting a specific urinary structure, observe 10 *fields*. A field is the circular area you observe when looking through the oculars of a microscope. When the low-power objective is in place, the area is referred to as a *low-power field* (lpf); when the high-power objective is in place, the area is called a *high-power field* (hpf). Count the number of structures in each field. After 10 fields are individually counted, add the numbers from the 10 fields and divide by 10 to find the average. Report this number on the request slip. As an alternate method you may report a range. To determine a range, note the lowest number seen in any field and the highest number seen in any field after examining 10 fields. Report the lowest number and the highest number followed by the power of the objective you used for the observation, for example, "10 to 15 per hpf." When the number of cells is so great that counting accurately is impossible, report the field as "packed" or "TNTC" (too numerous to count). Casts are reported in terms of low-power fields. Erythrocytes, leukocytes, and epithelial cells are reported in terms of high-power fields.

Table 13–2 **Plus System for Quantifying Urinary Sediment**

+	1–10
++	11–20
+++	21–30
++++	More than 30

Other Urinary Sediment

Methods for reporting the other organized sediment (bacteria, yeast, etc.) and unorganized sediment (crystals) vary considerably depending on the laboratory. Bacteria are often reported as negative, light, moderate, and heavy. Crystals are sometimes recorded as rare, occasional, few, moderate, and many. Other terms used to report unorganized sediment include occasional, few, many, abundant, innumerable, packed, and TNTC. Some laboratories use a plus system (Table 13–2). The method of reporting may vary from laboratory to laboratory, but it must be consistent within a single laboratory.

REFERENCE VALUES

As with most laboratory tests, there is no distinct value at which the physician defines pathology, and there is no precise definition of normalcy. For example, many authors define the presence of 0 to 3 RBCs per hpf as falling within the normal reference range. However, the presence of 4 RBCs does not conclusively define a pathological state. A complete clinical picture is needed before any conclusions can be reached. As you read different reference material, this becomes more apparent. Some texts list one set of reference values as normal, other texts list slightly different values. You should remain flexible while learning reference ranges. Table 13–3 summarizes reference ranges for microscopic elements in urine.

QUALITY CONTROL

Specimen Integrity

Changes that mask or alter results can occur in specimens that are not fresh or properly preserved. Large quantities of bacteria can appear in the specimen even though they are not present in the bladder. They metabolize urea to form ammonia, which elevates the pH of the specimen. Erythrocytes, leukocytes, epithelial cells, and urinary casts often disintegrate upon standing, especially in dilute urines with an elevated pH. Therefore, these important elements are not observed during the microscopic examination and go unrecorded. See Chapter 7 for more information.

Table 13–3 **Reference Ranges for Microscopic Elements in Urine**

Microscopic Structure	Normal Value
WBC/hpf	0–4
RBC/hpf	0–3
Epi/hpf	Few squamous
Casts/lpf	Occasional hyaline
Bacteria/hpf	Few
Crystals/hpf	Urates, uric acid, calcium oxalate in acidic urine; and triple phosphate, calcium carbonate, and ammonium biurate in alkaline urine

lpf = low-power field; hpf = high-power field; RBC = red blood cell; WBC = white blood cell; Epi = epithelial cell

Standardization

The microscopic examination is the least standardized and most time-consuming portion of the routine urinalysis. Procedural variations, methods of specimen preparation, types of equipment, and manner of reporting all contribute to inconsistencies in test results. By using a set volume of urine, discarding the supernatant to leave a standardized amount of urine specimen for examination, and not touching the coverslip after it has been placed on the sample, you provide a degree of standardization within a laboratory.

The Kova System (ICL Scientific, Fountain Valley, Calif.), the Fisherbrand Urisystem (Fisher Scientific, Pittsburgh, Pa.), and the Count-10 system (V-Tech, Inc., Palm Desert, Calif.) are commercial products that bring standardization to microscopic evaluation. The Kova System is discussed in further detail.

KOVA SYSTEM

The Kova system offers a consistent, simplified method for the complete standardization of the microscopic examination. It includes Kova Tubes, Kova Kap, Kova Petter, and Kova slides (Fig. 13–2). The Kova Tube is a graduated 12-mL centrifuge. It standardizes sample size. The Kova Kap is used to prevent spillage and to eliminate aerosol contamination during transportation and centrifugation. In the Kova system, the sample of urine is centrifuged at a relative **centrifugal force** (rcf) of 400 for 5 minutes. This eliminates variations that occur when different centrifuges are used. The Kova system of 400 rcf for 5 minutes equates to approximately 1500 rpm for 5 minutes using a centrifuge with a 6-inch radius rotor. The Kova Petter is a disposable plastic transfer pipette that locks into position on the centrifuge tube after centrifugation. When it is locked into position, it retains 1 mL of urine above the sediment as 11 mL of the sample is **decanted.** In this way the sediment is resuspended in an exact amount of urine. A drop of Kova Stain

> **Centrifugal force:** *the force that impels solid particles outward from the center of rotation*

> **Decant:** *pour off*

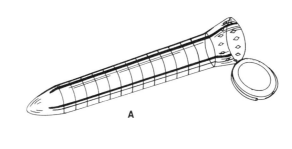

A

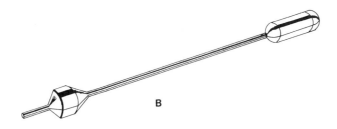

B

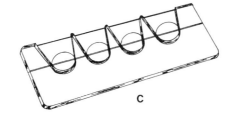

C

Figure 13–2 The Kova system. *(A)* Kova tube and cap. *(B)* Kova petter. *(C)* Kova slide.

may be added to the sediment. The sediment is resuspended into a homogeneous mixture by squeezing the Kova Petter bulb several times. A small sample of the resuspended sediment is transferred to the Kova slide using the Kova Petter. The design of the Kova slide controls the amount of the sample that is observed during the microscopic examination. With the Kova system there is a standardized method for reporting urinary sediment.

SUMMARY

The purpose of the microscopic examination is to detect, identify, and quantify solid structures present in urine. Both biologic and chemical sediments are reported. Some of the components found during the microscopic examination are clinically important to diagnosis, while others have no significance at all.

Since specimen collection and handling are essential to accurate results, you must adequately instruct the patient on urine collection and preservation (see Chapter 7). The results of the microscopic examination of a urine specimen must correlate with the findings in the physical and chemical analysis of urine. By becoming familiar with normal urine structures, you are able to identify abnormal results and bring them to the attention of the physician.

PATIENT EDUCATION

- The microscopic examination provides the most accurate results when you use a first morning midstream sample.
- Menstruating females should use a fresh tampon prior to collecting a specimen for microscopic examination.
- When urine samples are brought from home, be sure that the transport container is clean and free of soap residue.

TECHNICAL CONSIDERATIONS

- The entire button of sediment must be resuspended in the supernatant to ensure that all sediment will be examined.
- Specially trained laboratorians perform the microscopic evaluation of urine.
- Use only the recording method approved by your laboratory director for enumerating urinary sediment.

SOURCES OF ERROR

- The Kova method provides a standardized alternative to the traditional microscopic urine examination.
- Stale urine or urine not properly maintained prior to the urinalysis gives inaccurate results.
- Improper handling or processing of the urine sample will give inaccurate results. Erythrocytes, leukocytes, epithelial cells, and urinary casts often disintegrate upon standing, especially in dilute urines with an elevated pH.

Procedure with Rationale

Microscopic Examination of Urine

EQUIPMENT AND SUPPLIES

Hand soap	Disposable transfer pipette
Microscope	Urine specimen
Centrifuge	Biohazard container
Centrifuge tube	Latex gloves
Glass slide	Lab absorbent towel for countertop
Coverslip	Surface disinfectant

Assemble equipment.

Wash hands with soap and water. Observe the OSHA Standard for this procedure.

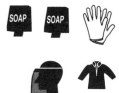

Using a well-mixed specimen, place the appropriate amount of urine in a centrifuge tube. ***Usually a sample size of about 10–15 mL will provide sufficient sediment for observation. The amount will be determined by your instructor.***

Balance the specimen in the centrifuge. ***Whenever the centrifuge is used, all specimens must be loaded in the instrument so that they balance. This may necessitate using a water blank for a balance when an uneven number of specimens are run.***

Set the speed and time for a urine sample as specified by the centrifuge manufacturer and centrifuge the specimen.

When the centrifuge has stopped spinning, remove the specimen. Use a disposable pipette to remove the supernatant. Leave 1 mL of urine in the centrifuge tube. ***By leaving 1 mL of specimen in the centrifuge tube the amount of urine for resuspending the sediment button has been standardized.***

Resuspend the entire sediment button in the urine remaining in the centrifuge tube. ***The centrifuge tube should be gently tapped until all of the sediment is resuspended. If the sediment is not completely resuspended, important urinary elements may remain behind and therefore will not be detected during the microscope examination.***

Using a disposable transfer pipette, place about two drops of urine on the slide and cover the specimen with a coverslip. Draw the coverslip to the drop of urine. After contact is made with the urine, the coverslip can be gently lowered onto the urine specimen. Do not touch the coverslip once it has been placed on the specimen. ***This technique reduces the chance that bubbles will become trapped under the coverslip. The weight of the coverslip provides a degree of standardization for the volume of specimen used for the microscopic examination.***

Focus the microscope using the low-power magnification (10×), and decrease the amount of light by adjusting the condenser and diaphragm. ***When unstained specimens are observed with the microscope, decreasing the amount of light generally enhances the contrast of the elements.***

If required by your instructor, observe for casts, especially around the edge of the coverslip. Examine 10 low-power fields, and find the average or range. If any casts are observed, switch to high power (40–50×) to identify type. Record your results. ***Because of their relatively large size, casts are usually found around the edge of the coverslip.***

Focus using high power (40–50×) and observe for other urinary sediment. Identify each type required by your instructor. Record your results.

Dispose of specimen following laboratory protocol.

Disinfect and wash all nondisposable equipment

Clean work area following laboratory protocol.

Remove gloves. Wash hands with soap and water.

Questions

Name _____ Date _____

1. What is urinary sediment? What constituents make up the organized and unorganized urinary sediment?

2. What steps should be taken when inconsistencies exist among the physical, chemical, and microscopic properties of urine?

3. Why is it necessary to centrifuge the urine sample before examination with the microscope?

4. How are casts formed? What is their clinical significance?

5. Name three types of epithelial cells that may be found in urine and give possible causes for each.

6. Explain the clinical significance of erythrocytes and leukocytes in a urine specimen.

7. List four normal crystals that may be found in urine. What crystals are likely to be present in alkaline urine? Acid urine?

8. Briefly explain the Kova system and describe its advantages over the standard method of performing a microscopic examination of urine.

9. Describe the various methods of quantitizing urinary structures.

Terminal Performance Objective

Microscopic Examination of Urine

Given a urine specimen and the necessary equipment, you will prepare a sample of urine for microscopic examination within 5 minutes. If required by your instructor, you will identify and record any microscopic elements found in the urine within 10 minutes and properly record your results. This procedure must be performed to a level of accuracy determined by your instructor.

INSTRUCTOR'S EVALUATION FORM

Name _____ Date _____

+ = SATISFACTORY   ✓ = UNSATISFACTORY

_____ Assemble equipment.

_____ Wash hands with soap and water. Observe the OSHA Standard for this procedure.

_____ Using a well-mixed specimen, place the appropriate amount of urine in a centrifuge tube.

_____ Balance the specimen in the centrifuge.

_____ Set the speed and time for a urine sample as specified by the centrifuge manufacturer and centrifuge the specimen.

_____ When the centrifuge has stopped spinning, remove the specimen. Use a disposable pipette to remove the supernatant. Leave 1 mL of urine in the centrifuge tube.

_____ Resuspend the entire sediment button in the urine remaining in the centrifuge tube.

_____ Using a disposable transfer pipette, place about two drops of urine on the slide and cover the specimen with a coverslip. Draw the coverslip to the drop of urine. After contact is made with the urine, the coverslip can be gently lowered onto the urine specimen. Do not touch the coverslip once it has been placed on the specimen.

_____ Focus the microscope using the low-power magnification (10×), and decrease the amount of light by adjusting the condenser and diaphragm.

_____ If required by your instructor, observe for casts, especially around the edge of the coverslip. Examine 10 low-power fields, and find the average or range. If any casts are observed, switch to high power (40–50×) to identify type. Record your results. Casts _____

_____ Focus using high power (40–50×) and observe for other urinary sediment. Identify each type as required by your instructor. Record your results.
RBCs _____   WBCs _____
EPI _____   Crystals _____
Other _____

_____ Dispose of specimen following laboratory protocol.

_____ Disinfect and wash all nondisposable equipment.

_____ Clean work area following laboratory protocol.

_____ Remove gloves. Wash hands with soap and water.

_____ The procedure was completed in the required time.

_____ The procedure was properly performed, and all required urinary sediment was correctly identified and recorded to a level of accuracy specified by your instructor.

_____ The results were properly recorded.

Final Competency Evaluation

_____ SATISFACTORY   _____ UNSATISFACTORY

Comments:

Instructor _____ Date _____

UNIT
IV

CLINICAL HEMATOLOGY AND CHEMISTRY

Introduction to Hematology

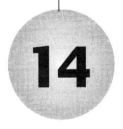

14

LEARNING OBJECTIVES

On completing this chapter, you will be able to:

COGNITIVE OBJECTIVES
- Describe the appearance of an erythrocyte and state its major function.
- List the five types of leukocytes found in blood and state their primary function.
- Describe the appearance and function of the platelet and identify the three essential steps of blood coagulation.
- List the major components of blood plasma.
- Define the term *hematopoiesis.*
- List the two types of blood specimens used for hematologic studies and the tests included in the complete blood count.

Hematology is the study of blood and the blood-forming organs. Because of the multitude of functions performed by blood, it is analyzed more than any other body fluid. Literally hundreds of different tests are performed using blood specimens. Chemistry analysis, **immunology** studies, and **immunohematology** tests all require a blood sample analysis. Hematology tests, however, focus chiefly on the study of erythrocytes, leukocytes, and platelets. Hematology involves counting, classifying, or otherwise studying the blood components and the blood-forming organs. Another important aspect of hematology is the investigation of **coagulation** abnormalities.

Blood (whole blood) is a body tissue composed of formed elements suspended in a liquid medium called *plasma.* The formed elements include red blood cells (RBCs), also called *erythrocytes,* white blood cells (WBCs), or *leukocytes,* and platelets, which are also known as *thrombocytes.* They are produced primarily in bone marrow. Plasma accounts for about 55 percent of the total blood volume; the other 45 percent is made up of the formed elements—blood cells and platelets (Fig. 14–1).

Blood transports nourishment, water, vitamins, electrolytes, hormones, gases, and

Immunology: *the study of antigen-antibody reactions*

Immunohematology: *the study of blood diseases including certain autoimmune disorders using antigen-antibody techniques*

Coagulation: *blood clotting; hemostasis*

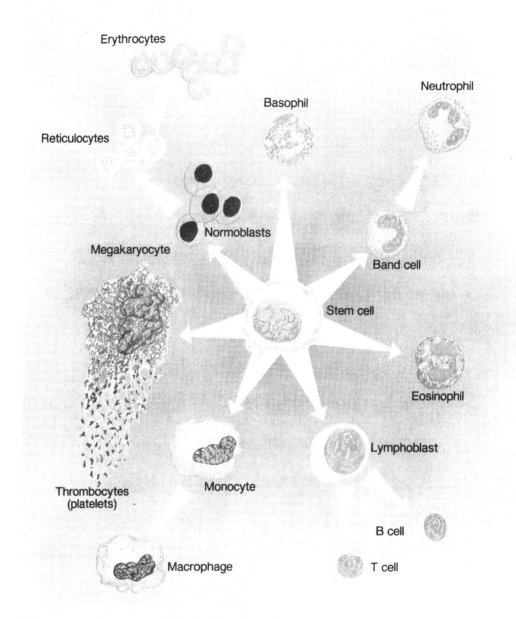

Figure 14-1 Components of blood and the relationship of blood to other body tissues. (Scanlon, VC, and Sanders, T: Essentials of Anatomy and Physiology, ed 2, FA Davis, Philadelphia, 1995, p 245, with permission.)

Immune substances: *primarily antibodies (immunoglobulins) that assist in defending the body against invasion by antigens (immunogens)*

immune substances to body tissues. It carries carbon dioxide (CO_2) from body tissues to the lungs for removal from the body. It carries waste products to the kidneys for disposal. It also serves as a heat regulator for the body.

ERYTHROCYTES

The most numerous blood cells are erythrocytes. There are approximately 500 RBCs for each WBC. Their major purpose is to carry oxygen to all tissues of the body. Erythrocytes contain a compound called hemoglobin. Hemoglobin is composed of an iron-containing portion (hematin) and a simple protein (globin). When erythrocytes pass through the lungs, the hemoglobin gains oxygen (it undergoes oxygenation) and blood becomes bright red in color. Saturated with oxygen, the RBCs return to the heart where they are pumped to the capillary beds found in all tissues of the body. In the capillary beds gases are exchanged. Body tissues trade their carbon dioxide, formed as a waste product of metabolism, for oxygen in the red cells. When this occurs, erythrocytes lose oxygen (they undergo deoxygenation) and become dark red as they take up carbon dioxide. Deoxygenated blood passes through the venous system to the heart. The heart pumps deoxygenated blood to the lungs for oxygenation, to repeat the cycle once again.

Mature erythrocytes have a bioconcave disk shape, flattened in the center and thicker at the edge—somewhat like tiny buttons. This shape gives them an increased surface area, which makes the cells more efficient at their job of gas transport. Each cell measures approximately 7.5 micrometers (μm) in diameter. Nuclei are found only in immature erythrocytes. Immature RBCs are not normally found in circulating blood. By the time the red blood cell matures enough to be released into circulation by the bone marrow, the red cell has lost its nucleus.

Erythrocytes live about 120 days and then rupture. **Reticuloendothelial cells** in the liver and spleen destroy the aged erythrocytes by splitting the hemoglobin molecule. Most iron is reused for new erythrocytes. The rest of the hemoglobin molecule is converted into other substances, which the body reuses or eliminates. Red blood cells are replaced by the bone marrow at a rate of approximately 140 million per minute.

Reticuloendothelial cells: *cells lining vascular and lymphatic channels capable of destroying cells, bacteria, and viruses*

Clinical Comment: Anemia

The most common pathologies associated with erythrocytes are anemias. In the broadest sense, *anemia* is the inability of blood to deliver an adequate supply of oxygen to body tissues. Anemias are usually diagnosed when there is a decrease in the number of erythrocytes, a decrease in the amount of hemoglobin in the cells, or a decrease in red cell volume. The signs and symptoms associated with most anemias include difficulty in breathing, weakness, rapid heart beat, paleness, low blood pressure, and, frequently, a low-grade fever. Hematology tests help to identify the type and extent of anemias.

LEUKOCYTES

Five major types of leukocytes are normally found in the circulating blood. They protect the body by controlling various disease conditions and tissue injury. They are identified by observing their staining characteristics, the shape of their nuclei, and the nature of their cytoplasm. You will find a more complete discussion of white cell **morphology** in Chapter 18.

Morphology: *the study of structure and form without regard to function*

Clinical Comment: Leukemia

Leukemia is a malignancy of the blood-forming organs. With this condition, healthy bone marrow cells are replaced by malignant cells. The various types of leukemias are identified by the duration of the disease from onset to death of the patient as being acute or chronic. In acute leukemias, death occurs in a few months; in chronic leukemias, life expectancy exceeds 1 year.

This disease is frequently categorized by the particular cell population that is affected, granulocytic (myelogenous) or lymphocytic.

Acute lymphocytic leukemia (ALL) is found primarily in children. Chronic myelogenous leukemia (CML) is associated with an abnormal chromosome called the Philadelphia (Ph[1]) chromosome. The onset of CML is between the ages of 40 and 50. Chronic lymphocytic leukemia (CLL) is found primarily in the older population, generally over 50 years of age.

Unlike erythrocytes, leukocytes do not necessarily remain in blood vessels. Most types of leukocytes leave the vascular system and wander through tissue spaces, never to return again. One type of leukocyte, the lymphocyte, enters the lymphatic system for a while and then returns to the vascular. The ability of leukocytes to move freely around the body in this manner makes them ideally suited for their job of surveying cells, tissues, and organs. It also places them at the site where they can defend the body or otherwise resolve disease, infection, or injury that threatens well-being.

Leukocytes are classified into two categories: the *granulocytes* (those containing granules in the cytoplasm) and the *agranulocytes* (those without granules), also called *mononuclear cells.* The granulocytes include neutrophils, basophils, and eosinophils. The agranulocytes include the monocytes and the lymphocytes. Each of these cell types provides specialized protection including:

- Phagocytosis
- Detoxification
- Inflammation
- Adaptive immune response

Table 14–1 summarizes the protection provided by the various types of leukocytes.

Phagocytosis

Phagocytosis: *the process whereby cells engulf and destroy particulate matter including bacteria*

One of the most important functions provided by leukocytes, especially neutrophils and monocytes, is **phagocytosis.** Bacteria or other foreign substances become fixed to the surface of the phagocytic cell. The cytoplasm of the phagocytic cell streams around and engulfs the foreign material, drawing it within its cytoplasm (Fig. 14–2). Specialized internal structures of the phagocyte then destroy the foreign material through enzyme action. Phagocytosis is so important to the defense of the host that if total phagocytic activity is lost by white cells, death of the host results.

Detoxification

Another protection afforded by leukocytes is the removal or neutralization of poisonous or harmful substances. This process is called *detoxification.* Eosinophils neutralize the effects of histamine in allergic reactions in order to control some of the adverse tissue changes that accompany the allergic response. Eosinophils also destroy certain parasitic worms that infest the body.

Table 14–1 **Protection Provided by Leukocytes**

Leukocyte	Type of Protection
Granulocytes	
Neutrophils	Phagocytosis
Eosinophils	Detoxification
Basophils	Mediation of inflammatory reaction
Agranulocytes	
Monocytes	Phagocytosis
Lymphocytes	Adaptive immune response

Phagocytosis

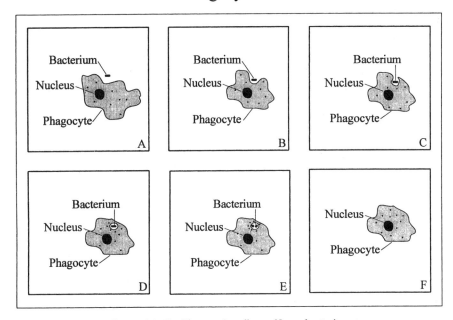

Figure 14–2   Phagocytic cell engulfing a bacterium.

Inflammation

Basophils help to **mediate** the various activities associated with inflammation. *Inflammation* is a vascular activity in which capillary walls found in tissues adjacent to an area of injury become "leaky." As a result, plasma, white cells, and dissolved substances escape from the capillary beds and enter the injured area. These components act together to produce a sequence of events to neutralize toxic products, eliminate offending agents, destroy **necrotic tissue,** and establish an environment necessary for tissue repair.

Basophils contain large amounts of histamine, which they release into injured tissue spaces to increase inflammation. Basophils also contain heparin, an anticoagulant, which inhibits blood clotting.

Mediate: *to initiate and synchronize a series of activities*

Necrotic tissue: *dead tissue*

Adaptive Immune Response

The adaptive immune response is a highly complex and specialized defense mechanism of the body. This intricate response involves the ability of the body to recognize substances that are different in some way from its own normal tissues. Once these substances are identified as foreign, this immune system destroys them, renders them harmless, or eliminates them from the body. Any foreign substance that can provoke this type of response from the adaptive immune system is called an **antigen** or **immunogen.** (Chapter 24 details information on the adaptive immune response.)

The adaptive immune system is so highly specific that it can identify extremely subtle molecular differences among the multitude of antigens to which the host is exposed. Each response to eliminate or destroy the antigen is unique and singular for that particular antigen.

Finally, a memory component of the adaptive immune response permits a recall of the actions that were taken in a previous exposure to destroy the antigen and then duplicate this action immediately. In most instances this response is so rapid that the host is immune to future bouts of illness caused by the same organism.

Antigen, Immunogen: *a substance, usually protein, that is identified as nonself and has the ability to elicit an immune response*

PLATELETS (THROMBOCYTES)

Megakaryocyte: *a large bone marrow cell that gives rise to platelets*

The smallest formed elements found in the blood are platelets, or thrombocytes. They are fragments of cytoplasm shed from the periphery of cells in the bone marrow called **megakaryocytes.** Like mature erythrocytes, platelets have no nuclei. They are important in *hemostasis,* the process by which the body spontaneously stops or controls bleeding by producing blood clots. Without the ability to form clots, an individual would hemorrhage to death with any major vascular injury. Equally important, blood must remain in the fluid state and not form blood clots while it circulates within blood vessels. Movement of blood clots through the vascular system is life-threatening.

The two major systems responsible for hemostasis are the fibrin-forming system *(coagulation)* and the fibrin-destroying system *(fibrinolytic system).*

Coagulation

Thromboplastin: *a complex substance found in tissue that is essential to the clotting process*

Coagulation begins when **thromboplastin,** released from injured tissue, reacts with various plasma proteins and factors released from platelets. This process consists of a chain of at least 13 interlinked reactions. If any of the interlinked reactions is absent or faulty, blood will not clot. Coagulation can be simplified and expressed in three essential steps.

- Platelet factors and thromboplastin released from injured tissues react with clotting substances in the plasma to form *prothrombin activator.*
- Prothrombin activator converts a blood protein called *prothrombin* to *thrombin.*
- Thrombin converts another blood protein called *fibrinogen,* a soluble protein, into *fibrin,* a stringy insoluble material.

The diagram that follows shows the formation of a clot.

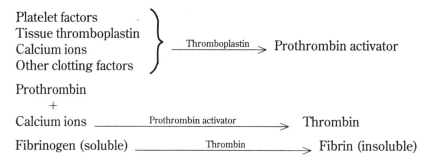

Fibrinolytic System

The fibrinolytic system is composed of *endothelial cells* that line the blood and lymphatic vessels, the heart, and other hollow organs. These cells prevent excessive pathological coagulation by releasing an anticoagulant, heparin. Basophils also release heparin thereby keeping blood in the fluid state while it circulates through the body. Another anticoagulant, produced in the liver and found in the blood, is *antithrombin.* This protein inactivates thrombin, thus destroying the ability of the blood to clot.

PLASMA

Plasma is the liquid component of whole blood that remains after the formed elements are removed. It is about 90 percent water. The remaining 10 percent includes the plasma proteins (albumins, globulins, and fibrinogen), the electrolytes, gases (CO_2, O_2, N_2), nutrients (glucose, amino acids, cholesterol, and fats), hormones, and excretory products (urea, uric acid, creatinine, and bile products). When blood is allowed to coagulate, the liquid remaining is called *serum* (see Chapter 8).

Plasma serves as the medium that maintains **homeostasis** for body cells. It continuously circulates in and out of blood vessels, transporting substances around the body. When it is found in tissue spaces, it is called *interstitial fluid* or *tissue fluid*. As tissue fluid, it delivers nutrients, vitamins, hormones, and many other products to the cells through which it is circulating. It also takes waste products from these cells. Tissue fluid directly reenters the vascular system or passes through lymphatic channels back to the vascular system. The vascular system carries waste products to the kidneys, lungs, and liver for disposal. The continuous delivery of products through blood vessels, intracellular spaces, and lymphatic channels keeps body cells in a state of homeostasis.

> **Homeostasis:** *the condition of a stable environment for cells and tissues maintained by a dynamic process of feedback and regulation*

HEMATOPOIESIS

All blood cell types originate from a single primitive blood cell, called the *stem cell*. Through a highly complex process, the stem cell becomes committed to the production of one or more cell lines. The formation and maturation of blood cells is called *hematopoiesis,* or *hemopoiesis*. Most blood cells are produced in the red bone marrow; however, the lymph nodes and spleen contribute to the formation of some of the cellular components of blood. In a healthy individual, mature or almost mature blood cells are released into the vascular system to replace old or worn out cells. A red blood cell showing a slight degree of immaturity is called a *reticulocyte*. Reticulocytes have small filaments of nuclear material, ribonucleic acid (RNA), in the cell. This nuclear material remains a short time after the nucleus is extruded. Reticulocytes are identified using a special stain that reacts with the nuclear material. These cells are then identified using a microscope. Reticulocytes normally constitute about 1 percent of the circulating erythrocytes. Elevation of the number of reticulocytes *(reticulocytosis)* is a sign that the body needs more erythrocytes. It is a symptom of some types of anemia, for example, hemolytic anemia. A lower than normal number of reticulocytes in circulating blood *(reticulocytopenia)* can be caused by defects in hematopoiesis or hemoglobin production.

Slightly immature neutrophils called *band cells* or *stab cells* occasionally enter the bloodstream. You can identify them by their C-shaped nuclei, which have not yet formed lobes. In a normal individual, about 5 percent of the neutrophils in peripheral circulation are band cells. This percentage increases during some infections. Figure 14–3 shows the development and maturation of the different cell lines from the stem cell.

SPECIMENS FOR HEMATOLOGIC STUDIES

Most hematologic tests performed in a physician's office require a capillary blood specimen (peripheral puncture) collected by a fingerstick or a venous blood specimen collected by phlebotomy. Ethylenediaminetetraacetic acid (EDTA) is the anticoagulant of choice when a venipuncture is performed for hematology studies. This particular anticoagulant preserves the shape and characteristics of cellular elements. When collecting blood using an anticoagulant, you must thoroughly mix the blood with the anticoagulant. Even the smallest clot present in a sample of whole blood invalidates the results of hematologic studies. Gently invert all Vacutainer tubes containing an anticoagulant at least eight times to mix the anticoagulant with the blood thoroughly.

COMPLETE BLOOD COUNT

The complete blood count (CBC) is a basic screening test and one of the most frequently performed procedures. The results of the CBC give information necessary to determine

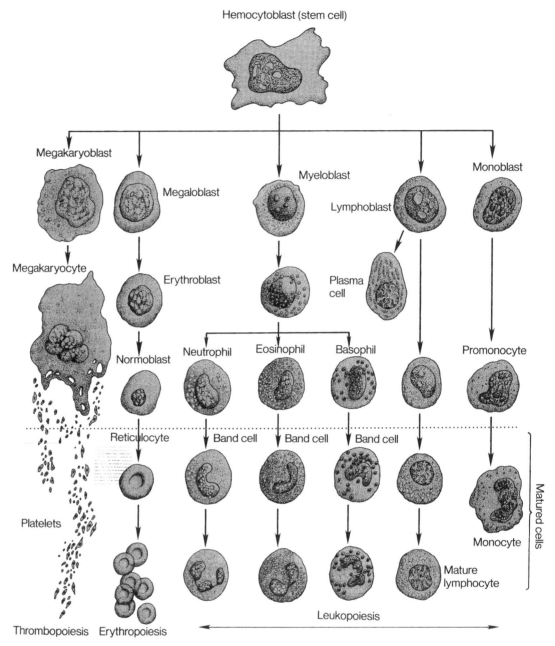

Figure 14–3 The maturation of blood cells—hematopoiesis. (From Gylys, B, and Wedding, ME: Medical Terminology: A Systems Approach, ed 3. FA Davis, Philadelphia, 1995, p 176, with permission.)

Diagnosis: *the term denoting the name of the disease or the syndrome a person has or is believed to have*

Prognosis: *prediction of the course or end of a disease*

the patient's **diagnosis,** response to treatment, and **prognosis.** The tests included in the CBC are:

- Hemoglobin (Hgb)
- Hematocrit (Hct)
- Red blood cell count (RBC)
- White blood cell count (WBC)
- Platelet count
- Red blood cell indices
- Differential blood cell count (Diff)

These tests are described in detail in the following chapters.

SUMMARY

Hematology tests involve classifying, evaluating, and enumerating the various blood cells. Coagulation studies are also included in hematologic testing. Most hematology tests are performed on whole blood, collected by a fingerstick (peripheral puncture) or by phlebotomy, using EDTA, an anticoagulant. This anticoagulant preserves the shape and morphologic features of blood cells.

Whole blood is composed of plasma, the liquid portion of blood, and the cellular components including erythrocytes, leukocytes, and platelets. Erythrocytes are the most numerous blood cells. They transport oxygen and carbon dioxide. The five major types of leukocytes are neutrophils, basophils, eosinophils, monocytes, and lymphocytes. Each of these cells provides specialized defenses and protection for the body including phagocytosis, detoxification, inflammation, and the adaptive immune response. White cell counts are usually elevated in infectious diseases. Platelets play an important role in blood coagulation and hemostasis. Blood coagulation is a complex process that involves several steps. If there is an interruption in any step, a clot does not form.

Questions

Name _____ Date _____

1. Describe the appearance of an erythrocyte and give its major function.

2. Name the five types of leukocytes and state the functions associated with these cells.

3. Briefly describe phagocytosis and tell which cells are associated with this process.

4. What is inflammation? What function does it provide for the body?

5. What is the adaptive immune response? What is the term used to describe the foreign substance that can provoke the adaptive immune response?

6. Briefly describe the process of blood coagulation. Briefly discuss the function of the fibrinolytic system.

7. What are the major components of plasma?

8. What two types of blood specimens are collected in a physician's office for hematologic studies?

9. List the tests included in the complete blood count.

Hemoglobin

15

Learning Objectives
Cognitive Objectives
Psychomotor Objectives
Affective Objectives

Method for Hemoglobin Determination

Conditions and Diseases Affecting Hemoglobin Levels

Conditions and Diseases that Alter Hemoglobin Values
Hyperbilirubinemia
Lipemia
Leukemia
Carotenemia

Hemoglobin Reference Values

Quality Control

Summary
Patient Education
Technical Considerations
Sources of Error

Procedure with Rationale
Hemoglobin Determination

Questions

Terminal Performance Objective
Hemoglobin Determination
  ○ Instructor's evaluation form

LEARNING OBJECTIVES

On completing this chapter, you will be able to:

COGNITIVE OBJECTIVES
- Explain the function of hemoglobin and describe where hemoglobin is found.
- Describe two methods of hemoglobin determination.
- Name four substances that affect the hemoglobin levels.
- List the hemoglobin reference values for adults and children.
- Describe methods used for quality control in hemoglobin determinations.

PSYCHOMOTOR OBJECTIVES
- Perform a hemoglobin determination following the Terminal Performance Objective presented in this chapter.
- Record the results of the hemoglobin.
- Record the normal and abnormal hemoglobin controls.

AFFECTIVE OBJECTIVES
- Show concern for yourself and your fellow workers by disposing of blood specimens according to the OSHA Standard.
- Assume responsibility for a clean and safe work environment.

Hemoglobin (Hgb) is the iron-containing portion of the red blood cell. Its function is to carry oxygen from the lungs to the cells and to remove carbon dioxide from the cells and carry it to the lungs for elimination from the body. All body cells require oxygen, which they can obtain only from hemoglobin in erythrocytes. Therefore, the hemoglobin content of the erythrocytes is of particular interest to physicians.

Since the oxygen-carrying capacity of the blood is directly related to the level of hemoglobin, its measurement is an excellent aid in diagnosing, evaluating, and monitoring the progression of diseased states, especially anemia.

The specimens for hemoglobin testing may be obtained by capillary puncture or venous whole blood collected in an evacuated tube with EDTA, an anticoagulant. Refer to Chapter 8 for specimen collection by finger puncture or venipuncture.

METHOD FOR HEMOGLOBIN DETERMINATION

Drabkin's reagent: *a solution of potassium ferricyanide and sodium cyanide that when combined with hemoglobin converts the hemoglobin to cyanmethemoglobin, a stable compound*

Assay: *the analysis of a substance to determine its composition and the quantity of its constituents*

There are many tests available for performing a hemoglobin determination. The most frequently used method is the cyanmethemoglobin test. In this test, the hemoglobin is converted to cyanmethemoglobin by adding **Drabkin's reagent,** a solution of potassium ferricyanide and sodium cyanide. This reagent is poisonous and must be handled as a hazardous material.

The Drabkin's reagent and hemoglobin combine to form a stable, colored, end product that can be **assayed** by using a spectrophotometer. Refer to Chapter 5 for using the spectrophotometer.

UNOHEME of the Unopette system can be used for measuring hemoglobin using the cyanmethemoglobin method. It is safer and more convenient because UNOHEME uses a premeasured amount of modified Drabkin's reagent, 4.98 mL, in a disposable, prefilled reservoir with a sealed diaphragm. It also has a 20-µL capillary pipette for collecting the blood from a finger puncture or a venous blood sample. See Figure 17–1 for an illustration of the Unopette system.

Hemoglobinometers are available for the POL that measures hemoglobin only. An example of such an instrument is the HemoCue. The HemoCue hemoglobin system gives a reliable quantitative blood hemoglobin determination that can be performed within 45 seconds. The microcuvette serves as a pipette, test tube, and measuring device. It automatically draws a precise amount of blood. The microcuvette does not require the mixing or dispensing of liquid reagents. It contains an exact quantity of a dry reagent, which yields a reaction when contact is made with the blood. The microcuvette is placed into the HemoCue photometer for a direct display of Hgb in g/dL (Fig. 15–1).

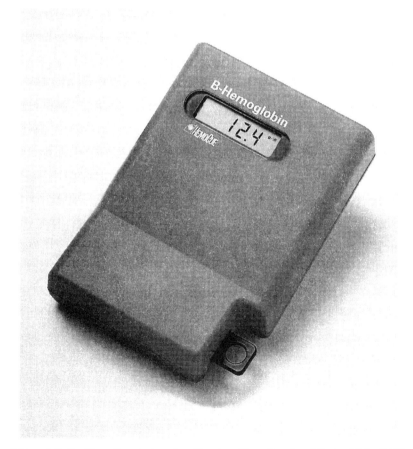

Figure 15–1 HemoCue photometer. (Courtesy HemoCue, Inc., Mission Viejo, Calif.)

Hemoglobin determinations are also performed by several automated hematology analyzers. Refer to Chapter 5 for discussion of some of these analyzers.

CONDITIONS AND DISEASES AFFECTING HEMOGLOBIN LEVELS

Diet, age, and gender have an effect on the blood hemoglobin concentration. Iron is a necessary ingredient in the formation of hemoglobin. Diets low in iron may cause a reduction in the hemoglobin concentration.

The hemoglobin levels are decreased in conditions such as anemia, hyperthyroidism, cirrhosis of the liver, severe hemorrhaging, Hodgkin's disease, leukemia, and hemolytic reactions. It may also decrease during pregnancy.

Clinical Comment: Hodgkin's Disease

Hodgkin's disease is characterized by painless, progressive enlargement of the lymph nodes, spleen, and lymphoid tissue. It is a lymph node neoplastic disease that begins in the cervical node on the side of the neck and spreads through the body. This disease is also known as Hodgkin's lymphoma.

Hemoglobin levels are increased in a condition called **polycythemia.** Hemoglobin increases as a result of the increased red blood cells. Hemoglobin levels also increase in **hemoconcentration** of the blood, chronic obstructive pulmonary disease, and congestive heart failure.

Polycythemia: *an excess of red blood cells*

Hemoconcentration: *a condition in which the number of red blood cells increases because of a decrease in the volume of plasma*

CONDITIONS AND DISEASES THAT ALTER HEMOGLOBIN VALUES

Hyperbilirubinemia

Hyperbilirubinemia in the blood produces **icteric** specimens. Specimens that are icteric impart a yellow color that interferes with the test results, leading to falsely elevated hemoglobin values. For every 1.0 mg/dL of bilirubin in the blood, the hemoglobin value will increase approximately 0.13 g/dL.

Hyperbilirubinemia: *an excessive amount of bilirubin in the blood*

Icteric: *pertaining to jaundice*

Lipemia

For best results, hemoglobin levels should not be determined on specimens with **lipemia.** Hemoglobin values are altered when blood has a high lipid or fat content. Some hemoglobinometers, such as the HemoCue hemoglobin system, correct the hemoglobin value for lipemia.

Lipemia: *having an abnormal amount of fat in the blood*

Leukemia

Leukemia is a disease characterized by unrestrained production of white blood cells. This interferes with the production of red blood cells, resulting in lower hemoglobin values. As a function of normal operation, the HemoCue hemoglobin system corrects the hemoglobin value for **leukocytosis.**

Leukocytosis: *an increase of leukocytes in the blood*

Carotenemia

Carotenemia is the presence of carotene in the blood, which interferes with the hemoglobin values. Carotene in the blood results from ingesting an excessive amount of

Table 15–1 **Hemoglobin Reference Values**

Newborn	14–24 g/dL	8.7–14.9 mmol/L
1 month	11–20 g/dL	6.8–12.4 mmol/L
6 months	10–15 g/dL	6.2–9.3 mmol/L
1–10 years	11–16 g/dL	6.8–9.9 mmol/L
Adult		
Man	13.5–18 g/dL	8.4–11.2 mmol/L
Woman	12–16 g/dL	7.4–9.9 mmol/L

Adapted from Watson, J, and Jaffe, MS: Nurse's Manual of Laboratory and Diagnostic Tests, FA Davis, Philadelphia, 1995, p 34, with permission.

carotene-containing foods or synthetic β-carotene. This condition usually produces a yellowing of the skin. Carotenemia may also occur in diabetes mellitus and in hypothyroidism.

HEMOGLOBIN REFERENCE VALUES

Reference values for hemoglobin vary according to age, sex, and locality. At birth the hemoglobin reading is normally quite high and decreases until age 12. Since the normal red blood cell count is higher in males than in females, the hemoglobin value is usually higher in males.

Geographic location also influences the hemoglobin values, especially with marked changes in higher altitudes. The body responds to the lack of oxygen at higher elevations by increasing the number of red blood cells, thereby increasing the concentration of hemoglobin. Physicians should establish regional reference values for the areas where their patients live. The reference values for hemoglobin are found in Table 15–1.

QUALITY CONTROL

Hemoglobin determinations are assayed with commercially prepared hemoglobin controls. Use normal and abnormal controls with each set of patient hemoglobin determinations. The controls should read within the values provided on the product insert. Be sure to log the lot number of the controls, the results of the controls, and the expected values in the daily log book.

Maintain a clean work environment for the safety of yourself and your fellow workers. Wash all counters with a disinfectant of 10 percent bleach. Dispose of all blood specimens in the biohazard container.

SUMMARY

Hemoglobin is the oxygen-carrying agent of the body. Since all cells require oxygen for survival, hemoglobin concentration in the blood has an important role in body mechanism. Hemoglobin deficiency anemias can be diagnosed and therapy monitored by hemoglobin determinations.

PATIENT EDUCATION

- No special preparation for the patient is necessary.
- Explain the procedure to the patient.

TECHNICAL CONSIDERATIONS

- Drabkin's reagent is a hazardous material and should be handled according to laboratory protocol.
- Calibrate the instrument for hemoglobin determination if appropriate.

SOURCES OF ERROR

- When performing a capillary puncture, never squeeze the finger near the puncture site. This will produce a sample high in tissue fluid and may give a false low reading.
- When performing a capillary puncture, make sure that no bubbles appear in the capillary tube or micropipette. If bubbles occur, results will be inaccurate. Discard the tube and begin again.
- Avoid touching the ends of the capillary tube or pipette tip since this will remove part of the blood sample and cause an error in the results.
- When using venous whole blood, failure to mix the blood sample before pipetting may cause the results to be inaccurate.

Procedure with Rationale

Hemoglobin Determination
EQUIPMENT AND SUPPLIES

Hand soap	Capillary or EDTA anticoagulated blood
Latex gloves	specimen
Hemoglobinometer or	Biohazard container
spectrophotometer	Surface disinfectant
Normal and abnormal	
controls	

Assemble equipment.

Wash hands with soap and water. Observe the OSHA Standard for this procedure.

Turn on the instrument and let it warm up for the time recommended by the manufacturer. *If the instrument is not allowed to warm up for the correct time, the results will be inaccurate.*

Calibrate or standardize the instrument according to the manufacturer's instructions, if appropriate.

Prepare a blood specimen for a hemoglobin determination according to the instructions provided by the manufacturer of your instrument. *If you are using a capillary pipette, be sure to fill the pipette without any air bubbles to ensure accurate results.*

Wipe the excess blood from the outside of the capillary tube. *Any residue blood will interfere with the accuracy of the end results.*

Mix the capillary blood with the diluent according to manufacturer's instructions, if appropriate.

Wait the exact time specified for the procedure used. *Timing is always critical when performing color photometry.*

Insert the cuvettes into the instrument and read the results.

Record the results of the controls.

Record the results of the specimens. *Be sure to include the correct unit of measurement for hemoglobin (g/dL).*

Clean work area following laboratory protocol.

Remove gloves. Wash hands with soap and water.

Questions

Name _____ Date _____

1. Describe the function of hemoglobin and tell where is it found.

2. Name two methods for hemoglobin determination and describe the process.

3. Name four conditions or diseases that affect the hemoglobin determination and give the reasons.

4. Name two pathological conditions that cause an increase in the hemoglobin level.

5. Name four pathological conditions that cause a decrease in hemoglobin levels.

6. Give the hemoglobin reference values for men and women.

Terminal Performance Objective

Hemoglobin Determination

Given the necessary equipment, you will be able to perform a hemoglobin determination. Record the results of the test and the normal and abnormal controls. This procedure must be performed within 10 minutes and read with a level of accuracy specified by your instructor.

INSTRUCTOR'S EVALUATION FORM

Name _____ Date _____

+ = SATISFACTORY   ✓ = UNSATISFACTORY

_____ Assemble equipment.

_____ Wash hands with soap and water. Observe the OSHA Standard for this procedure.

_____ Turn on the instrument and let it warm up for the time recommended by the manufacturer.

_____ Calibrate or standardize the instrument according to the manufacturer's instructions, if appropriate.

_____ Prepare a blood specimen for a hemoglobin determination according to the instructions provided by the manufacturer of your instrument.

_____ Wipe the excess blood from the outside of the capillary tube.

_____ Mix the capillary blood with the diluent according to manufacturer's instructions, if appropriate.

_____ Wait the exact time specified for the procedure used.

_____ Insert the cuvettes into the instrument and read the results.

_____ Record the results.

RESULTS _____

_____ Record the results of the controls.

NORMAL _____ ABNORMAL _____

_____ Clean work area following laboratory protocol.

_____ Remove gloves. Wash hands with soap and water.

_____ The procedure was completed within 10 minutes.

_____ The reading was to the level of accuracy specified by your instructor.

_____ The results were properly recorded.

Final Competency Evaluation

_____ SATISFACTORY   _____ UNSATISFACTORY

Comments:

Instructor _____ Date _____

Microhematocrit

LEARNING OBJECTIVES

On completing this chapter, you will be able to:

COGNITIVE OBJECTIVES
- Explain the purpose of determining a microhematocrit.
- Describe the method of performing a microhematocrit.
- List the three interfaces used to interpret the microhematocrit.
- Identify pathological conditions that cause changes in the microhematocrit reading.

PSYCHOMOTOR OBJECTIVES
- Perform a microhematocrit following the Terminal Performance Objective presented in the chapter.
- Record the results of the microhematocrit.

AFFECTIVE OBJECTIVES
- Show concern for your coworkers by disposing of blood specimens according to laboratory protocol.
- Assume responsibility for a clean and safe work environment.

Spinning a tube of anticoagulated whole blood specimen in a high-speed centrifuge separates the blood components into three distinct layers. The erythrocytes, or red blood cells (RBCs), collect at the bottom of the tube in a layer called the packed RBCs. The other formed elements (leukocytes and platelets) create a layer on top of the RBCs. This thin, light-colored layer is called the *buffy coat*. The clear amber fluid at the top is the plasma layer, the liquid portion of blood (Fig. 16–1).

Dividing the amount of the packed RBC layer by the amount of all three layers gives the percentage of packed RBCs in the whole blood sample—the **hematocrit.** This measurement is an important part of the complete blood count (CBC). The hematocrit tells the physician how much of the patient's blood is composed of RBCs, which is an indication of the oxygen-carrying capacity of the blood. Refer to Chapter 14 for information on the complete blood count.

> **Hematocrit:** *the volume of RBCs packed by centrifugation in a given volume of blood*

Centrifuged Whole Blood

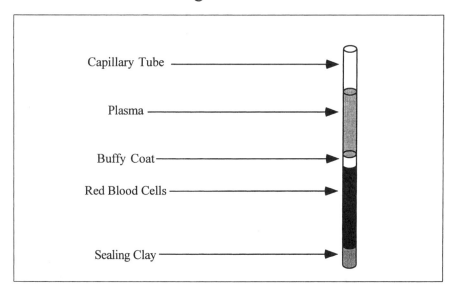

Figure 16-1 Diagram of a centrifuged capillary tube of whole blood.

MICROHEMATOCRIT SPECIMEN COLLECTION

In the physician's office hematocrits are usually performed using the microhematocrit method. The reference values for venous and capillary blood samples using the microhematocrit are consistent with the venous blood values of a hematocrit.

For laboratories using the evacuated-tube system, the blood sample is drawn in a lavender-stoppered tube containing the anticoagulant EDTA. A capillary tube is filled from the evacuated tube, after it has been well mixed by gently inverting. The measurement can also be obtained from very small samples using two or three drops of blood from a capillary puncture. Refer to Chapter 8 for the collection of blood samples by venipuncture or finger puncture.

METHOD OF PERFORMING THE MICROHEMATOCRIT

Capillary Tube Selection

The microhematocrit requires high-speed centrifugation of an anticoagulated blood sample in special capillary tubes. These are very small diameter glass tubes that are open at both ends. The tubes have a colored line etched into the glass at one end. A red line indicates that the tube contains heparin, an anticoagulant, and a blue line indicates that the tube contains no anticoagulant.

Capillary blood will clot without the anticoagulant heparin, rendering the sample useless. Therefore, use red-lined tubes containing heparin when collecting blood from a capillary puncture for a microhematocrit. Use plain tubes when blood has been collected in an EDTA-anticoagulated evacuated-tube system.

Filling Capillary Tubes

To fill the capillary tube from either a finger puncture or tube of venous blood, hold it horizontally downward, and bring the lined end into contact with the surface of the blood sample (Figs. 16-2 and 16-3). Capillary attraction and gravity cause the blood to flow into the tube when it is placed in a horizontal position against the drop of blood.

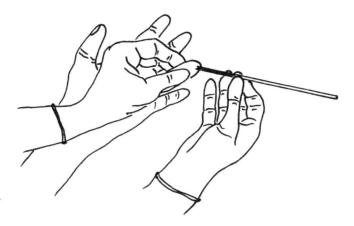

Figure 16-2 Filling a capillary tube from a capillary puncture.

Clinical Comment: Capillary Attraction

Capillary attraction is the effect of the surface tension of a liquid that causes it to be drawn up into a tube by the attraction of the molecules of the liquid for each other and for the molecules of the tube.

Before filling a capillary tube with blood from a capillary puncture, wipe away the first drop of blood after the finger stick. The first drop of blood may contain alcohol and tissue fluids, which may distort the accuracy of the microhematocrit reading.

Before filling a capillary tube with blood from a venous sample, mix the venous sample by gently inverting the tube several times. RBCs tend to settle out of solution in a standing whole-blood sample. A capillary tube filled with an unmixed sample will give an inaccurate microhematocrit reading.

When the microhematocrit tube is three-quarters full, pull the tube away from the blood source. At the same time cover the opposite end of the tube with your gloved finger to prevent the blood from flowing back out of the tube. While keeping your gloved finger over the end of the tube, gently wipe off any residue blood on the outside of the microhematocrit tube and tilt the blood away from the end before inserting the cleaned end into sealing clay (Fig. 16-4). The procedure is done this way so that the clay does not become contaminated with blood, which would necessitate disposal of the tray in the biohazard container. Dried blood on the microhematocrit tube will also obscure the microhematocrit reading.

The special sealing compound, which acts as a tiny stopper, is commercially available in trays with numbered sections. The numbered position on the tray in which the tube has been placed enables you to identify the sample.

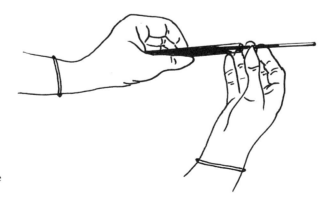

Figure 16-3 Filling a capillary tube from an evacuated tube of blood.

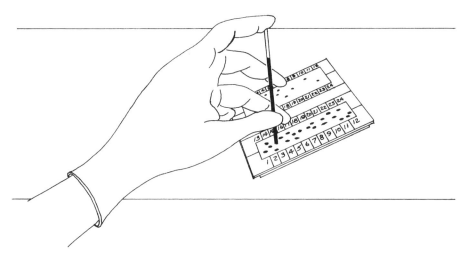

Figure 16-4 Securing the capillary tube with sealing clay.

Always prepare two capillary tubes for each patient sample. This is referred to as *running in duplicate*. It provides a backup in case one breaks and, more importantly, provides quality control for the test. Both tubes will be centrifuged, and the final microhematocrit will be the average of the two readings. If the readings vary from each other by more than ±2 percent, the test is invalid and must be repeated.

Centrifuging Capillary Tubes

Once the tubes are filled, wiped, and sealed, identify the sample by recording the numbers from the sealing clay tray on the request forms. Place the capillary tubes into the high-speed microhematocrit centrifuge (Fig. 16-5). Place the sealed ends of the capillary tubes toward the outside, against the rubber gasket, and keep the open ends facing

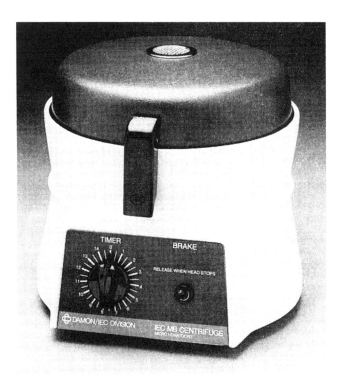

Figure 16-5 Microhematocrit centrifuge. (Courtesy International Equipment Co. [IEC].)

Capillary Tube Placement

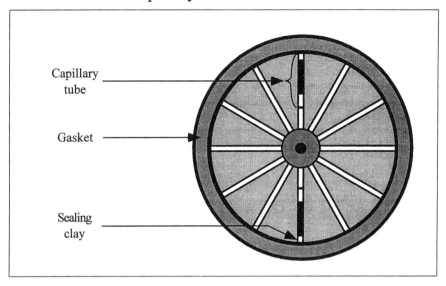

Capillary tube

Gasket

Sealing clay

Figure 16–6 Proper placement of sealed capillary tubes in the microhematocrit centrifuge.

toward the center (Fig. 16–6). If the open ends face outward, the blood will spin out of the tubes. Use the numbers on the circumference of the centrifuge to identify the samples. Secure the inner cover before closing the lid of the centrifuge. Start the centrifuge by setting the timer for 3 to 5 minutes or as specified by the manufacturer of the centrifuge.

Interpreting the Microhematocrit Results

As soon as the centrifuge stops, remove the capillary tubes one at a time. Use a microhematocrit reader to determine the hematocrit reading and immediately record the results on the request slip.

There are several types of microhematocrit readers. Most are based on the principle of the sliding scale that locates three **interfaces** and produces a numerical reading based on their relative positions. The three interfaces are (1) the bottom of the packed RBC layer, (2) the top of the packed RBC layer, and (3) the **meniscus** of the plasma at the top of the tube.

Figure 16–7 shows a circular microhematocrit reader. It is a metal disk with a transparent radial arm into which the capillary tube fits so that the bottom of the packed RBC layer touches a line etched on the disk near the center. To use this type of reader, rotate the disk until the meniscus of the plasma layer lines up with a line that spirals from the center of the disk to its outer edge. Then rotate the reader until the spiral line crosses the top of the packed RBC layer. A line on the end of the radial arm points to the correct microhematocrit value on a numbered scale at the circumference of the disk.

Figure 16–8 shows a different type of microhematocrit reader. To use this reader, place the capillary tube with the bottom of the RBC layer on the line marked 0. Then slide the tube along the scale until the meniscus of the plasma layer touches the line marked 100. The number marked on the line that crosses the top of the RBC layer is the microhematocrit reading. In this figure, the microhematocrit reading is 45 percent.

Because the tubes are so small, putting identification on them is impossible. Throughout the centrifugation and reading steps, take care to identify the two samples by the numbers on the side of the clay tray and the numbers in the microhematocrit centrifuge.

Interface: *a plane forming the common boundary between two parts, e.g., plasma and RBCs*

Meniscus: *the curved upper surface of a liquid in a container*

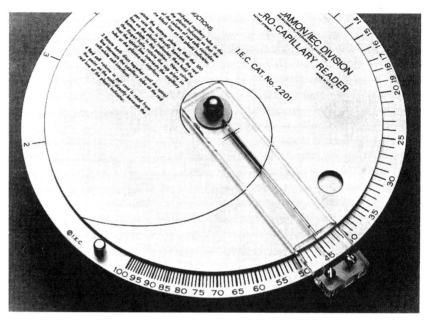

Figure 16-7   Microhematocrit reader. (Courtesy International Equipment Co. [IEC].)

CONDITIONS AFFECTING THE MICROHEMATOCRIT

Dehydration: *condition resulting from excessive loss of body fluid*

Low microhematocrit values are found in anemia, leukemia, and bleeding disorders. High microhematocrit values are found in polycythemia and **dehydration.** *Polycythemia vera* is a chronic, life-shortening condition in which there is an abnormal increase in red blood cell mass and hence an increase in hemoglobin concentration. Dehydration results from diarrhea, vomiting, or excessive sweating. The hematocrit reference values vary with the patient's sex and age. Table 16-1 gives the reference range of hematocrit values.

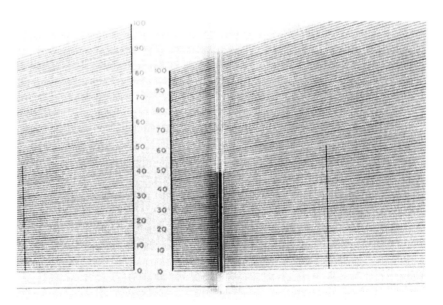

Figure 16-8   Microhematocrit capillary tube reader. (From Frew, MA, Lane, K, and Frew, D: Comprehensive Medical Assisting: Competencies for Administrative and Clinical Practice, ed 3, FA Davis, Philadelphia, 1995, p 804, with permission.)

Table 16–1 **Hematocrit Reference Values**

Newborn	44–64%
1 month	35–49%
6 months	30–40%
1–10 years	35–41%
Adult	
Man	40–54%
Woman	38–47%

Adapted from Watson, J, and Jaffe, MS: Nurse's Manual of Laboratory and Diagnostic Tests, FA Davis, Philadelphia, 1995, p 33, with permission.

QUALITY CONTROL

Quality control is achieved by running the microhematocrit in duplicate. The results of the microhematocrits should be within ±2 percent of each other. Under normal conditions, the microhematocrit is approximately three times the value of the hemoglobin. Refer to Chapter 15 for information on the hemoglobin.

Dispose of blood samples and contaminated clay trays in the biohazard containers. Clean the rubber gasket of the microhematocrit centrifuge with a solution of 10 percent bleach. Remember to maintain a clean and safe environment for yourself and your coworkers.

AUTOMATION

Instruments that automatically calculate the hematocrit are available for the medical office. They use small amounts of blood, and the results are more accurate and reliable.

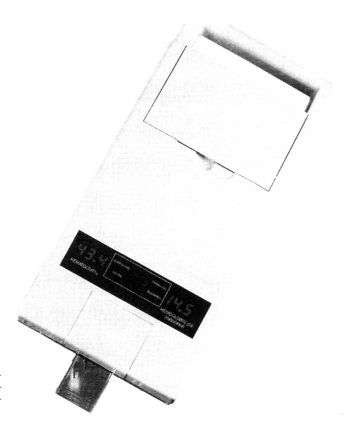

Figure 16–9 Stat-Crit hematocrit/hemoglobin measuring instrument. (Courtesy Wampole Laboratories, Cranbury, NJ.)

QBC by Becton Dickinson is an example of such an instrument. The Stat-Crit instrument from Wampole Laboratories measures the hematocrit of whole blood in 30 seconds (Fig. 16–9). Two illuminated digital displays on the instrument provide a direct reading of hematocrit in percent and a calculation of hemoglobin concentration expressed in grams per deciliter (g/dL). The test is performed on blood from a capillary puncture or on venous blood collected in an EDTA-anticoagulated vacuum tube.

SUMMARY

The hematocrit is a simple test that gives the physician information regarding the volume of packed red blood cells in whole blood. The microhematocrit is a commonly used variation of the hematocrit because it requires only a small specimen of blood, which can be obtained by a finger puncture or from an anticoagulated whole-blood sample. The reference values of the microhematocrit are consistent with the reference values of the hematocrit.

PATIENT EDUCATION

- Explain the procedure to the patient.
- Hold the finger of the patient firmly during the finger puncture.

TECHNICAL CONSIDERATIONS

- Use the appropriate microhematocrit tube for the type of sample collected.
- When measuring the microhematocrit value from the microhematocrit reader, check that all layers are accurately placed on the reader.

SOURCES OF ERROR

- If the finger is squeezed too tightly during a capillary puncture, too much tissue fluid enters the blood sample. This diluted sample may result in a false low reading.
- Failure to wipe away the first drop of blood from a finger puncture may lead to erroneous results.
- Failure to gently invert the tube containing a whole-blood anticoagulated specimen before filling the capillary tube may result in an inaccurate microhematocrit reading.
- Failure to follow the directions of the manufacturer of the microhematocrit centrifuge regarding time and speed may also give erroneous results.
- Many types of microhematocrit readers are available and the method of use varies with each reader. Failure to follow directions correctly for the reader can result in inaccurate readings.

Procedure with Rationale

Performing the Microhematocrit

EQUIPMENT AND SUPPLIES

Hand soap	Microhematocrit centrifuge
Capillary tubes (plain/heparinized)	Microhematocrit reader
Sealing clay	Latex gloves
Capillary or EDTA-anticoagulated blood sample	Biohazard container
	Surface disinfectant

Assemble equipment.

Wash hands with soap and water. Observe the OSHA Standard for this procedure.

Fill two capillary tubes three-quarters full using free-flowing blood from a finger puncture or a well-mixed EDTA anticoagulated whole-blood sample. *When using a finger puncture, make sure to wipe away the first drop of blood. When using a whole-blood sample, mix by inverting several times, so that red blood cells will not settle to the bottom of the vacuum tube, resulting in erroneous readings.*

After tilting the blood away from the end of the tube, remove the blood on the outside of the tube, and seal the ends of each capillary tube with soft sealing clay. *If the clay is hard the tube may break.*

Place the capillary tubes into the microhematocrit centrifuge against the rubber gasket with the sealed ends facing outward. *The sealed ends must face outward so the blood will not be spun out of the tubes.*

Place the inner cover on the centrifuge before closing the lid and spin for the time recommended by the manufacturer. *If the inner cover is not secured on the centrifuge, the microhematocrit tubes will break.*

Remove the tubes, one at a time, from the microhematocrit centrifuge as soon as it has stopped. Read the microhematocrit values and record your results in volume percentage. *The microhematocrit must be read immediately or the dimension of the packed red-cell layer will change, distorting the results.*

Clean work area following laboratory protocol.

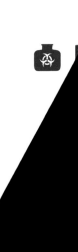

Remove gloves. Wash hands with soap and water.

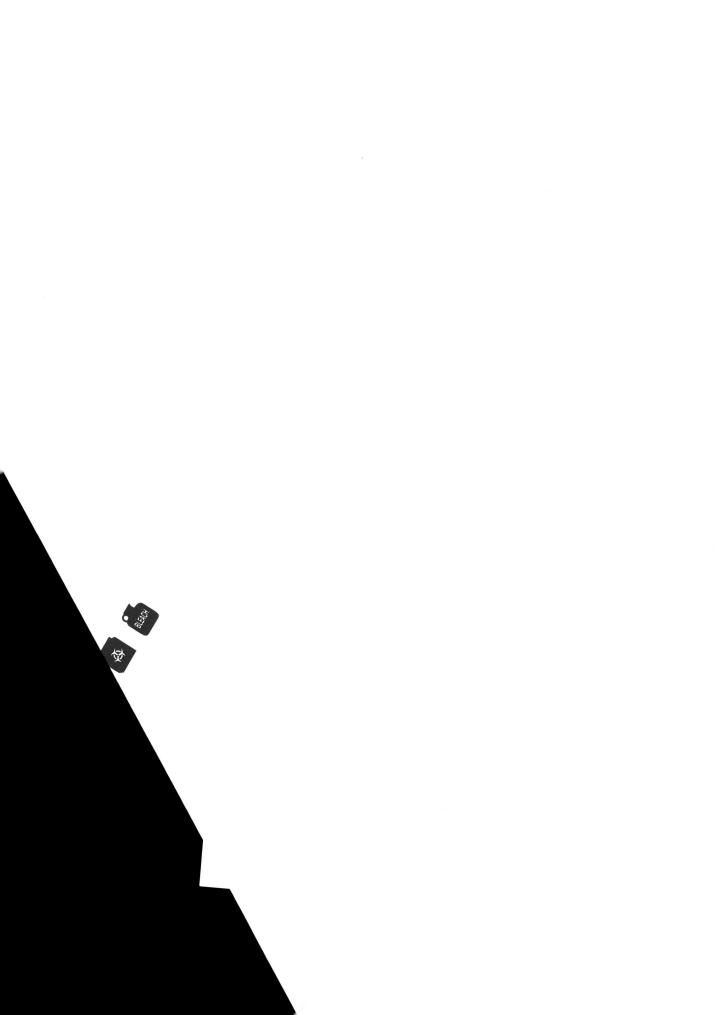

Questions

Name _____   Date _____

1. List the three layers into which whole blood separates after centrifugation. Tell what component of blood constitutes each layer.

2. Two types of microhematocrit tubes are available. One contains an anticoagulant and one does not. Explain when each is used and give a reason.

3. Give the three interfaces located in the microhematocrit tube that are used to obtain the hematocrit reading.

4. Name three pathological conditions that cause a decrease in the microhematocrit.

5. Name two pathological conditions that cause an increase in the microhematocrit.

6. Give the hematocrit reference values for men, women, and infants.

7. List three sources of error in microhematocrit determinations.

Terminal Performance Objective

Performing the Microhematocrit

Given the necessary equipment, you will be able to perform a microhematocrit test and record the results of the test. This procedure must be performed within 10 minutes and read with a level of accuracy within ±2 percent of your instructor's reading.

INSTRUCTOR'S EVALUATION FORM

Name _____ Date _____

+ = SATISFACTORY   ✓ = UNSATISFACTORY

_____ Assemble equipment.

_____ Wash hands with soap and water. Observe the OSHA Standard for this procedure.

_____ Fill two capillary tubes three-quarters full using free-flowing blood from a finger puncture or a well-mixed EDTA anticoagulated whole-blood sample.

_____ Seal both capillary tubes with sealing clay.

_____ Place capillary tubes into the microhematocrit centrifuge.

_____ Place inner cover on the centrifuge before closing the lid and spin.

_____ Remove the tubes one at a time. Read the microhematocrit values and record your results.   RESULTS _____

_____ Clean work area following laboratory protocol.

_____ Remove gloves. Wash hands with soap and water.

_____ The procedure was completed within 10 minutes.

_____ The reading was correct to within ±2 percent of your instructor's reading.

_____ The results were properly recorded.

Final Competency Evaluation

_____ SATISFACTORY   _____ UNSATISFACTORY

Comments:

Instructor _____ Date _____

Blood Cell Counts

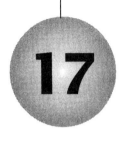

17

LEARNING OBJECTIVES

On completing this chapter, you will be able to:

COGNITIVE OBJECTIVES
- Explain the purpose of performing a complete blood cell count (CBC).
- List the normal values of white blood cell counts, red blood cell counts, and platelets.
- Describe the manual method using the Unopette to determine a blood cell count.
- List several sources of errors when performing a manual blood cell count.

PSYCHOMOTOR OBJECTIVES
- Perform a white blood cell count following the Terminal Performance Objective presented in this chapter.
- Record the results of the white blood cell count.

AFFECTIVE OBJECTIVES
- Take responsibility for maintaining the integrity of the white blood cell count by controlling the conditions affecting the count.
- Follow laboratory protocol regarding the disposal of blood for the safety of yourself and your coworkers.

The complete blood count (CBC) is the hematology test most frequently ordered for laboratory studies. The CBC is the laboratory test performed in the diagnosis of disease states of the **hematopoietic system**. It gives information on many disorders of the body.

A blood cell count enumerates the number of blood cells in a given amount of blood. It is usually expressed as the number of cells in a cubic millimeter of blood, for example, 5.0 million red blood cells per cubic millimeter ($5.0 \times 10^6/mm^3$).

> **Hematopoietic system:**
> *the organs pertaining to the production and development of blood cells*

231

Table 17–1 **Abnormal Results of WBCs by Degree of Severity**

	Elevations	Decreases
Slight	11,000–20,000	3,000–4,500
Moderate	20,000–30,000	1,500–3,000
Severe	>50,000	<1,500

Adapted from Watson, J, and Jaffe, MS: Nurse's Manual of Laboratory and Diagnostic Tests, FA Davis, Philadelphia, 1995, p 45, with permission.

FORMED ELEMENTS IN BLOOD

The white blood cells (WBCs), red blood cells (RBCs), and platelets are the formed elements found in the circulating blood.

White Blood Cells

The white blood cell is responsible for the body's defense against invasion by foreign substances, such as bacteria and viruses. An above-normal white blood cell count, *leukocytosis*, usually indicates infection, inflammation, or parasitic infestation. An extremely high white blood count may be characteristic of leukemia.

Leukopenia, a decrease in WBCs, occurs with some viral infections, drug therapy, and especially during chemotherapy and radiation therapy. The reference range of WBCs for adults is 5,000 to 10,000 WBC per mm^3. Abnormal results may be classified by degree of severity as indicated in Table 17–1.

Red Blood Cells

The function of the RBCs in the circulatory system is to transport oxygen to the tissues and to remove carbon dioxide from the tissues to be exchanged in the lungs. This function is important for life-sustaining metabolism.

Increased levels of RBCs, *polycythemia*, occur in polycythemia vera and dehydration. People living at higher elevations may also have an RBC higher than people living at lower elevations. The concentration of oxygen decreases as elevation increases, and the exchange of oxygen is therefore less efficient. The body produces more RBCs to make up for that inefficiency. Elevated RBC counts may happen in people with heart and lung disease, in certain malignancies, and in people who smoke.

A decrease in the number of RBCs, *erythropenia*, may occur in the various types of anemias. Along with the hemoglobin and hematocrit, physicians use the RBC count to determine the type and the severity of anemias.

Decreased values of RBCs may also occur from excessive blood loss, *hemorrhage*, or excessive blood cell destruction, *hemolysis*, with the release of hemoglobin into the plasma. In addition, decreased blood cell formation is associated with leukemia, nutritional deficiencies, and chronic inflammatory diseases. Rheumatoid arthritis and systemic lupus erythematosus (SLE) are examples of chronic inflammatory diseases that result in erythropenia.

Clinical Comment: Lupus

Lupus is a chronic autoimmune disease in which the body's immune system forms antibodies that attack healthy tissues and organs. There are several types of lupus. Discoid lupus affects the skin, causing a rash and lesions across the face and upper part of the body. SLE can attack any body organ or system, such as joints, kidneys, brain, heart, and lungs. If not controlled, SLE can be life-threatening. Another form of this disease is drug-induced lupus, caused by reaction to medication. When the medication is discontinued, the symptoms disappear. There is no cure for lupus, but medical treatment can usually control the disease.

An RBC count can be performed manually using the Unopette system or automatically by a hematology analyzer. The manual method requires skills beyond the scope and practice of a medical assistant.

Normal values of RBCs depend on the patient's sex and age. Men usually have slightly higher values for RBCs than women. Table 17–2 lists the reference ranges of the RBCs.

Platelets

Platelets, the smallest formed elements or fragments of a cell present in circulating blood, are responsible for hemostasis and blood clot formation. Platelets activate the factors that produce the fibrin clot necessary for **coagulation** to occur. Platelets are manually counted using the Unopette system, but most hematology analyzers give an automated platelet count. Manual platelet counting requires skills beyond the scope of a medical assistant. Platelets are also known as *thrombocytes*.

An increase of platelets in the blood, *thrombocytosis*, can occur with polycythemia vera; posthemorrhagic and iron deficiency anemias; surgical procedures, especially **splenectomy**; and chronic leukemias.

A decrease of platelets, *thrombocytopenia*, occurs in vitamin B–folic acid deficiencies, acute leukemias, viral infections, **anaphylactic shock**, certain hemorrhagic diseases, and during chemotherapy and radiation therapy. The reference range of platelet counts is 150,000 to 350,000 per mm^3, with 250,000 per mm^3 as an average count.

Coagulation: *the process of clotting*

Splenectomy: *surgical excision of the spleen*

Anaphylactic shock: *severe allergic reaction*

SPECIMEN COLLECTION FOR BLOOD CELL COUNTS

For manual performance of blood cell counts, use whole blood collected by capillary puncture or EDTA-anticoagulated evacuated venous blood collected by venipuncture. Refer to Chapter 8 for capillary puncture and venipuncture collection of blood. Dilute the capillary or venous whole blood with an appropriate diluting fluid.

For WBC counts, use acetic acid, which destroys RBCs and preserves WBCs. The dilution of the blood to diluting fluid is 1:20. Diluting fluids used for RBC counts are Hayem's, Gowers', or isotonic saline. For RBC counts, use a 1:200 dilution of blood to the diluting fluid.

Table 17–2 **Reference Ranges of RBCs**

Newborn	$4.8–7.1 \times 10^6$/mm^3 or 10^{12}/L
1 month	$4.1–6.4 \times 10^6$/mm^3 or 10^{12}/L
6 months	$3.8–5.5 \times 10^6$/mm^3 or 10^{12}/L
Adult	
Man	$4.6–6.2 \times 10^6$/mm^3 or 10^{12}/L
Woman	$4.2–5.4 \times 10^6$/mm^3 or 10^{12}/L

Adapted from Watson, J, and Jaffe, MS: Nurse's Manual of Laboratory and Diagnostic Tests, FA Davis, Philadelphia, 1995, p 32, with permission.

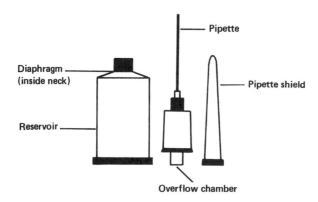

Figure 17–1 The Unopette system, consisting of a reservoir containing a diluent, a pipette used to deliver the specimen into the reservoir, and a pipette shield used to puncture the plastic seal of the reservoir and as a cap for the pipette to prevent evaporation. (From Frew, MA, Lane, K, and Frew, D: Comprehensive Medical Assisting: Competencies for Administrative and Clinical Practice, ed 3, FA Davis, Philadelphia, 1995, p 732, with permission.)

The Unopette system (Fig. 17–1) is an example of a disposable blood-diluting pipette with a prefilled reservoir containing a premeasured diluting fluid. Unopettes are available for counting WBCs, RBCs, and platelets. With Unopettes, the diluting fluid is premeasured and the capillary tube for the collection of blood is standardized. Carefully follow the manufacturer's directions for blood collection with the Unopette system (Fig. 17–2).

MANUAL METHOD OF BLOOD CELL COUNTING

Hemacytometer

A hemacytometer is a specially designed counting chamber of uniform dimensions used in counting blood cells (Fig. 17–3). It has two identically ruled areas, called *chambers*, to allow the performance of blood cell counts in duplicate. Each chamber consists of lines of specific dimensions etched into the chamber. The most frequently used hemacytometer is the Neubauer-type, which has nine squares of equal size. Each square is equivalent to 1 mm^2.

Charging or Filling the Hemacytometer

In order to charge or fill a hemacytometer, use a specially designed cover glass with uniform dimensions. Place the cover glass over the ruled area of the hemacytometer. Fill the hemacytometer with a properly prepared, diluted sample of blood. If using the Unopette system for WBC counting, allow 10 minutes for the acetic acid to destroy the RBCs before charging the hemacytometer (Fig. 17–4).

Expel four to five drops from the pipette before filling the chamber. Place the dispensing tip of the pipette at the end of the hemacytometer where the cover glass ends. Dispense a small amount of fluid directly under the cover glass. Completely fill the surface under the glass with the cell suspension. Make sure the chamber is free of air bubbles and contains no liquid in the channels surrounding the rule area. The distribution of the cells must be uniform over the ruled area.

Wait 2 minutes to allow the cells to settle, then count them using the microscope. Using the low-power objective (10×), count the WBCs. Using the high-power objective (40×), count the RBCs.

Thoroughly clean the hemacytometer and coverslip with 70 percent isopropyl alcohol so that dirt and finger smudges do not interfere with an accurate count. Replace any damaged or unclean cover glasses.

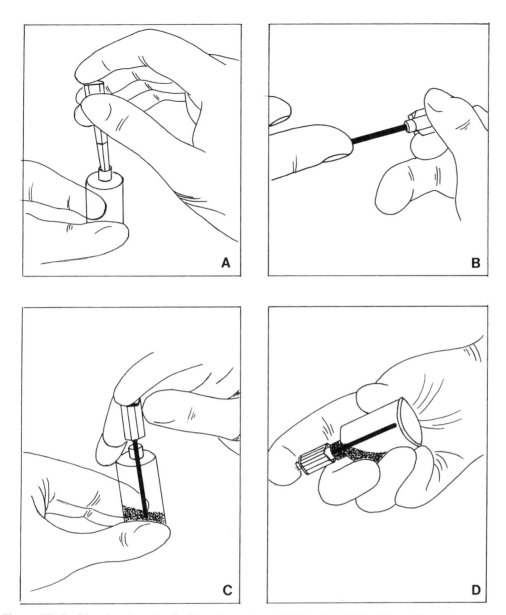

Figure 17-2   Directions for using the Unopette system. *(A)* Using the shield of the capillary pipette, puncture the diaphragm of the reservoir. *(B)* Fill the capillary with a sample from a finger prick. *(C)* Transfer the sample to the reservoir by squeezing the reservoir slightly to force out some air. Do not expel any liquid. Cover the opening of overflow chamber with the index finger. Maintain pressure until the pipette is secured in the reservoir neck. Squeeze reservoir several times to rinse capillary bore without expelling any liquid. *(D)* Place index finger over upper opening and gently invert several times to thoroughly mix sample with diluent.

White Blood Cell Count

When performing a WBC count manually using a hemacytometer, the outer four squares of the counting chamber are counted (Fig. 17-5). Each of these squares is divided again into 16 smaller squares. Count only WBCs within these 16 squares and those situated on the left and top border (Fig. 17-6).

Locate these squares using low-power magnification. To help verify accuracy, focus on the other chamber and follow the same procedure. This provides two counts on the same sample. The two counts should not vary by more than ±10 cells. If the count is within ±10 cells, divide the total number of cells by 2 to give an average number of leukocytes. Multiply the average by the factor 50 to give the actual WBC count.

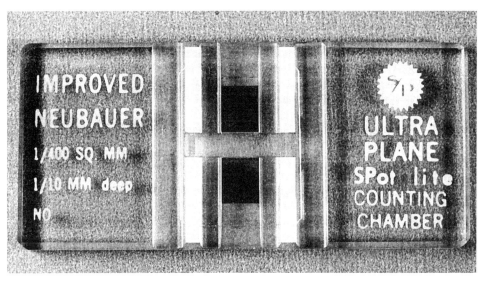

Figure 17-3 Hemacytometer with cover glass.

Each area counted has a depth of 0.1 mm; therefore, the depth factor is 10. The dilution used for WBCs is 1:20, so the dilution factor is 20. The final factor is derived by multiplying the depth factor of 10 by the dilution factor of 20 and dividing by the area counted, 4 mm². Each WBC area is 1 mm². The formula for the WBC factor is

$$\frac{10 \times 20}{4} = 50.$$

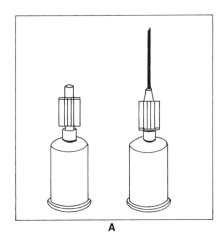

A

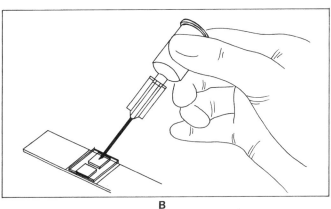

B

Figure 17-4 Charging the hemacytometer using the Unopette System. *(A)* Convert to dropper assembly by withdrawing pipette from reservoir and securing it in the reverse position. *(B)* Invert reservoir and discard first three or four drops. Charge hemacytometer by gently squeezing reservoir to expel contents until chamber is properly filled.

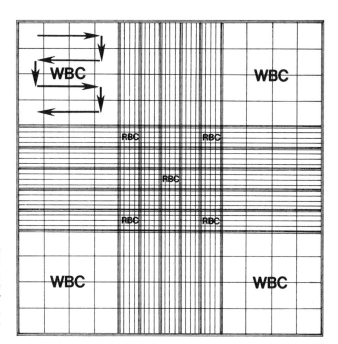

Figure 17–5 Spencer Bright-Line double counting system with improved Neubauer ruling. (From Frew, MA, Lane, K, and Frew, D: Comprehensive Medical Assisting: Competencies for Administrative and Clinical Practice, ed 3, FA Davis, Philadelphia, 1995, p 806, with permission.)

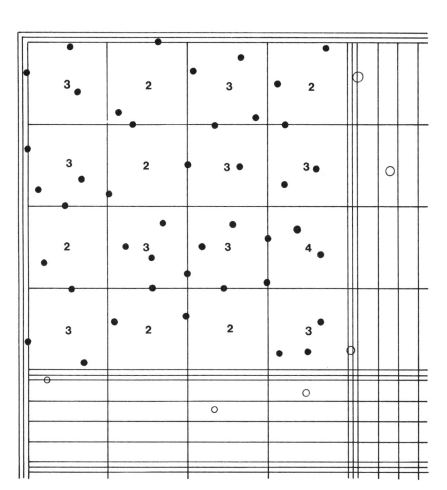

Figure 17–6   A sample count in one square of a WBC counting area.

Red Blood Cell Count

The RBC count uses the center square of the hemacytometer for counting. Each center square has 25 smaller squares. Using the high-power objective, count the five squares illustrated in Figure 17–5. Count only the cells in the four corner squares and the center square for RBC counts. Count only the RBCs that fall on the left and top border of these squares.

Repeat the procedure on the other side of the hemacytometer and divide the number obtained by 2 to give the average cell count. Multiply the average by the factor 10,000.

Each area counted has a depth of 0.1 mm; therefore, the depth factor is 10. The final factor is derived by multiplying the depth factor of 10 by the dilution factor 200, divided by the area of the five squares counted, 0.2 mm². Each RBC square is 0.04 mm².

The formula for the RBC factor is

$$\frac{10 \times 200}{0.2} = 10,000.$$

Platelet Cell Count

A platelet count can be obtained manually by using a hemacytometer. Although platelet counts are routinely performed in hospital laboratories, this test is not usually performed in the physician's office. Today, many of the hematology analyzers automatically count the platelets, and some of these analyzers are found in POLs.

CALCULATING RBC INDICES

Indices are mathematical calculations of the RBC count, hematocrit, and hemoglobin. They estimate the approximate size of an average RBC, the amount of hemoglobin in an average RBC, and the concentration of hemoglobin per unit volume of an RBC. The indices are within the reference ranges when all three factors are normal. RBC indices are used by the physician to identify the various types of anemias.

Mean Corpuscular Volume

Femtoliter (fL): *a unit of volume; 10^{-15} L*

Mean corpuscular volume (MCV) is a measure of the average volume of RBCs per liter. It is expressed in **femtoliters** (fL) using the hematocrit percentage and the RBC count. The formula is:

$$MCV = \frac{Hct \times 10}{RBC \text{ count in millions/mm}^3} = fL$$

Mean Corpuscular Hemoglobin

Picogram (pg): *micro-microgram; 10^{-12} gram*

Mean corpuscular hemoglobin (MCH) is a measure of the average hemoglobin content of an RBC. It is calculated from the hemoglobin and RBC count and expressed in **picograms** (pg). The formula is:

$$MCH = \frac{Hgb \times 10}{RBC \text{ count in millions/mm}^3} = pg$$

Mean Corpuscular Hemoglobin Concentration

Mean corpuscular hemoglobin concentration (MCHC) is a measure of the average hemoglobin concentration (weight) per unit volume of RBCs. It is calculated using the hemoglobin and the hematocrit values and expressed in g/dL or percent.

Table 17–3 **Red Blood Indices Reference Range**

	Man	Woman	Newborn
MCV	80–94 fL	81–99 fL	96–108 fL
MCH	27–31 pg	27–31 pg	32–34 pg
MCHC	32–36%	32–36%	32–33%

MCV = mean corpuscular volume
MCH = mean corpuscular hemoglobin
MCHC = mean corpuscular hemoglobin concentration
Adapted from Watson, J, and Jaffe, MS: Nurse's Manual of Laboratory and Diagnostic Tests, FA Davis, Philadelphia, 1995, p 35, with permission.

The formula is:

$$MCHC = \frac{Hgb \times 100}{Hct} = g/dL \text{ or } \%$$

Values in newborn infants are slightly different, but adult levels are achieved within 1 month of age. Table 17–3 lists the reference ranges for red cell indices.

AUTOMATION

Because cost-effective equipment is available, most blood cell counts are processed by automatic cell counters, even in POLs. Manual counts are necessary only when the equipment fails.

Most automated cell counters operate on two principles. First, the cells to be counted are diluted in a fluid that conducts electrical current. The cells are aspirated through a very small opening called an *aperture*. As the cells are drawn into the opening, they interrupt the electric current across the aperture. This interruption is noted and counted as a cell.

The second method aspirates the diluted blood sample into a special opening so narrow only one cell at a time passes through. The cell interrupts a laser beam and each interruption is counted as a cell.

SUMMARY

The CBC is the most important test of all hematology studies. Physicians diagnose many disease conditions from the results of CBCs. Along with the hemoglobin and hematocrit, the RBC count provides the information for calculating RBC indices. Using indices values, physicians can classify the various types of anemia and determine other diseased states.

PATIENT EDUCATION

- No special preparation of the patient is necessary.
- Explain the procedure to the patient.

TECHNICAL CONSIDERATIONS

- When using the microscope, focus on the hemacytometer with low power before switching to high power.
- Count only cells that fall on the left and top border of the appropriate squares.

Box continues on following page

- Count both chambers of the hemacytometer, divide by 2, and multiply by the appropriate factor to obtain the count.

SOURCES OF ERROR

- When using the Unopette system for cell counting, failure to use the appropriate amount of diluting fluid may lead to erroneous results.
- When using the Unopette system for WBC cell counting, not waiting 10 minutes before filling the hemacytometer may result in an inaccurate count.
- Failure to thoroughly mix the Unopette before filling the hemacytometer may lead to erroneous results.
- Failure to expel a few drops of the Unopette's diluting fluid before filling the hemacytometer may lead to erroneous results.
- Do not flood the chamber with diluting fluid or use too little fluid. Too much fluid results in a higher blood count, whereas too little fluid results in a low count.

Procedure with Rationale

White Blood Cell Count

EQUIPMENT AND SUPPLIES

Hand soap	Microscope
Latex gloves	70 percent isopropyl alcohol
Hemacytometer and cover glass	Gauze
Unopette system	Hand counter
Capillary or EDTA-anticoagulated	Surface disinfectant
blood specimen	Biohazard container
Lens paper	

Assemble equipment.

Wash hands with soap and water. Observe the OSHA Standard for this procedure.

Prepare a blood specimen for a white blood cell count using the Unopette system according to the manufacturer's directions.

After 10 minutes have elapsed, mix and fill the hemacytometer using the capillary tube of the Unopette system. ***The time is critical for the lysing of the erythrocytes.***

Place a clean coverslip over the counting chamber.

Before filling the hemacytometer, expel a few drops of dilution onto dry gauze. ***Expelling a few drops is necessary to ensure a sample typical of the dilution in the Unopette reservoir.***

Hold the tip of the pipette to the edge of the coverslip and fill the chamber. ***Be sure there are no bubbles and that fluid does not overflow into the grooves, thus producing inaccurate results.***

Place the hemacytometer with cover glass under the microscope and focus using low-power objective (10×).

Count the four outer squares of the counting chamber on both sides of the hemacytometer. Count only cells within the 16 squares and those cells that fall on the left and top border of each square.

Calculate and record the number of leukocytes by multiplying the average of both chambers by the factor 50.

Clean work area following laboratory protocol.

Remove gloves and wash hands with soap and water.

Questions

Name _____ Date _____

1. Explain the function of the white blood cell and the purpose of performing a WBC count.

2. Explain the function of the red blood cell and the purpose of performing an RBC count.

3. Name three conditions associated with leukocytosis and three conditions of leukopenia.

4. Name the conditions associated with polycythemia.

5. Name three pathological conditions that cause a decrease in platelets.

6. Describe the manual method of WBC counting using the Unopette system.

7. List at least four sources of errors when performing the manual method of WBC counting.

8. List the reference values of the WBC count and platelet count.

9. Give the reference range of RBCs for adult men and women.

10. Calculate the MCV, MCH, and MCHC using the following information: Hct = 45 percent, Hgb = 15.0 g/dL, RBC = 5.0×10^6/mm^3.

Terminal Performance Objective

White Blood Cell Count

Given the necessary equipment, you will be able to perform a white blood cell count and record the results. This procedure must be performed within 30 minutes and with a level of accuracy as specified by your instructor.

INSTRUCTOR'S EVALUATION FORM

Name _____ Date _____

+ = SATISFACTORY   ✓ = UNSATISFACTORY

_____ Assemble equipment.

_____ Wash hands with soap and water. Observe the OSHA Standard for this procedure.

_____ Prepare the Unopette with capillary blood or an EDTA-anticoagulated whole blood specimen.

_____ After 10 minutes have elapsed, mix and fill the hemacytometer using the capillary tube of the Unopette system.

_____ Place a clean coverslip over the counting chamber.

_____ Before filling the hemacytometer, expel a few drops of dilution onto dry gauze.

_____ Hold the top of the pipette to the edge of the coverslip and fill the chamber.

_____ Place the hemacytometer with cover glass under the microscope and focus using the low-power objective.

_____ Count the four outer squares of the counting chamber on both sides of the hemacytometer.

_____ Calculate and record the number of leukocytes per cubic millimeter.
RESULTS _____

_____ Clean work area following laboratory protocol.

_____ Remove gloves and wash hands with soap and water.

_____ The procedure was completed within 30 minutes.

_____ The results were at the level specified by your instructor.

_____ The results were properly recorded.

Final Competency Evaluation

_____ SATISFACTORY   _____ UNSATISFACTORY

Comments:

Instructor _____ Date _____

Blood Smear Preparation and Differential Blood Count

18

Learning Objectives
Cognitive Objectives
Psychomotor Objectives
Affective Objectives

Preparing a Blood Smear
Type of Specimen
Applying the Blood to the Slide
Staining

Criteria for a Properly Made Blood Smear
Macroscopic
Microscopic

Performing a Differential Blood Count
Leukocyte Morphology
Erythrocyte Morphology
Platelet Estimate

Absolute Values
Reference Ranges

Summary
Patient Education
Technical Considerations
Sources of Error

Procedure with Rationale
Blood Smear Preparation and Differential
  Blood Count

Questions

Terminal Performance Objective
Blood Smear Preparation and Differential
  Blood Count
  ○ Instructor's evaluation form

LEARNING OBJECTIVES

On completing this chapter, you will be able to:

COGNITIVE OBJECTIVES

- List the criteria for a properly made blood smear.
- Name the five types of leukocytes, and describe how each is identified when stained with Wright's stain.
- Tell what other information, besides the differential, is obtained when a blood smear is observed microscopically.
- State the reference range for each white blood cell type in the differential.
- List four pathological conditions that cause variations from the normal differential.

PSYCHOMOTOR OBJECTIVES

- Prepare and stain a blood smear suitable for a differential blood count following the Terminal Performance Objective presented in this chapter.
- Identify all blood cell types required by your instructor.
- Calculate the absolute number of each type of leukocyte when the leukocyte blood cell count is known.

AFFECTIVE OBJECTIVES

- Recognize the importance of referring to manufacturer's directions regarding the proper application of hematology stains.
- Understand that only specially trained personnel are permitted to perform the leukocyte differential count.

247

A *differential white blood cell count* (differential, or diff) is an important part of the complete blood count. It provides the percentage of each of the five major types of leukocytes found in circulating blood. The test has three distinct components:

- Preparing a blood smear on a glass slide and staining it
- Classifying a minimum of 100 white blood cells according to type using a microscope
- Evaluating the general **morphology** of the formed elements in the sample

Medical assistants frequently prepare and stain blood smears as part of their laboratory duties. Like all skills, practicing the procedure over and over helps to develop the technique until it becomes second nature.

Physicians, medical technologists, or specially trained technicians classify 100 white blood cells according to their type and evaluate the formed elements in the specimen. This part of the differential requires a knowledge of normal, abnormal, and immature forms of various cells that are found in blood. Although medical assistants do not normally perform this part of the differential, they should be able to identify all normal blood cells and know the values that constitute the reference range for the complete blood count.

Morphology: *shape and structure*

PREPARING A BLOOD SMEAR

Blood smears for each patient should be prepared in duplicate. In this way there is a reserve slide in case one is broken or there is a need to verify results. You need two glass slides for each blood smear. They must be clean and dry, with edges that are chip-free.

Type of Specimen

Blood from a fingerstick or venous blood collected using an EDTA (lavender top) tube can be used for preparing the blood smear. When blood from a venipuncture is used, gently invert the tube at least eight times to resuspend the cells completely before making the smear. Transfer a small drop of blood from the test tube to the slide using a transfer pipette, an applicator stick, or a hematocrit tube. Be sure to make the slides within 1 hour of the draw, because changes occur in the morphology and staining of the cells. When blood from a capillary puncture is used, lightly touch the slide to the drop of blood but avoid touching the patient's finger since skin oil leaves smudges on the slide.

Applying the Blood to the Slide

Place a small drop of blood on one side of the slide and set the slide on a firm surface with the drop of blood upward. Place a second slide called the "spreader slide" in front of the drop of blood at about a 45° angle. Draw the spreader slide into the drop and allow the blood to flow evenly across the width of the spreader slide almost to its edges. In a swift, even motion spread the blood across the length of the slide (Fig. 18–1). The thickness of the smear can be varied by altering the angle of the spreader slide and the size of the drop of blood. Increasing the angle of the spreader slide will produce a shorter smear; decreasing the angle of the spreader slide will produce a longer smear. Evaluate each blood smear as soon as it is made. If it is not suitable for the differential, immediately make another slide. This is especially important when making a smear from a peripheral puncture and the puncture site is still yielding free-flowing blood. If the slide appears well made, fan it in the air to speed drying. This minimizes cell distortion. Do not blow on the slide, since this may cause lysis of the cells. Immediately label the slide by writing the patient's identification on the frosted edge of the slide or in the thick portion of the smear. Use a lead pencil.

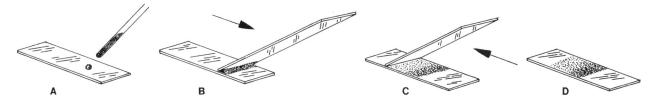

Figure 18-1 Preparing a blood smear. *(A)* Place a drop of blood at one end of a clean, chip-free glass slide. *(B)* Draw the spreader slide back into the drop of blood and allow the blood to travel almost the entire width of the slide. *(C)* In a single smooth motion, spread the drop of blood across the slide. *(D)* Properly identify the slide by placing the name of the patient on the frosted area, or write the name directly in the thick end of the blood using a lead pencil.

Staining

Stain the blood smear as soon as possible after it dries. Many commercial stains are available, but the most common stain for a differential is Wright's stain. This *polychromatic stain* consists of several dyes, each having a different staining characteristic. Cellular structures accept different dyes, based on their pH. Some cellular structures are stained with an alkaline dye; others are stained with an acid dye. Wright's stain contains two dyes, methylene blue (basic or alkaline stain) and eosin (acid stain). Each of these dyes will react with different cellular structures. In order to stain a blood smear, position the slide on a staining rack, and apply stain directly to the blood smear. Follow the directions from the manufacturer. Some processes require application of a stain only and rinsing with distilled water. Others require the use of a **buffer solution** during the staining process. Package inserts provide specific directions on the proper use of the stain. After staining, place the slide in a vertical position and allow it to air dry. Examine the slide microscopically using oil-immersion (95–100×) magnification and assess its quality.

> **Buffer solution:** *a solution that helps maintain a constant pH even when additional acid or alkaline products are added*

CRITERIA FOR A PROPERLY MADE BLOOD SMEAR

Macroscopic

A well-made blood smear has the following characteristics:

- Smooth appearance
- Feathered edge
- Slight margin on either side of the length of the slide

Maintain an even pressure on the spreader slide as you spread the blood over the slide to produce a smooth appearance. The weight of the spreader slide is sufficient. A feathered edge at the thin end of the smear is essential. As the name implies, the edge of the smear will resemble a bird's feather. If you do not have a feathered edge, you must prepare another slide. A feathered edge ensures that you will have an area that is acceptable for the differential blood count, with an even distribution of cells. Without a feathered edge the blood film may be so long that it extends the entire length of the slide and cells are "pushed over" the opposite end of the slide, or it may be so short that the cells "pile up" in an abrupt ending. In the first situation the WBCs are deposited over the edge of the slide where they cannot be counted or classified. In the second situation, the leukocytes are deposited in a pile of blood so thick that the hematologist cannot see distinguishing features of the cells. A properly made blood film does not extend the entire width of the slide. Rather, there is a small margin on either side of the blood film. Again, this ensures that the entire blood sample is available on the slide and cells are not lost by being "pushed over the edge" (Figs. 18–2 and 18–3). Slides that do not have a margin need not be rejected for the differential blood count if all other criteria are met.

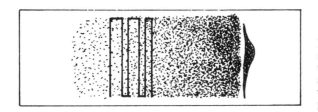

Figure 18-2 A properly made blood smear shows a slight margin on both sides of the length of the smear, a feathered edge, and a smooth appearance. The line indicates where the differential is performed and the pattern that is followed.

Microscopic

After staining the smear, evaluate it with the microscope using the oil-immersion lens (95-100×). A properly prepared blood smear will have about 0.5 inch of blood where the hematologist performs the differential white cell count. This is the *examination area.* Cells in this area of the slide should have the following features:

> **Monolayer:** *a layer composed of cells only one layer thick*

- Distributed in a **monolayer**
- Stained so that distinguishing characteristics are clearly visible
- Free of excessive distortion

In a properly prepared smear, the cells in the examination area appear as a monolayer, one cell lying adjacent to another. You should not see any clusters of white cells or more white cells at the edges of the slide. The cells must not be stacked one upon the other as found in the first portion of the smear, nor so sparse that empty spaces appear between the cells, as found at the feathered edge (Fig. 18-4).

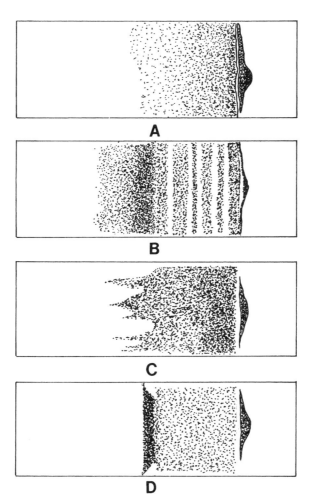

Figure 18-3 Improperly made blood smears. *(A)* Too short, no margin. *(B)* Irregular pressure. *(C)* Too short, jagged end rather than a feathered edge. *(D)* An abrupt edge lacking a feathered appearance.

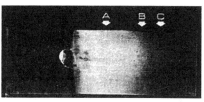

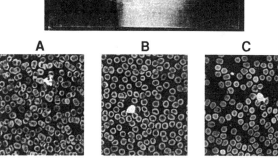

Figure 18–4 Microscopic evaluation of a blood smear. *(A)* Thick end of the slide shows clumping of the cells. *(B)* Monolayer where cells almost touch each other. *(C)* Thin end of the slide where cells are far apart. Erythrocytes tend to lose their central pallor and show atypical staining. (Rapaport, SI: Introduction to Hematology, ed 2, JB Lippincott, Philadelphia, 1987, with permission.)

After you have evaluated the slide for cell distribution, examine it for the quality of the stain. Erythrocytes should appear a pinkish-red color, and the granules of the granulocytes should show proper coloration: pink and lilac in the neutrophils, orange in the eosinophils, and purple in the basophils. Evaluate only the examination area since erythrocytes tend to lose their central pallor and appear atypical in the feathered edge and leukocytes do not show proper coloration: in the thick part of the slide.

Finally, the cells should appear round and intact. When improper technique is used in preparing the slide, blood cells are broken and show distortion.

PERFORMING A DIFFERENTIAL BLOOD COUNT

The hematologist performs the differential blood count where the cells appear in a monolayer using oil-immersion magnification. In most POLs, 100 cells are classified. A device called a differential counter keeps a running tally of the cell types (Fig. 18–5). To ensure that no cell is counted twice, a pattern for examination is followed (Fig. 18–2).

Leukocyte Morphology

Leukocytes are divided into two major categories, granulocytes and agranulocytes, which are also called **mononuclear** cells. Granulocytes are further divided into three groups—neutrophils, eosinophils, and basophils. These three cells are characterized by the presence of granules within the cytoplasm. Their names are derived from the se-

Mononuclear: *having only one nucleus; generally refers to monocytes and lymphocytes*

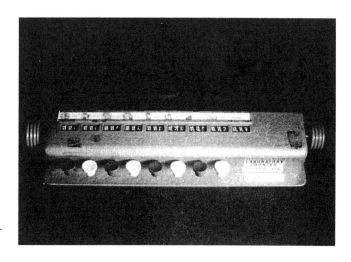

Figure 18–5 White cell differential counter.

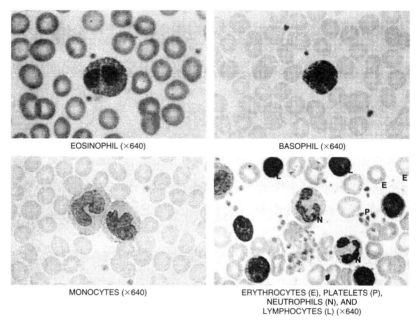

EOSINOPHIL (×640)　　　　　　　　BASOPHIL (×640)

MONOCYTES (×640)　　　　　　ERYTHROCYTES (E), PLATELETS (P),
　　　　　　　　　　　　　　　　NEUTROPHILS (N), AND
　　　　　　　　　　　　　　　　LYMPHOCYTES (L) (×640)

Figure 18–6　Types of blood cells.

lective staining characteristics of their granules after staining with Wright's stain. Their granules accept either a basic dye (methylene blue) or an acidic dye (eosin); hence their names, basophils and eosinophils. The neutrophils contain granules that react with both acid and basic dye and exhibit a neutral staining reaction selecting both eosin and methylene blue.

Mature granulocytes have lobed or multilobed nuclei, which are called *polymorphonuclear.* Upon close observation there are small **chromatin** strands joining the lobes. The nuclei of all three granulocytes stain a deep purple.

Immature neutrophils show a nucleus that has not yet formed lobes. Rather, the nucleus appears as a large "comma" within the cytoplasm. This immature cell is called a *band* cell.

Agranulocytes characteristically contain few or no granules in their cytoplasm. They are chiefly identified by their nuclei. Lymphocytes have a flattened, dark-staining nucleus, and monocytes have a lacy, netlike nucleus. Figure 18–6 shows the morphology of the five types of leukocytes. Unlike granulocytes, the nuclei of the agranulocytes do not typically form lobes but exist as a single mass within the cytoplasm, hence, they are often referred to as mononuclear leukocytes. Table 18–1 summarizes the appearance of the various leukocytes. The descriptions are brief and general. Variations occur, especially in pathology (see also Fig. 14–3).

Erythrocyte Morphology

In addition to the enumeration of different white cells, the blood smear provides an opportunity to observe erythrocytes for obvious abnormalities. During the differential, the trained hematologist identifies and reports abnormal erythrocytes. A normal red blood cell is *normochromic* when it appears to contain the normal amount of hemoglobin and *normocytic* when it falls within the normal size range. Erythrocytes have a tendency to absorb acid stains. The depth of staining gives an approximate guide as to the amount of hemoglobin in the cell. In normochromic cells the central area is pale and the periphery stains pinkish red. By observing the depth of color and the size of central **pallor,** a quali-

Chromatin: *deeply staining substance present in the nucleus; contains the genetic material*

Pallor: *paleness*

Table 18-1 **Leukocyte Morphology**

Cell Type	Cytoplasm	Nucleus
Neutrophil	Pink, containing lilac and pink granules	Usually 3 lobes, darkly stained, granular and clumped chromatin
Eosinophil	Pink, containing large orange granules	Usually 2 lobes, darkly stained, granular and clumped chromatin
Basophil	Pink, containing dark purple granules, frequently covering the nucleus	Usually 2 lobes, darkly stained
Lymphocyte	Usually light blue, sometimes dark blue (azurophilic); occasional pink granules	Solid, flat, usually round or oval
Monocyte	Blue-gray, sometimes vacuoles and pseudopods	Lacy, often kidney-shaped or oval to round

tative judgment can be made about the relative amount of hemoglobin present within the erythrocytes. Erythrocytes that appear lightly stained with only a very small margin of color around the edge have decreased amounts of hemoglobin and are called *hypochromic.*

Red blood cells that are larger than normal are called *macrocytes;* smaller than normal, *microcytes.* Marked variation in the size of the erythrocytes is called *anisocytosis.* When RBCs are shaped other than the normal biconcave disk, the abnormality is called *poikilocytosis.* Sickle cell anemia produces a form of poikilocytosis. The cells have bizarre shapes that resemble sickles or clubs.

Some RBCs show a variation in color when stained, causing them to appear blue-gray. This is referred to as *polychromasia* or *polychromatophilia.* It is often indicative of very active bone marrow. Figure 18–7 shows variations in red cell morphology.

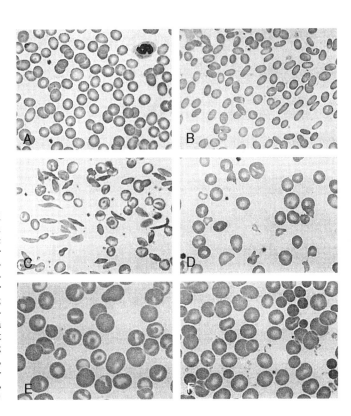

Figure 18–7 Abnormal red cell morphology: The blood smear can provide important morphologic clues to red cell disease. A number of important morphologic abnormalities are shown in this composite, including *(A)* normal smear (for comparison); *(B)* elliptocytosis; *(C)* sickle cells; *(D)* red cell fragmentation from a patient with a heart valve prosthesis; *(E)* target cells and uniform macrocytosis; *(F)* spherocytosis. (From Hillman, RS, and Finch, CA: Red Cell Manual, ed 5, FA Davis, Philadelphia, 1985, pp 44–45, with permission.)

Clinical Comment: Erythrocyte Distribution

Rouleaux formation is an alteration in erythrocyte distribution on a stained peripheral smear. The erythrocytes appear as stacks of coins. When rouleaux appear in the thick end of the smear, it is of little significance. However, when the rouleaux are found in the thin end of the slide, this may be associated with pathology, especially diseases associated with elevations in blood protein levels.

Platelet Estimate

An approximate estimate of the platelet count is also undertaken during the differential count. Using the oil-immersion objective, the hematologist examines the monolayer area of the blood smear. It is normal to see about 5 to 15 platelets in each oil-immersion field. When they are found only with great difficulty, the platelet count is probably decreased. On the other hand, when many platelets are observed in each field, the platelet count is probably elevated.

Clinical Comment: Platelet Estimation

For the platelet estimation to be valid, there must be approximately 200 cells per oil-immersion field. This can be assessed by counting approximately 50 cells in a quadrant of the field.

ABSOLUTE VALUES

The differential white blood count indicates the relative number (percentage) of each type of leukocyte per cubic millimeter (mm^3) of blood. Physicians use the results from the differential in conjunction with the total white blood cell count to obtain the absolute number of the various white blood cells. The total white cell count is multiplied by the relative number of each of the cells counted in the differential to determine the actual number of each cell type.

Total leukocyte count (cells/mm^3) $\times$ relative value (percent)
= absolute value (leukocytes/mm^3)

For example,

Total leukocyte count = 6000
Neutrophils (relative value) = 50 percent
$$\text{Absolute value} = 6000 \times \frac{50}{100} = 3000 \text{ per mm}^3$$
$$\text{SI units} = 3.0 \times 10^9/\text{L}$$

Table 18–2 **Reference Ranges for Relative and Absolute White Blood Cell Count**

Cell Type	Relative Value (%)	Absolute Value (cells/mm^3)	Absolute Cell Value ($\times 10^9$/L)
Neutrophils	45–75	1500–8000	1.5–8.0
Basophils	0–1	25–100	0.03–0.1
Eosinophils	1–3	50–700	0.05–0.7
Lymphocytes	20–45	800–3200	0.8–3.2
Monocytes	0–9	50–800	0.05–0.8
Band Cells	0–5	50–500	0.05–0.5

Table 18–3 **Possible Causes for Variations from Reference Values**

Leukocyte Cell Type	Pathological Causes for Abnormal Differentials
Neutrophils	Bacterial infections, inflammatory disorders, stress, some drugs
Basophils	Blood dyscrasias, certain forms of leukemia, radiation exposure
Eosinophils	Allergic disorders, parasitic infections
Lymphocytes	Viral infections (measles, rubella, chickenpox, infectious mononucleosis)
Monocytes	Severe infections, bacterial endocarditis, some forms of arthritis

Reference Ranges

Table 18–2 lists the reference ranges for the relative and absolute values for leukocytes. These values vary somewhat depending on age. Table 18–3 provides some possible causes for variations from normal reference values.

SUMMARY

The differential white blood cell count gives the relative percentage of each type of leukocyte in a sample of peripheral blood. It is performed on a blood smear that has been stained so that distinguishing characteristics are observable. Physicians correlate the information from the differential blood count with the white blood count to determine the actual number of each cell type.

Although the differential is often performed by specially trained personnel, medical assistants and other health-care personnel prepare and stain blood smears. Like most skills, this technique is perfected through practice. With much additional training, some medical assistants perform the differential count. All medical assistants should be familiar with the normal values for the complete blood count and be able to identify normal blood cells.

It is the physician's responsibility to interpret the differential blood count. Actual diagnosis of disease can be undertaken only when the physician considers a complete clinical picture.

PATIENT EDUCATION

- No specific patient education is required for this test.
- Reassure any patient who shows undue concern about obtaining the blood specimen.

TECHNICAL CONSIDERATIONS

- An improper angle of the spreader slide, or the improper size of the drop of blood, may result in slides that are too thick or too thin for proper evaluation.
- Applying pressure to the spreader slide produces smears that are inadequate for microscopic evaluation.
- Water splashes on unstained blood smears will wash away the specimen, rendering the smear invalid for the differential count.

SOURCES OF ERROR

- Dirty, chipped slides or poor quality slides produce poor quality smears that may be unacceptable for testing.
- Failure to thoroughly resuspend cells after collection via venipuncture produces inaccurate results.

Procedure with Rationale

Blood Smear Preparation and Differential Blood Count
EQUIPMENT AND SUPPLIES

Hand soap	Microscope
Glass slides (4)	Immersion oil
Blood specimen (capillary or venous)	Latex gloves
Wright's stain	Disinfectant
Staining rack	Biohazard container
Distilled water	

Assemble equipment.

Wash hands with soap and water. Observe the OSHA Standard for this procedure.

Apply a drop of blood (capillary puncture or venipuncture) to a clean, chip-free glass slide. *Dirty or chipped slides will adversely affect the quality of the smear.*

Center it about 0.5 inch from the right edge of the slide (or left edge if you are left-handed).

Hold a spreader slide at about a 45° angle to the first slide. *The angle of the spreader slide affects the thickness of the blood film.*

Place the spreader slide about 1 inch from the right edge of the slide (or left edge if you are left-handed).

Draw the spreader slide into the drop of blood and wait until the blood travels almost its entire width. *This makes a smear wide enough for proper examination and produces a slight margin the length of the slide after the smear has been made.*

Spread the blood across the slide using only the weight of the spreader slide to provide pressure.

Macroscopically examine the slide for:
- Smoothness
- Feathered edge
- Slight margin

Prepare a second slide as a backup.

If the slides meet the macroscopic criteria, quickly dry them by fanning them in the air. *This keeps cell distortion to a minimum.*

Write the patient's name and the date in the thick end of the film or on the frosted end of the slide using a pencil.

Place the slide on a staining rack and stain the smear following the manufacturer's directions. *Because of the differences in stain types, always read and follow the directions supplied by the manufacturer.*

Place the slides in a vertical position to let them air dry.

When the slides are dry, examine them using the oil-immersion lens (95–100×) to assess the microscopic quality of the smear for:

- Monolayer
- Stain
- Cells intact

Identify all cells required by instructor.

Clean work area following laboratory protocol.

Remove gloves and wash hands with soap and water.

Questions

Name _____ Date _____

1. What is a differential blood count? What are the three components of the differential?

2. Name the five types of white blood cells. Briefly describe their appearance after staining with Wright's stain.

3. What is a polychromatic stain? What is the name of the stain commonly used for differentials?

4. Give three microscopic and three macroscopic criteria for a properly prepared blood smear.

5. Besides the differential count, what other relevant information is obtained from the microscopic examination of the blood smear?

6. How are absolute values obtained for the different types of white cells?

7. Give the reference range for the differential blood cell count.

Terminal Performance Objective

Blood Smear Preparation and Differential Blood Count

Given a blood sample and the necessary equipment, you will prepare and stain two blood smears that meet the microscopic and macroscopic criteria identified in this chapter. Your instructor will determine whether the slide meets these criteria. This procedure must be completed within 20 minutes. If required by your instructor, you will also identify and record all blood cell types and record your observations, within 5 additional minutes.

INSTRUCTOR'S EVALUATION FORM

Name _____ Date _____

+ = SATISFACTORY   ✓ = UNSATISFACTORY

_____ Assemble equipment.

_____ Wash hands with soap and water. Observe the OSHA Standard for this procedure.

_____ Apply a drop of blood (capillary puncture or venipuncture) to a clean, chip-free glass slide.

_____ Center it about 0.5 inch from the right edge of the slide (or left edge if you are left-handed).

_____ Hold a spreader slide at about a 45° angle to the first slide.

_____ Place the spreader slide about 1 inch from the right edge of the slide (or left edge if you are left-handed).

_____ Draw the spreader slide into the drop of blood and wait until the blood travels almost its entire width.

_____ Spread the blood across the slide using only the weight of the spreader slide to provide pressure.

_____ Macroscopically examine the slide for:
   ____ Smoothness
   ____ Feathered edge
   ____ Slight margin

_____ Prepare a second slide as a backup.

_____ If the slides meet the macroscopic criteria, quickly dry them by fanning them in the air.

_____ Write the patient's name and the date in the thick end of the film or on the frosted end of the slide using a pencil.

_____ Place the slide on a staining rack and stain the smear following the manufacturer's directions.

_____ Place the slides in a vertical position to let them air dry.

When the slides are dry, examine them using the oil-immersion lens (95–100×) to assess the microscopic quality of the smear for:
   ____ Monolayer
   ____ Stain
   ____ Cells intact

_____ Identify and record all cells required by instructor.

erythrocyte _____   neutrophil _____

basophil _____   eosinophil _____

monocyte _____   lymphocyte _____

platelet _____

_____ Clean work area following laboratory protocol.

_____ Remove gloves and wash hands with soap and water.

_____ The procedure was completed within 20 minutes.

_____ The blood smear met the macroscopic and microscopic criteria identified in this chapter. All required cells were properly identified and recorded (5 additional minutes).

Erythrocyte Sedimentation Rate

LEARNING OBJECTIVES

On completing this chapter, you will be able to:

COGNITIVE OBJECTIVES
- Explain the purpose of performing an erythrocyte sedimentation rate (ESR).
- Identify the factors that influence the ESR.
- Describe three methods of performing an ESR.
- List several technical factors affecting the accuracy of the ESR.

PSYCHOMOTOR OBJECTIVES
- Perform an ESR that meets the Terminal Performance Objective presented in this chapter.
- Record the results of the ESR.

AFFECTIVE OBJECTIVES
- Take responsibility for maintaining the integrity of the ESR by controlling the conditions affecting the ESR.
- Follow the OSHA Standard regarding the disposal of blood for your safety and that of your coworkers.

The *erythrocyte sedimentation rate* (ESR), also known as the *sed rate,* is a nonspecific laboratory test that determines the rate at which erythrocytes separate from plasma and settle to the bottom of a tube. Sed rate results do not give the physician information about a specific disease, but they indicate a general condition such as the presence of acute or chronic inflammation. A series of sed rates allows the physician to evaluate a course of treatment by following the progress of an inflammatory condition.

Sedimentation: *substances settling at the bottom of a liquid; red blood cells settling at the bottom of plasma*

Sedimentation is the process of solids settling out of a liquid in which they have been dissolved or suspended. The most numerous solids in whole blood are erythrocytes, and when an anticoagulated sample of whole blood is allowed to stand, the erythrocytes gradually settle to the bottom of the container. In normal individuals, the rate at which this occurs—the erythrocyte sedimentation rate—is fairly slow. In patients with inflammatory disease, RBCs fall more quickly. This increase of the sedimentation rate is usually in proportion to the severity of the inflammation. The more severe the disease, the faster the erythrocytes settle out of solution.

FACTORS THAT INFLUENCE THE ERYTHROCYTE SEDIMENTATION RATE

The speed at which the erythrocytes settle out of plasma in a blood sample depends on four factors:

- Size of the erythrocytes
- Concentration of the erythrocytes
- Shape of the erythrocytes
- Composition of the plasma proteins

Size

Macrocyte: *an abnormally large erythrocyte that exceeds 10 microns in diameter*

Microcyte: *an unusually small erythrocyte that is less than 5 microns in diameter*

RBCs settle out of plasma because of their density. The rate at which RBCs settle in plasma is directly proportionate to their density. Large RBCs are usually denser than smaller RBCs; therefore they settle out of solution faster than smaller-sized cells. **Macrocytes** have a higher sedimentation rate than **microcytes.**

Concentration

The concentration of the RBCs in plasma affects the ESR. Fewer RBCs reduce the erythrocyte-to-plasma ratio, such as occurs in anemia, causing an elevated rate of sedimentation. A higher than normal concentration of erythrocytes in the blood, such as in polycythemia, has the opposite effect on the sedimentation rate and results in lower ESRs.

Shape

Rouleau: *a group of red blood cells arranged like a roll of coins*

Spherocytes: *erythrocytes that assume a spheroid shape*

Some diseases cause changes in the shape of RBCs that increase or decrease the sedimentation rate. In sickle cell anemia, for instance, the sickle shape of the erythrocytes makes them resistant to **rouleau** formation, which results in lower sedimentation rates. **Spherocytes** also settle at a slower rate (see Fig. 18–7).

Clinical Comment: Sickle Cell Anemia

Sickle cell anemia is a hereditary, chronic form of hemolytic anemia characterized by large numbers of sickle-shaped RBCs circulating in the blood. The RBCs have a reduced life span and are a crescent or sickle shape. The shape is a result of an abnormality in the hemoglobin causing deformed RBCs. Sickle cell disease is found almost exclusively in persons of African and Mediterranean descent. Some scientists believe that sickle cell disease developed as a defense against malaria. Malarial parasites do not grow in sickle-shaped RBCs.

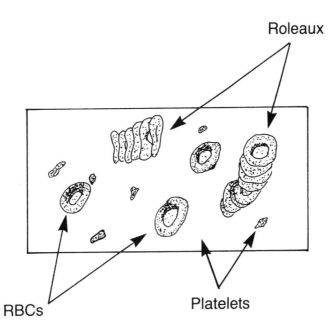

Figure 19–1 Erythrocyte aggregates in rouleau formation.

Plasma Proteins

The rate of sedimentation depends on the amount of protein present in plasma. Plasma proteins include fibrinogen, globulin, and albumin. Fibrinogen and globulin increase during acute infections, inflammation, and tissue injury, but albumin decreases. Increased fibrinogen and globulin cause the surfaces of RBCs to become sticky. The erythrocytes stick together in stacks, like rolls of coins or poker chips, called rouleaux (Fig. 19–1).

These clumps of erythrocytes are called **aggregates.** Because they are larger and heavier, aggregates tend to settle out of solution more quickly and elevate the ESR. An increase in the level of albumin has an opposite effect and slows the rate of sedimentation of red blood cells.

> **Aggregate:** *red blood cells that cluster or come together*

METHOD OF PERFORMING THE ERYTHROCYTE SEDIMENTATION RATE

One method for determining ESR is the *Wintrobe method.* This system uses a Wintrobe sedimentation tube and a long-stemmed Pasteur-type pipette (Fig. 19–2). A *Wintrobe tube* is a glass cylinder, 1 mm in diameter, with a capacity of 1 mL. The tube is graduated from 0 to 100 mm from top to bottom on one side of the scale and from bottom to top on the other side. The system includes a special rack that holds the tube in a vertical position.

To determine the ESR, collect a venous whole blood sample in a lavender-stoppered tube containing EDTA. See Chapter 8 for collecting a venous blood sample. Using the long-stemmed pipette, fill the Wintrobe tube to the 0-mm line with the well-mixed blood sample (Fig. 19–3). Place the tube into the rack and let the tube stand undisturbed for exactly 1 hour (Fig. 19–4). The erythrocytes and plasma will separate, leaving the plasma at the top of the tube, above the red cells that have settled to the bottom of the tube. Measure the sed rate by noting the number (reading down from 0) at which the meniscus of RBCs crosses the scale etched on the Wintrobe tube (Fig. 19–5). That number is recorded in millimeters per hour.

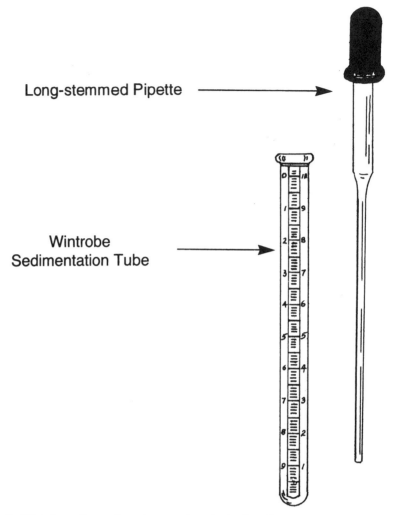

Long-stemmed Pipette

Wintrobe
Sedimentation Tube

Figure 19-2 Wintrobe sedimentation tube, a graduated tube that allows precise measurement of the sedimentation rate, and a 9-inch long-stemmed pipette used to fill the Wintrobe tube.

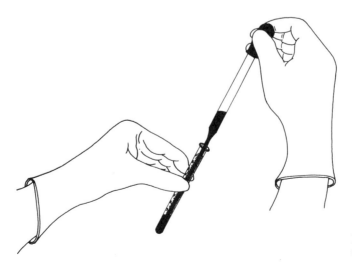

Figure 19-3 Filling a Wintrobe sedimentation tube.

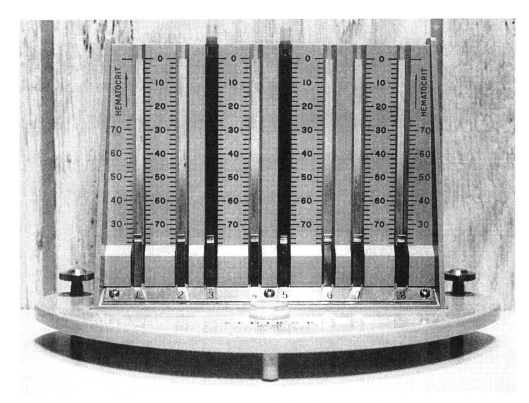

Figure 19–4   Wintrobe tubes in sedimentation rack.

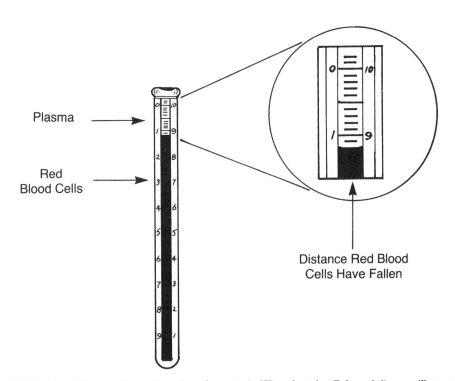

Plasma

Red
Blood Cells

Distance Red Blood
Cells Have Fallen

Figure 19–5   After 1 hour, sedimentation of erythrocytes in Wintrobe tube. Enlarged diagram illustrates a sedimentation rate of 12 mm/h.

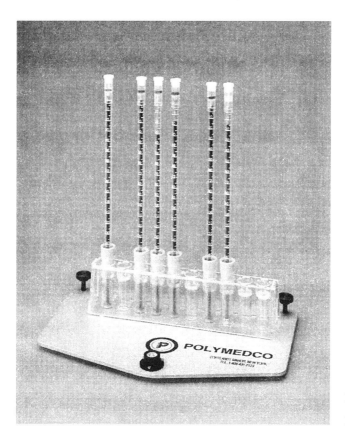

Figure 19-6 Sediplast ESR System. (Courtesy Polymedco, Inc., Cortlandt Manor, NY.)

The Westergren ESR is another method for measuring the sedimentation rate. This method uses a pipette graduated from 0 to 200 mm and a rack for holding the calibrated pipettes. The Westergren test is more sensitive than the Wintrobe and more complex to perform, because it requires the blood to be diluted with 3.8 percent of sodium citrate.

The test has been modified in recent years and kits are available that have closed systems with self-filling disposable pipettes and premeasured diluent. Sediplast ESR System is an example of the modified Westergren method (Fig. 19-6). These kits eliminate the biohazard conditions of the original Westergren technique and have disposable pipettes.

In the Sediplast ESR System, anticoagulated whole blood is mixed with the premeasured diluent (3.8 percent sodium citrate) in the sedivial. Thoroughly mix the whole blood sample before transferring to the sedivial. Insert the calibrated pipette into the vial with a twisting motion until the pipette reaches the bottom of the sedivial. The column of blood will automatically zero itself, and any extra blood overflows into the sealed reservoir. The sedivial with the pipette is placed in the rack for 1 hour (Fig. 19-7). Set the timer for 1 hour.

After 1 hour, immediately read the results and record them on the request slip. The distance the red cells have fallen, according to the markings on the pipette, is then reported in millimeters and represents the ESR.

Another measurement comparable to the ESR is the zeta sedimentation ratio (ZSR). This method is especially useful for pediatric patients because it uses a small blood sample. It is performed with a small-bore capillary tube filled with blood from a finger puncture. The capillary tube is spun in a special centrifuge called the Zetafuge made by Coulter Diagnostics. The tube is read on a special reader to obtain a value called the *zetacrit*. The zetacrit, which represents the percent of sedimented erythrocytes, is divided into the hematocrit value and the results are expressed as a percentage.

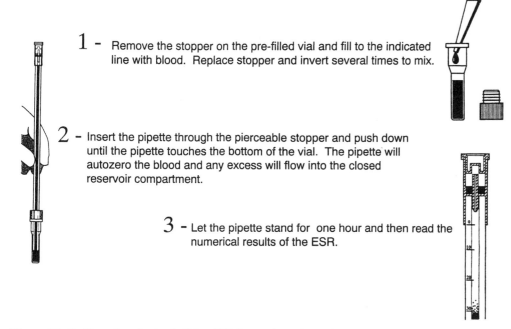

1 - Remove the stopper on the pre-filled vial and fill to the indicated line with blood. Replace stopper and invert several times to mix.

2 - Insert the pipette through the pierceable stopper and push down until the pipette touches the bottom of the vial. The pipette will autozero the blood and any excess will flow into the closed reservoir compartment.

3 - Let the pipette stand for one hour and then read the numerical results of the ESR.

Figure 19-7   Procedure for the Sediplast ESR System from the package insert. (Courtesy Polymedco, Inc., Cortlandt Manor, NY.)

CONDITIONS AFFECTING THE ERYTHROCYTE SEDIMENTATION RATE

Most inflammatory diseases cause an increase of the erythrocyte sedimentation rate. Acute infections, inflammatory disorders, severe anemias, renal disease, acute myocardial infarction, and collagen disorders such as systemic lupus erythematosus (SLE) and rheumatoid arthritis elevate the sed rate. For some time after recovery from infectious diseases, the ESR is elevated before slowly returning to normal. The defense mechanisms of the body are active long after the clinical symptoms disappear.

TECHNICAL FACTORS AFFECTING THE ERYTHROCYTE SEDIMENTATION RATE

Several technical factors affect the settling process and may introduce errors in the results of the test. These include the following:

- The slightest variation from a vertical position in the sedimentation tube can increase the ESR. Adjust the special rack for holding the Wintrobe tube so that it is precisely level. A variation as small as a 3° angle can increase the ESR by 30 percent.
- Timing is critical; taking the reading before or after the specified time gives a result that is too low or too high.
- Any movement of the sample during the test period can increase the ESR. The counter or bench on which the rack holding the calibrated pipettes rests during the test must be free from vibration. Do not operate a centrifuge on the same bench or counter during the test.
- Do not jar or move the rack holding the sedimentation tube.
- Blood that has been drawn more than 2 hours before the test or blood that has

Table 19–1   **Reference Values for ESR**

	Wintrobe (mm/h)	Westergren and Sediplast (mm/h)
Man		
<age 50 years	0–7	0–15
>age 50 years	5–7	0–20
Woman		
<age 50 years	0–15	0–20
>age 50 years	25–30	0–30

Adapted from Watson, J, and Jaffe, MS: Nurse's Manual of Laboratory and Diagnostic Tests, FA Davis, Philadelphia, 1995, p 39, with permission.

not been properly mixed with the correct anticoagulant will not yield a true ESR. Use a fresh, well-mixed EDTA-anticoagulated whole-blood sample for the test. If necessary, the blood sample may be stored at 4°C for up to 6 hours. Bring it to room temperature before using for testing.

- Changes in environmental temperature can cause changes in ESR. Make sure room temperature is constant (20°C–25°C) during the test.
- The rate of sedimentation will vary with any change in the size, shape, or dimensions of the sedimentation tube. Therefore, use only the calibrated pipette specified for the method used.
- Even a small variance in volume affects the measurement of the ESR. Be careful to fill the tube completely to the top of the scale, with no bubbles in the sample.

The ESR is very sensitive to technical error. Observe all technical requirements so that results are accurate and quality assurance is maintained. Wintrobe and Westergren tubes are disposable and must be put into the biohazard containers along with the blood samples for your safety and that of your fellow workers.

REFERENCE VALUES FOR THE ERYTHROCYTE SEDIMENTATION RATE

ESR reference values vary with age, sex, and method of testing. Elderly patients and pregnant women often show an elevated ESR. Table 19–1 gives the reference values of ESR for the Wintrobe and Westergren methods.

The ZSR is calculated from the hematocrit and zetacrit and reported as a percentage. The ZSR value is corrected for RBC volume; therefore, it has the same values for men and women and all ages. Table 19–2 gives the reference values for the ZSR.

Table 19–2
Reference Values for ZSR (all ages)

Normal	40–51%
Borderline	51–54%
Elevated	≥55%

SUMMARY

The ESR is a simple, nonspecific test that helps the physician determine the presence and follow the progression of inflammatory disorders. It also helps the physician to monitor conditions such as anemias, renal disease, acute myocardial infarction, and collagen disorders.

Although sedimentation rates do not assist the physician in diagnosing a disease state, they are helpful in monitoring the progression of disease. The ESR is especially useful as an indicator of obscure infections such as tuberculosis, systemic lupus erythematosus, and subacute bacterial endocarditis.

PATIENT EDUCATION

- No special preparation is necessary for this test.
- Explain the procedure to the patient.

TECHNICAL CONSIDERATIONS

- Carefully follow the instructions recommended for each method used by the manufacturer of the sed rate tubes.
- Keep the room temperature constant while performing the ESR.
- Use only an EDTA-anticoagulated blood sample for the Wintrobe ESR.

SOURCES OF ERROR

- Not filling the narrow sedimentation calibrated pipettes all the way to the 0-mm line will give erroneous results.
- Air bubbles in the sedimentation calibrated pipettes will cause erroneous results.
- Not reading the sedimentation results at exactly 1 hour may produce inaccurate results.

Procedure with Rationale

Erythrocyte Sedimentation Rate

EQUIPMENT AND SUPPLIES

Hand soap	Timer
Wintrobe tubes	Latex gloves
Sedimentation rack	Biohazard container
Pasteur pipettes (9 inch)	Surface disinfectant
Whole blood sample collected with EDTA	

Assemble equipment.

Wash hands with soap and water. Observe the OSHA Standard for this procedure.

Check the leveling device of the sedimentation rack and make any needed corrections. *Inaccurate readings may result if the rack is not level.*

Invert the blood sample several times before filling the Pasteur pipette. *Upon standing, the red blood cells settle to the bottom of the blood collecting tube.*

Fill the Wintrobe tube to the 0-mm line using the Pasteur pipette and place the tube into the sedimentation rack.

After exactly 1 hour has elapsed, read and record the distance the erythrocytes have settled in millimeters per hour using the scale on the Wintrobe tube. *Time is critical and the reading must be taken at exactly 1 hour to ensure accurate results.*

Clean work area following laboratory protocol.

Remove gloves and wash hands with soap and water.

Questions

Name _____ Date _____

1. Explain the purpose of performing an ESR.

2. Name four factors that have an effect on the sedimentation rate and explain their influence.

3. Explain rouleau formation and how it affects the sedimentation rate.

4. List four pathological conditions that cause an increase in ESR.

5. List the ESR normal values for men, women, and children using the Wintrobe, Westergren, and ZSR methods.

6. Name five technical factors affecting the performance of the ESR and give the rationale.

Terminal Performance Objective

Erythrocyte Sedimentation Rate

Given the necessary equipment, you will be able to perform an erythrocyte sedimentation rate and record the results. This procedure must be completed within 75 minutes and read to a level of accuracy within ±1 mm of your instructor's reading.

INSTRUCTOR'S EVALUATION FORM

Name _____ Date _____

+ = SATISFACTORY   ✓ = UNSATISFACTORY

_____ Assemble equipment.

_____ Wash hands with soap and water. Observe the OSHA Standard for this procedure.

_____ Check the level of the sedimentation rack.

_____ Invert the blood sample several times before filling the Pasteur pipette.

_____ Fill the Wintrobe tube to the 0-mm line using the Pasteur pipette and place the tube into the sedimentation rack.

_____ After exactly 1 hour has elapsed, read and record the distance the erythrocytes have settled in mm/h using the scale on the Wintrobe tube.
       RESULTS: _____

_____ Clean work area following laboratory protocol.

_____ Remove gloves and wash hands with soap and water.

_____ The procedure was completed within 75 minutes.

_____ The reading was correct to within ±1 mm of your instructor's reading.

_____ The results were properly recorded.

Final Competency Evaluation

_____ SATISFACTORY   _____ UNSATISFACTORY

Comments:

Instructor _____ Date _____

Introduction to Clinical Chemistry

20

Learning Objectives
Cognitive Objectives

Blood Chemistry Analytes
Glucose
Cholesterol
Lipoproteins
Blood Urea Nitrogen (BUN)

Blood Chemistry Profiles
Renal Profile
Liver Profile
Lipid Profile
Cardiac Profile

Summary

Questions

LEARNING OBJECTIVES

On completing this chapter, you will be able to:

COGNITIVE OBJECTIVES
- Explain chemical analysis and name the body fluids on which it may be performed.
- Name the reasons for an increased level of glucose in the blood.
- Describe cholesterol and give the reference ranges for total cholesterol found in the blood.
- Describe nitrogen found in the blood and give the reference range for blood urea nitrogen.
- Name several tests performed in a chemistry panel and tell what conditions they determine.
- Define the term "chemistry profile" and name four types of profiles.

Clinical chemistry is the study of the chemical analytes and enzymes found in the body. Chemistry tests are performed on whole blood, serum, plasma, urine, spinal fluid, **synovial fluid**, **pleural fluid**, and pericardial fluids. Most chemistry tests are performed on serum. Serum is the liquid portion of *coagulated* blood. After centrifuging, the blood separates into serum and a red blood cell clot (Fig. 20–1).

Some chemistry tests may be performed on plasma, the liquid portion of *uncoagulated* blood. After centrifuging, blood that has been treated with an anticoagulant separates into plasma, a layer called the **buffy coat**, and a layer of packed red blood cells (Fig. 20–2).

Some chemistry tests are performed on whole blood, that is, capillary or venous blood to which an anticoagulant has been added but which has not been centrifuged. Without an anticoagulant the whole blood will coagulate within 3 to 5 minutes if not tested immediately upon capillary or venous blood collection (see Chapter 8).

> **Synovial fluid:** *the lubricating fluid of the joints*

> **Pleural fluid:** *a serous secretion from the pleural cavity that reduces friction during respiratory movements of the lungs*

> **Buffy coat:** *cellular portion of the blood containing white blood cells and platelets*

BLOOD CHEMISTRY ANALYTES

Glucose

Glucose is a simple six-carbon sugar that cells and tissue use for energy. It is a by-product from the digestion of carbohydrates. Excess glucose is stored in the liver in the form of

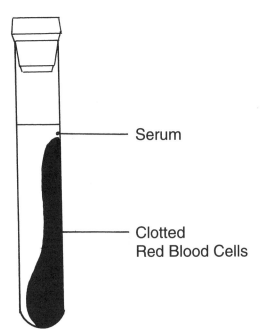

Figure 20–1 After centrifuging, the *coagulated* blood sample separates into serum and clotted red blood cells.

Permeability: *the ability to be penetrated or passed through*

Metabolism: *the sum of all physical and chemical changes that take place within an organism, including all energy and material transformations that occur within living cells*

glycogen. Glycogen is converted into glucose when additional energy is needed by the body.

Two of the many hormones that regulate blood glucose are *glucagon* and *insulin.* Glucagon accelerates the breakdown of glycogen stored in the liver, thereby increasing glucose levels in the blood. Insulin increases the **permeability** of the cell's membrane to glucose, allowing it to be transported into the cells for **metabolism**, thereby decreasing glucose levels in the blood.

When the blood glucose test detects levels outside the reference range, it may be the result of one of the following:

- Inability of the beta cells of the pancreas to produce insulin
- Inability of the intestines to absorb glucose

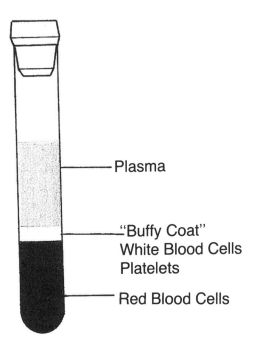

Figure 20–2 After centrifuging, the *uncoagulated* whole blood sample separates into plasma, buffy coat, and packed red blood cells.

- Inability of the liver to accumulate and break down glycogen
- Increased amounts of hormones

Clinical Comment: Diabetes Mellitus

Diabetes mellitus is a chronic disorder of carbohydrate metabolism, characterized by **hyperglycemia** and **glycosuria** resulting from inadequate production or use of insulin. Patients having these symptoms are classified as having type I, insulin-dependent diabetes mellitus (IDDM), or type II, non-insulin-dependent diabetes mellitus (NIDDM). In type I, there is little or no insulin secretion. Type I was previously called juvenile-onset, ketotic, or brittle diabetes. In type II, insulin is produced, but additional insulin is needed to control hyperglycemia. Older terms for type II are maturity-onset, nonketotic, or stable diabetes.

Hyperglycemia: *an increase above the normal level of blood glucose*

Glycosuria: *glucose in the urine*

For more information on blood glucose, refer to Chapter 21.

Cholesterol

Cholesterol is one of several fatty compounds manufactured by the body. It is found in bile, blood, and brain tissue and in the liver, kidneys, and adrenal glands. It is essential for a number of vital body functions, including the manufacture of cell membranes and the protective sheaths of nerve fibers and the production of sex hormones, vitamin D, and bile. Your body produces all the cholesterol it needs, but some additional cholesterol is absorbed from what you eat, particularly if your diet includes foods containing saturated fats.

Cholesterol is a steroid alcohol found in all fat of animal origin, including the fats in meat, in egg yolks, and in milk and other dairy products. In general, the more saturated a fatty acid, the harder or more solid it is at room temperature. The highly saturated animal and butter fats are solid at room temperature; the monounsaturated and polyunsaturated fats found in various vegetable, nut, and seed oils are liquid at room temperature. Saturated fats tend to raise the level of blood cholesterol, whereas monounsaturated fats, such as olive and canola, have been shown to lower the level of blood cholesterol. Polyunsaturated fats, the oils found in corn, sunflower, and safflower seeds and many fish, tend to lower blood cholesterol levels. Too high a cholesterol level is a major risk factor for developing coronary heart disease (CHD).

Clinical Comment: Coronary Heart Disease

Fatty deposits called *plaque* may build up along the inside walls of blood vessels. This may lead to hardening of the arteries (atherosclerosis). This accumulation may decrease or block the flow of blood in the coronary arteries, the vessels that serve the heart. The heart muscle is deprived of oxygen and nutrients. CHD is the largest cause of death in the United States.

Lipoproteins

Recent studies have found that cholesterol circulates in the blood in several different forms. Since water and fat do not mix, cholesterol, a fatty substance, must be carried in blood, a watery substance, by a special protein called a *lipoprotein*. Lipoproteins are manufactured in the liver. Three types of lipoproteins are instrumental in transporting cholesterol in the body. They are classified on the basis of density.

One type, high-density lipoproteins or HDL cholesterol, has the lowest fat content of all the lipoproteins. It seems to protect against atherosclerosis, the accumulation of fatty deposits on blood vessel walls. HDL is known as the "good cholesterol." It removes excess cholesterol from the walls of the blood vessels and carries it to the liver to be excreted. A higher level of HDL has been shown to reduce the risk of CHD.

The other two types, low-density and very low-density lipoproteins (LDL and VLDL cholesterol, respectively), are higher in fat content and are thought to be responsible for the development of atherosclerosis. LDL is known as the "bad cholesterol." It removes cholesterol from ingested saturated fat and from the liver and deposits fat on the walls of the blood vessels causing a build up of plaque. A higher than normal LDL is known to be a risk factor for CHD.

Some people seem to have a genetic predisposition to a higher HDL level, whereas others have a genetic predisposition to a higher LDL level. Vegetarians and people who consume a low-fat diet usually have higher levels of HDL cholesterol. Premenopausal women have higher levels of HDL than men. Athletes, particularly long-distance runners, and others who regularly participate in very vigorous exercise, have higher HDL cholesterol levels.

Total cholesterol levels become higher than normal during the following conditions:

- Bile duct obstruction
- Untreated diabetes mellitus
- **Familial hypercholesterolemia**
- **Hypothyroidism**
- Certain types of kidney disease

Increased levels of cholesterol are associated with increased risk for coronary heart disease. The National Institutes of Health (NIH) has established guidelines on safe levels of cholesterol. The NIH recommends that adults do not exceed a blood cholesterol level of 200 mg/dL (5.2 mmol/L). This is desirable for reducing the risk of CHD. The National Cholesterol Education Program (NCEP) was established to educate the public about desirable levels of blood cholesterol. A recent update of the NCEP's report, presented by the Adult Treatment Panel, emphasizes the importance of LDL cholesterol as a primary risk factor for CHD. Table 20–1 shows cholesterol risk categories and recommendations. Table 20–2 shows the risk categories and recommendations for HDL and LDL levels.

Familial: *with reference to disease, one occurring more frequently in a family than would be expected by chance*

Hypercholesterolemia: *a condition in which there is an excessive amount of cholesterol in the blood*

Hypothyroidism: *a condition caused by a deficiency of thyroid secretion, resulting in a lowered basal metabolism*

Table 20–1 **Cholesterol Risk Categories and Recommendations**

Total Cholesterol Level	Recommendation
Desirable level	
Less than 200 mg/dL (5.2 mmol/L)	Recheck level every 5 years
Borderline high	
200 to 239 mg/dL (5.2–6.2 mmol/L)	Dietary control; recheck level annually
Borderline high with risk factors	
Family history of premature coronary heart disease; cigarette smoking; hypertension; low level of high-density lipoprotein; diabetes; history of stroke; severe obesity	For men with one risk factor, women with two risk factors, or anyone with coronary heart disease, determine level of low-density lipoprotein and initiate stringent dietary program for lowering cholesterol; further treatment with drugs if necessary
High	
240 mg/dL (6.2 mmol/L) or higher	Same as above

Adapted from Taber's Cyclopedic Medical Dictionary, ed 17, FA Davis, Philadelphia, 1993, p 377.

Table 20–2 **HDL and LDL Cholesterol Risk Categories and Recommendations**

Desirable level	HDL 35 mg/dL (0.9 mmol/L) or above
	LDL below 130 mg/dL (3.4 mmol/L)
Borderline high	HDL below 35 mg/dL (0.9 mmol/L)
	LDL 130–159 mg/dL (3.4–4.1 mmol/L)
Borderline high with two or more risk factors	HDL below 35 mg/dL (0.9 mmol/L)
	LDL 130–159 mg/dL (3.4–4.1 mmol/L)
High	HDL below 35 mg/dL (0.9 mmol/L)
	LDL 160 mg/dL (4.1 mmol/L) or above

Adapted from the NCEP Adult Treatment Panel II Report, JAMA 269:3015, 1993.

The concentration of cholesterol in the blood may be below normal in conditions such as **hyperthyroidism**, as well as when levels of estrogen are increased and during malnutrition. The total cholesterol reference values are found in Table 20–3.

Blood Urea Nitrogen (BUN)

Blood urea nitrogen (BUN) is nitrogen found in the blood in the form of urea. The test for BUN measures the nitrogen portion of urea. Urea is formed in the liver and is the end product of protein **catabolism**. Blood carries urea to the kidneys, where it is filtered and excreted into the urine. The amount of urea in the blood is an indication of kidney function, glomerular function, and the liver's ability to produce urea. Higher than normal BUN levels are indicative of serious renal disease and may occur during the following conditions:

- Kidney disease
- Urinary obstruction
- An enlarged prostate
- High fever
- Shock
- Heart failure
- Dehydration
- Infection
- Diabetes

Lower than normal BUN levels occur in liver disease and malnutrition. The reference range for BUN is 6 to 20 mg/dL (2.1–7.1 mmol/L).

Hyperthyroidism: *a condition caused by excessive secretion of the thyroid glands, which increases the basal metabolic rate*

Catabolism: *the process by which complex substances are converted by living cells into simpler substances, with the release of energy*

Table 20–3 **Reference Values for Total Cholesterol**

Age	Values in mg/dL	(mmol/L)
< 25 years	125–200	(3.2–5.2)
25–40 years	140–250	(3.6–6.5)
40–50 years	160–260	(4.1–6.7)
50–65 years	170–265	(4.4–6.9)
> 65 years	175–280	(4.5–7.2)

Note: Values for total cholesterol may vary according to the laboratory performing the test. In addition, values have been found to vary according to sex, race, income level, level of physical activity, dietary habits, and geographic location, as well as in relation to age as shown here.

From Watson, J, and Jaffe, MS: Nurse's Manual of Laboratory and Diagnostic Tests, FA Davis, Philadelphia, 1995, p 183, with permission.

Table 20–4 **Common Laboratory Tests and Indicated Conditions**

Test	Disease or Condition
Acetone	Metabolic acidosis
Acid phosphatase	Prostatic cancer
Alkaline phosphatase	Liver disease
Alanine aminotransferase (ALT)	Liver disease
Amylase and lipase	Acute pancreatitis
Aspartate aminotransferase (AST)	Heart or liver disease
Bilirubin and alkaline phosphatase	Liver function
Blood urea nitrogen (BUN)	Kidney disease
Calcium (Ca), phosphorus (P)	Parathyroid function
Creatine kinase (CK)	Heart disease, myocardial infarction
Cholesterol/triglycerides	Atherosclerosis, CHD
Gamma glutamyl transferase (GGT)	Liver disease, hepatitis
Glucose (FBS), 2 h PPBS, hemoglobin A (glycated hemoglobin)	Diabetes mellitus
Glucose tolerance test (GTT)	Hypoglycemia, diabetes mellitus
Lactate dehydrogenase (LD)	Myocardial infarction, liver disease
Sodium (Na), potassium (K)	Fluid, electrolyte balance
Chloride (Cl), carbon dioxide (CO), blood pH, PO_2, PCO_2	Acid-base balance, respiratory function
Total protein, albumin, globulin, albumin/globulin (A/G) ratio	Cirrhosis, hepatitis, nephrosis, multiple myeloma
Thyroid-stimulating hormone (TSH), triiodothyronine (T_3), thyroxine (T_4)	Thyroid function
Uric acid	Gout

Adapted from Frew, MA, Lane, K, and Frew, D: Comprehensive Medical Assisting: Competencies for Administrative and Clinical Practice, ed 3, FA Davis, Philadelphia, 1995, p 708.

BLOOD CHEMISTRY PROFILES

Test results that deviate from the reference range for a given analyte may indicate abnormalities, a particular disease, or disease conditions. A single blood chemistry test may alert the physician to a possible condition, but usually a set of blood tests called a *profile* or *panel* is necessary to confirm abnormal findings. A chemistry profile is performed on a specimen to identify a disease process or support a clinical diagnosis of a specific disease. Analyzing the results of several chemistry tests assists the physician in diagnosing disease conditions. Table 20–4 lists several laboratory tests and their related disease or condition.

Clinical laboratories have several instruments capable of analyzing these different blood chemistries. See Chapter 5 for more information regarding blood chemistry instruments.

Renal Profile

Electrolytes: *ionized salts in blood, tissue fluids, and cells, including salts of sodium, potassium, and chlorine*

The *renal profile* is a panel of tests for assessing kidney function. The kidneys eliminate waste products, maintain water and **electrolyte** balance, and maintain pH balance of the blood. Renal profiles include such tests as:

- Blood urea nitrogen
- Uric acid
- Creatinine
- Calcium
- Phosphorus
- Sodium
- Potassium
- Chloride

- Total protein
- Albumin
- Albumin/globulin (A/G) ratio

Liver Profile

A *liver profile* is a panel of tests to determine liver function. The liver is important in carbohydrate metabolism, changing glycogen to glucose. The liver is a storage organ for iron, glycogen, vitamins, and other substances. Almost all plasma proteins are produced in the liver, such as albumin, fibrinogen, and lipoproteins. Cholesterol is produced in the liver and used to form bile acid, which emulsifies fats for digestion. The tests in a liver profile include:

- Total cholesterol
- Alkaline phosphatase
- Total bilirubin
- Total protein
- Albumin
- Globulin
- Albumin/globulin (A/G) ratio
- Aspartate aminotransferase (AST), formerly serum glutamic-oxaloacetic transaminase (SGOT)
- Alanine aminotransferase (ALT), formerly serum glutamic-pyruvic transaminase (SGPT)
- Lactate dehydrogenase (LD)

Lipid Profile

A *lipid profile* is a panel of tests for determining the fat content in the blood. Lipids are a group of fats or fatlike substances characterized by their insolubility in water and solubility in organic solvents such as alcohol, ether, and chloroform. Lipids are easily stored in the body and serve as a source of fuel. They are important constituents of cell structure and serve other biological functions. The tests included in the lipid profile are the following:

- Glucose
- Total cholesterol
- Total lipids
- Triglycerides
- Phospholipids
- Lipoprotein fractions HDL/LDL

Cardiac Profile

The *cardiac profile* is a panel of tests for assessing cardiac risk factors for CHD. It also assesses the function of the heart's muscle and the increased level of enzymes following a **myocardial infarction**. The tests included in a cardiac profile are the following:

- Total cholesterol
- HDL cholesterol
- LDL cholesterol
- VLDL cholesterol
- HDL/LDL ratio
- Triglycerides
- Aspartate aminotransferase (AST)
- Lactate dehydrogenase (LD)
- Creatine kinase (CK)

Myocardial infarction: *condition caused by partial or complete occlusion of one or more coronary arteries*

SUMMARY

Blood chemistry tests are very important to the physician for establishing a diagnosis of a disease state and following the course of treatment. Individual chemistry tests are used to screen blood for abnormalities. A profile of tests is performed to assess a patient's health condition. These tests assist the physician in determining a diagnosis by correlating the clinical symptoms with any laboratory test results that are outside the reference range. The medical assistant should know the different chemistry tests and how laboratory test results support the clinical diagnosis of a disease state or condition.

Questions

Name _____   Date _____

1. Differentiate between serum and plasma.

2. Define glucose and name a condition with an increased level of glucose in the blood.

3. Define cholesterol and give the cholesterol risk categories and recommendations.

4. What effect do HDL, LDL, and VLDL cholesterol have on the formation of atherosclerosis?

5. Define blood urea nitrogen and give five reasons for an increased level of blood urea nitrogen.

6. Name 10 tests performed in a chemistry profile and tell what conditions are determined.

Blood Glucose Testing

21

LEARNING OBJECTIVES

On completing this chapter, you will be able to:

COGNITIVE OBJECTIVES
- Explain the function of glucose in the body and describe where it is stored.
- List the two conditions most frequently associated with abnormal blood glucose levels.
- Describe the two major types of diabetes mellitus.
- Explain the glucose tolerance test (GTT).
- Describe the test for glucose from a finger puncture specimen using a glucose monitoring system.
- Explain quality control when testing for blood glucose.

PSYCHOMOTOR OBJECTIVES
- Perform a blood glucose test in accordance with the Terminal Performance Objective presented in the chapter.
- Record the results of the blood glucose test.
- Record the results of the normal and abnormal controls.

AFFECTIVE OBJECTIVES
- Follow the OSHA Standard for disposing of blood samples for the safety of yourself and your coworkers.
- Assume responsibility for a safe laboratory environment.

Glucose, a simple sugar, is the most important carbohydrate in body metabolism and one of the **monosaccharides.** It is required for the production of energy, and it provides fuel for most cells and tissue functions. Glucose is found naturally in many foods. The other monosaccharides are fructose, found in fruit and honey, and lactose, found in milk. Galactose, another monosaccharide, is derived from lactose. Glucose is also called dextrose.

Excess glucose in the body is stored in the liver and muscles as **glycogen,** a carbohydrate, or converted to fat and stored as adipose tissue. When blood glucose levels are low, the stored glycogen is converted back to glucose and returned to the bloodstream.

Monosaccharides: *simple, six-carbon sugars found in many foods*

Glycogen: *the form in which carbohydrate is stored in the body for future conversion into sugar*

Homeostasis: *the condition of a stable environment for cells and tissues*

Hyperglycemia: *an increase above the normal level of blood glucose*

Hypoglycemia: *a decrease below the normal level of blood glucose*

Glycosuria: *glucose in the urine*

Insulin: *a hormone secreted by the beta cells of the islets of Langerhans of the pancreas*

This process is known as *glycogenolysis.* Glycogenolysis is regulated by the hormone *glucagon,* produced by the alpha cells of the islets of Langerhans in the pancreas.

Maintaining **homeostasis** requires control of the level of glucose in the bloodstream. Too high a glucose level results in **hyperglycemia,** and too low a glucose level results in **hypoglycemia.** The blood glucose tests described in this chapter help physicians diagnose and manage disorders that result in hypoglycemia and hyperglycemia. The most prevalent disorder associated with hyperglycemia is diabetes mellitus.

DIABETES MELLITUS

Diabetes mellitus is a disorder of carbohydrate metabolism characterized by hyperglycemia and **glycosuria** resulting from inadequate production or utilization of **insulin.** It occurs when the pancreas is unable to produce enough effective insulin to allow glucose to enter body cells to be used for energy.

Insulin is a hormone produced by the beta cells of the islets of Langerhans in the pancreas. It controls the level of glucose by stimulating cellular uptake of glucose. Insulin is essential for the proper metabolism of glucose and for maintenance of the blood glucose level. Inadequate secretion of insulin results in hyperglycemia. About 5 percent of the population in the United States is afflicted with diabetes mellitus, one of the leading causes of death.

Types of Diabetes Mellitus

There are two types of diabetes mellitus: type I, insulin-dependent diabetes mellitus (IDDM), and type II, non-insulin-dependent diabetes mellitus (NIDDM). Only 5 to 10 percent of diagnosed diabetics are type I. The remaining 90 to 95 percent are type II. Relatives of diabetic patients have a hereditary predisposition to develop diabetes mellitus, and the risk of acquiring diabetes increases in proportion to the number of relatives affected, the severity of their disease, and the closeness of the individual's relationship to the diabetic patient.

Autoimmune disease: *disease in which the body produces antibodies against its own cells*

Retinopathy: *any noninflammatory disease of the retina*

Ketoacidosis: *excessive acidity of body fluids due to an excess of ketone bodies*

Type I diabetics have an **autoimmune disease** involving the destruction of the pancreatic islet beta cells, which results in a lack of sufficient insulin secretion. Their blood glucose levels must be carefully controlled by insulin injection, diet, and exercise. The onset of symptoms may occur early in life. The long-term complications of this form of diabetes include kidney disease, heart attack, stroke, blindness due to diabetic **retinopathy,** and gangrene of the extremities due to narrowing of blood vessels.

Patients with IDDM are more prone to **ketoacidosis.** Since glucose cannot get into the cells because of the lack of insulin, fat cells are used for energy. This breakdown of fat cells produces metabolic by-products called ketone bodies. These acids collect in the bloodstream and contribute to ketoacidosis, which is toxic to the brain.

Type II diabetics generally produce sufficient insulin to prevent ketoacidosis, but not enough to prevent hyperglycemia. It is believed that the beta cells of the pancreas get sluggish and can't release the right amount of insulin at the right time. It is also possible that some kind of antagonist in the blood prevents insulin from helping the cells absorb glucose. Another theory assumes that some cells of the body become resistant to the action of insulin, which prevents the cellular absorption of glucose.

Type II diabetic patients have the tendency to develop the disease after the age of 25. They are frequently obese. There is a higher incidence of NIDDM diabetes among persons who lead a sedentary lifestyle and have a high caloric intake. Treatment includes diet management, exercise, and possibly the use of oral hypoglycemic medication or insulin. Table 21–1 compares the two types of diabetes mellitus.

Insulinoma: *tumor of the islets of Langerhans of the pancreas*

Transient diabetes, such as diabetes that occurs during pregnancy *(gestational diabetes),* acute illness, or steroid therapy, usually lasts only as long as the condition or treatment continues and then subsides. Several medical conditions, such as **insulinoma,** acute hepatic failure, and chronic renal failure, may cause hypoglycemia.

Table 21–1 **Comparison of Type I and Type II Diabetes Mellitus**

	Type I	Type II
Age at onset	Usually under 25	Usually over 25
Type of onset	Abrupt	Gradual
Insulin in blood	Little to none	Usually some
Symptoms	**Polyuria, polydipsia, polyphagia,** weight loss, ketoacidosis	Polyuria, polydipsia, pruritus, peripheral neuropathy
Control	Insulin and diet	Generally diet, sometimes insulin
Vascular and neural changes	Eventually develop	Usually develop
Stability of condition	Fluctuates, difficult to control	Fairly stable, usually easy to control

Polyuria: *excessive secretion and discharge of urine*

Polydipsia: *excessive thirst*

Polyphagia: *excessive food intake*

BLOOD GLUCOSE SCREENING TESTS

Physicians use several different types of blood glucose tests to screen for diabetes mellitus. *Fasting blood sugar (FBS)* tests are performed on blood taken from patients who have been fasting for 12 to 14 hours. The 2-hour *postprandial blood sugar (PPBS)* test is performed on a specimen drawn 2 hours after the patient has eaten a breakfast or lunch of at least 100 g of carbohydrates. Table 21–2 gives the reference values for these blood glucose levels.

A random specimen is one collected from a patient at any time of day without fasting or special diet instructions. A specimen with 200 mg of glucose is indicative of possible diabetes mellitus. A glucose tolerance test (GTT) is performed when values are elevated.

Clinical Comment: Glycated Hemoglobin Test

The *glycated hemoglobin (glycohemoglobin) test* is performed to detect increased levels of glucose. When hemoglobin is exposed to high levels of glucose, the hemoglobin molecule permanently changes, forming hemoglobin A (Hb A_{1c}). This change does not affect the oxygen-carrying ability of hemoglobin and lasts only as long as the red cell lives, approximately 120 days. In diabetes mellitus, when the blood glucose levels are normal and carefully regulated over a long period, the Hb A_{1c} level is normal. If the blood glucose levels have not been monitored and have remained high, the Hb A_{1c} levels will be elevated. The Hb A_{1c} test is an excellent indicator of a diabetic patient's adherence to controlling his or her blood glucose levels over a period of time.

Table 21–2 **Reference Values for Blood Glucose Screening Tests**

	Child	Adult
Fasting Blood Glucose, Values in mg/dL (mmol/L)		
Whole blood	50–90 (2.8–5.0)	60–100 (3.3–5.5)
Serum or plasma	60–105 (3.3–5.8)	70–100 (3.9–5.5)
Two-Hour Postprandial Blood Glucose, Values in mg/dL (mmol/L)		
Whole blood	120 (6.6)	Up to 120 (6.6)
Serum or plasma	150 (8.3)	Up to 140 (7.7)

Values may vary depending on the laboratory method used.
Adapted from Watson, J, and Jaffe, MS: Nurse's Manual of Laboratory Tests, FA Davis, Philadelphia, 1995, pp 148 and 150.

Glucose Tolerance Test (GTT)

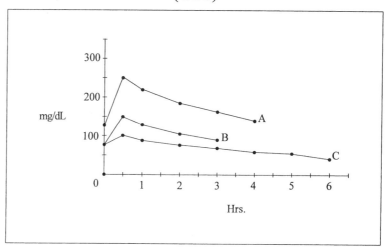

Figure 21–1 Glucose tolerance test curve, showing *(A)* hyperglycemic results, *(B)* normal results, and *(C)* hypoglycemic results.

GLUCOSE TOLERANCE TEST

The *glucose tolerance test* is a series of blood glucose tests that measures the body's response to the ingestion of a large amount of glucose. The patient ingests 1.75 g of glucose per kilogram of body weight or the standard adult dose of 100 g. The GTT includes glucose tests on a fasting specimen taken before the ingestion of a 100-g dose of glucose, on a specimen taken a half hour after taking the glucose, and on 1 to 6 hourly specimens taken thereafter. Urine samples are collected and tested for glycosuria at the same time as the blood samples are drawn.

The number of hourly specimens tested depends on the suspected diagnosis. If hyperglycemia is suspected, the physician orders a 3-hour GTT. If the physician suspects hypoglycemia, he or she orders a 5- or 6-hour GTT. In a patient with hypoglycemia, the glucose challenge triggers the production of insulin, which results in a decrease in the blood glucose. This is demonstrated in the GTT from 4 to 6 hours following the ingestion of glucose (Fig. 21–1).

Clinical Comment: Glycosuria

> Glycosuria occurs when glucose levels are above the **renal threshold,** approximately 160 mg/dL (8.8 mmol/L) to 180 mg/dL (9.9 mmol/L). If glycosuria occurs in the absence of elevated blood glucose levels, renal function abnormalities may exist.

Renal threshold: *the blood concentration at which a substance not normally excreted by the kidneys appears in the urine, e.g., glucose*

The medical assistant administering the GTT should watch the patient for signs or symptoms, such as feeling faint or nauseous. Ask the physician for instructions for terminating the test. Specific instructions regarding termination of the GTT should be established in the medical office and followed exactly.

DETERMINING GLUCOSE LEVELS FROM FINGER PUNCTURE SPECIMENS

Blood glucose may be determined by using only one drop of whole blood from a finger puncture and a blood glucose monitor (BGM). The use of a BGM in the physician's office gives immediate feedback on blood glucose control. The physician may alter the medical regimen at the time of the patient's visit.

Patients also monitor their own blood glucose levels at home using BGMs. It is the responsibility of the medical assistant to teach the patient the proper use of the blood glucose monitoring instrument. It is important for the proper management of the diabetic patient that instructions are thorough and include the use of controls.

One of the instruments used by clinical laboratories, physicians' offices, and outpatient clinics is the HemoCue (Fig. 21–2). The HemoCue blood glucose system measures the total glucose concentration in whole blood and is not influenced by low hemoglobin or hematocrit values. The photometer displays the results within 45 to 240 seconds, depending on blood glucose concentration.

Most instruments are **reflectance photometers.** Refer to Chapter 5 for more information on reflectance photometry. Several models of glucose monitors are available for home use. The Glucometer Elite and Encore Diabetes Care Systems (Fig. 21–3) are available from Bayer Corporation. Other examples of blood glucose monitors are the Accu-Chek Easy and Accu-Chek Advantage (Fig. 21–4) manufactured by Boehringer Mannheim Corporation. The Accu-Chek Easy system is a nonwipe, blood glucose monitor that gives results with time and date in 15 seconds. The Advantage system uses new sensor technology and gives results in 40 seconds. No cleaning is required. The OneTouch system by Lifescan, Inc. (Fig. 21–5) includes everything the patient needs. No timing, wiping, blotting, or washing is necessary and results are displayed in 45 seconds.

Reflectance photometer: *an instrument that detects color changes in the reagent pads*

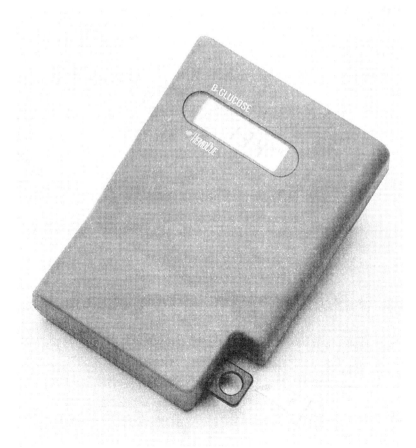

Figure 21–2 HemoCue blood glucose system. (Courtesy HemoCue, Inc., Mission Viejo, Calif.)

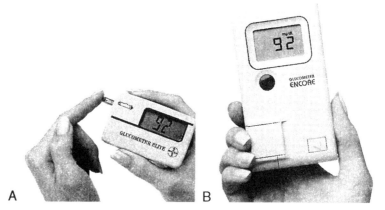

Figure 21–3 *(A)* GLUCOMETER ELITE Diabetes Care System and *(B)* GLUCOMETER ENCORE Diabetes Care System. (Courtesy Bayer Corporation, Diagnostics Division, Elkhart, Ind.)

PATIENT PREPARATION

Instructing the patient in preparation for the blood glucose test and the GTT is the responsibility of the medical assistant. Frequently, the physician recommends a special diet prior to blood glucose determinations. This diet is designed to supply the proper amounts of nutrients needed to obtain an accurate test of how efficiently the body uses carbohydrates. It is important for the patient to be instructed to eat at least the minimum amounts shown on the diet.

QUALITY CONTROL

Quality control includes correct specimen collection, correct identification, accurate reporting of results, and proper maintenance of the glucose monitors. Using normal and abnormal controls for specimen testing and calibrating the instrument verify that the reagents and equipment are working properly. This supports accuracy and checks the performance of the medical assistant. The results of the controls should be entered into a daily log to document quality assurance for the entire process.

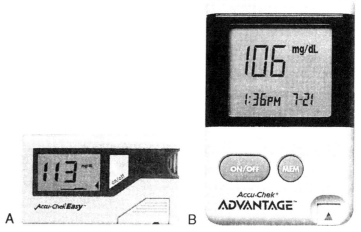

Figure 21–4 *(A)* Accu-Chek Easy and *(B)* Accu-Chek Advantage systems. (Courtesy Boehringer Mannheim Corporation, Indianapolis, Ind.)

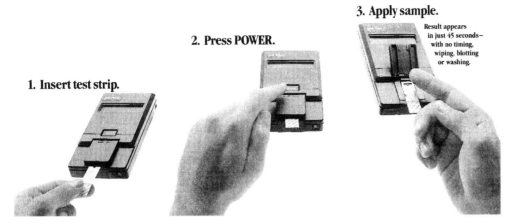

3. Apply sample.

Result appears in just 45 seconds— with no timing, wiping, blotting or washing.

2. Press POWER.

1. Insert test strip.

Figure 21–5 One Touch Profile System. (Courtesy Johnson & Johnson, Mountain View, Calif.)

SUMMARY

Glucose is an important energy source for cell metabolism. The amount of glucose in the blood is regulated by two hormones, glucagon and insulin. Patients with diabetes mellitus are unable to produce enough effective insulin or use the insulin properly to allow cellular absorption of glucose. The result of this imbalance is an elevated blood glucose level. Severe complications develop from too high a level of blood glucose.

PATIENT EDUCATION

- Instruct the patient regarding fasting and special diets for the FBS, 2-hour PPBS, and GTT.

TECHNICAL CONSIDERATIONS

- Calibrate instruments before performing blood glucose determination.
- Use normal and abnormal controls when performing blood glucose determinations.
- If signs or symptoms of fainting or nausea occur during a GTT, follow the protocol for terminating the test.

SOURCES OF ERROR

- Failure to properly store reagent strips and kits or use them before the expiration date may give erroneous results.
- Failure to dry the puncture site after wiping with alcohol may dilute the blood specimen and give erroneous results.

Procedure with Rationale

Blood Glucose Determination

EQUIPMENT AND SUPPLIES

Hand soap	Blood glucose monitor
Latex gloves	Test strips
Automatic lancet	Normal and abnormal controls
Alcohol pad and dry gauze	Biohazard container
Whole blood sample	Surface disinfectant

Assemble equipment.

Wash hands with soap and water. Observe the OSHA Standard for this procedure.

Turn on the instrument.

Calibrate test instrument according to the manufacturer's directions and program the instrument. *Calibrating the test instrument ensures that it is working properly.*

If appropriate, record normal and abnormal control lot number and the test reagent strip lot number. *Recording the lot numbers assures reliability of the testing procedure, a necessary aspect of quality control.*

Perform a blood glucose test on both normal and abnormal controls according to the manufacturer's instructions. *Using normal and abnormal controls verifies that the reagents and equipment are working properly and you are performing the test correctly.*

Record the results of the normal and abnormal controls.

Obtain a large hanging drop of blood from a finger puncture. *If using an alcohol pad, make sure the site is dry before puncturing.*

Bring the reagent strip to the finger and cover the test zones with blood.

Press the timer if appropriate.

Wait the appropriate time according to the manufacturer's directions.

If necessary, wipe or blot the reagent strip with a tissue according to the manufacturer's instructions. *All blood residues must be wiped from the test strips for accuracy of testing, but not too much as to cause inaccurate results.*

Insert the reagent pad into the instrument.

Wait for the appropriate time according to the manufacturer's directions.

Read the blood glucose value from the digital display screen on the instrument and record the results.

Remove the reagent strip and dispose of the sample into a biohazard container.

Turn off the instrument and clean according to the manufacturer's instructions. *Turning off the instrument preserves the batteries.*

Clean work area following laboratory protocol.

Remove gloves and wash hands with soap and water.

Questions

Name _____ Date _____

1. Describe the source and function of insulin.

2. Name a condition characterized by an abnormally low level of blood glucose.

3. Name a condition characterized by an abnormally high level of blood glucose.

4. Give a brief description of the two types of diabetes mellitus.

5. Name the different kinds of glucose tests used to screen for diabetes mellitus.

6. Describe the glucose tolerance test.

7. Describe a method of glucose determination using whole blood from a finger puncture.

8. Describe quality control when testing for blood glucose.

Terminal Performance Objective

Blood Glucose Determination

Given the necessary equipment, you will be able to perform a blood glucose determination and record the results of the test as well as the normal and abnormal controls. This procedure must be completed within 15 minutes and with a level of accuracy within ±5 mg/dL of your instructor's results.

INSTRUCTOR'S EVALUATION FORM

Name _____ Date _____

+ = SATISFACTORY   ✓ = UNSATISFACTORY

_____ Assemble equipment.

_____ Wash hands with soap and water. Observe the OSHA Standard for this procedure.

_____ Turn on the instrument.

_____ Calibrate test instrument according to manufacturer's directions and program the instrument.

_____ If appropriate, record normal and abnormal control ranges, control lot number, and the test reagent strip lot number.
RECORD: _____

_____ Perform blood glucose tests on both normal and abnormal controls.

_____ Record the results of the normal and abnormal controls.
RESULTS: _____

_____ Obtain a large hanging drop of blood from a finger puncture.

_____ Bring the reagent strip to the finger and cover the test zones with blood.

_____ Press the timer if appropriate.

_____ Wait the appropriate time.

_____ If necessary, wipe or blot the reagent strip with a tissue.

_____ Insert the reagent strip into the instrument.

_____ Wait for the appropriate time.

_____ Read the blood glucose value from the digital display screen on the instrument and record the results.   RESULTS: _____

_____ Remove the reagent strip and dispose of the sample into a biohazard container.

_____ Turn off the instrument and clean according to manufacturer's instructions.

_____ Clean work area following laboratory protocol.

_____ Remove gloves and wash hands with soap and water.

_____ The procedure was completed within 15 minutes.

_____ The results were within ±5 mg/dL of the results of your instructor.

_____ The results were properly recorded.

Final Competency Evaluation

____ SATISFACTORY ____ UNSATISFACTORY

Comments:

Instructor _____ Date _____

UNIT
V

MICROBIOLOGY AND IMMUNOLOGY

Introduction to Microbiology

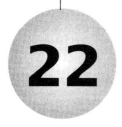

22

Learning Objectives
Cognitive Objectives

Bacterial Nomenclature

Equipment

Culture Media
Additives
Agar
Types of Culture Media

Bacterial Culturing
Pure Culture

Methods of Identification
Bacterial Morphology and Staining
  Characteristics
Biochemical Testing

Colony Counts
Method

Quality Control

Summary

Questions

LEARNING OBJECTIVES

On completing this chapter, you will be able to:

COGNITIVE OBJECTIVES

- Name and briefly describe the organisms of medical interest that are included in the study of microbiology.
- Identify the sites where normal flora reside in the body.
- Describe the procedure for flaming an inoculating loop or needle using a Bunsen burner.
- Explain the function of agar regarding isolating a pure culture.
- Explain the procedure and necessity for isolating a pure culture from a biologic specimen before identification is undertaken.
- Generally describe the morphology of the three major types of bacteria.
- Explain how a colony count is performed and relate this information to urinary tract infections.

Microbiology is the study of all organisms that are too small to be seen with the naked eye. *Medical microbiology* includes all microbial organisms that are capable of causing human diseases. Included in this area of study are **viruses, fungi** (singular, fungus), and **bacteria.**

Viruses are strict intracellular parasites that can replicate only within a living cell. This complex viral requirement precludes POLs from culturing viruses. However, immunologic methods of laboratory testing are quite simple and some tests for viral diseases can be performed in POLs (Chapter 24).

Fungi are infrequent causes of disease, but their importance should not be minimized. Some fungal diseases have a high mortality rate. Moreover, they are often misdiagnosed because they resemble bacterial diseases. Historically, laboratories offered little more than minimal **mycological** services. However, the emergence of HIV infections and the growing number of procedures that cause a suppression of the immune system have increased medical interest in fungal diseases.

> **Viruses:** *minute organisms that are entirely dependent on another cell for nutrient and reproductive needs, without which they are considered nonliving*

> **Fungi:** *A class of plant-like organisms that includes molds and yeast*

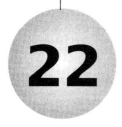

305

Bacteria: *one-celled organisms that lack a nuclear membrane and have a cell wall that provides a consistency of form*

Mycological: *pertaining to the study of fungi*

Sign: *any objective evidence or manifestation of an illness*

Symptom: *any perceptible change in the body or its functions that indicates disease*

Genus: *a taxonomic division between the species and the family*

Species: *the taxonomic group just below genus*

Sterilized: *rendered free from microorganisms, including spores*

Bunsen burner: *a gas burner that has an adjustable flame that can be regulated by altering the amount of air that is mixed with gas*

Incineration: *destruction by fire*

POLs perform relatively few procedures regarding the diagnosis of fungal infections except for direct examination of clinical specimens using wet mount preparations (Chapter 9) and collection of mycological specimens for transport.

Medical bacteriology is the science that is concerned with the isolation, identification, and control of bacteria that cause human diseases. Bacteria include a variety of single-cell microscopic organisms (microorganisms) found virtually everywhere. Some types of bacteria reside in and on a human host. Most have a neutral effect, neither helping nor harming the host. Some of them are beneficial and essential to life. Neutral and "friendly" bacteria residing in or on a host are called *flora,* or *normal flora.* Flora are found on the skin and mucous membranes and in some parts of the respiratory, gastrointestinal, and genitourinary systems. As long as each type of flora remains in the area where it is normally found and as long as their number remains within acceptable limits, no harm comes to the host. When either of these conditions changes, pathology may result.

Organisms capable of causing disease are called *pathogens.* Some microbial diseases manifest characteristic features in their host called **signs** and **symptoms.** Frequently, diagnosis is based on identifying these signs and symptoms. Some microbial diseases produce signs and symptoms that are very general or that mimic other diseases. Thus, the only way to determine the cause of the disease is to identify the pathogen.

BACTERIAL NOMENCLATURE

Bergey's Manual of Determinative Bacteriology (edited by Krieg and Holt) is the definitive source in naming and classifying bacteria. As with other living organisms, only the **genus** and **species** names are used to designate a given bacterium. For example, a common bacterium of the colon is *Escherichia coli; Escherichia* is the genus name, and *coli* is the species name. The genus and species names are either underlined or italicized. The genus name begins with a capital letter, and the species name begins with a lowercase letter. Frequently, just the initial of the genus is given, followed by the species name, for example, *E. coli.*

EQUIPMENT

Special wires called *inoculating loops* and *inoculating needles* are used to transfer specimens for bacterial studies. They are made of platinum or nicrome wire inserted into a handle. They can be **sterilized** by passing the loop or needle through the flame of a **Bunsen burner.**

A Bunsen burner produces a blue flame with a colorless cone in the center. The blue portion of the flame is extremely hot and may cause spattering of live bacteria into the air. This most frequently occurs when moist material is on the loop as it is placed in the blue flame. This can be very dangerous when working with pathogens. The cone is much cooler and does not cause spattering. Instead, bacteria are destroyed by heat-drying, followed by the actual **incineration** of the bacteria in the blue portion of the flame. Follow the steps listed below to flame an inoculating loop or wire properly using a Bunsen burner.

- Place the loop in the colorless cone of the flame for a few seconds to heat-kill live bacteria.
- When all the microorganisms have been heat-killed, pass the loop into the blue portion of the flame to incinerate any residual material (Fig. 22–1).
- Next hold the wire approximately perpendicular in the blue flame so that most of the wire glows red.
- Finally, allow the loop to cool momentarily before you use it for additional transfers.

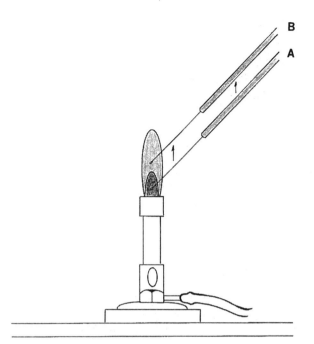

Figure 22–1 To avoid spattering of live bacteria, *(A)* insert the loop into the cone to heat-kill any bacteria. *(B)* Next, move loop to blue portion of flame to incinerate any remaining material.

Some states require the use of electric incinerators rather than Bunsen burners. These devices protect against spattering that occurs if the flaming procedure is not properly performed. Sterile, prepackaged disposable loops are available that can be discarded after a single use. This is especially convenient in small offices or offices that are not fitted with gas outlets for Bunsen burners.

CULTURE MEDIA

Culture media (singular, medium) are nutrient substances used to grow bacteria for laboratory studies. They must contain all the essential nutrients required by the organism for it to grow and reproduce. Culture media may be either in a liquid state (broth) or solid state. A general nutrient broth used to culture bacteria contains meat extracts, **peptone,** and mineral salts (sulfates, chlorides, and calcium and sodium phosphates). Most pathogenic bacteria require carbohydrates and a source of nitrogen along with some **micronutrients** in order to survive outside the host.

Peptone: *water-soluble nitrogen compound*

Micronutrients: *small quantities of substances necessary for metabolism*

Additives

Bacteria differ widely in their nutritional requirements. Some are very **fastidious** and additional substances must be added to the media. Others require only a very simple medium for growth. *Escherichia coli* is a nonfastidious organism. It has simple nutritional needs. It can synthesize most of its metabolic requirements from media that contain ammonium sulfate, glucose, and salts. On the other hand, *Neisseria gonorrhoeae* is a fastidious organism. In addition to the above nutrients, it requires blood serum, various amino acids, vitamins, and an atmosphere high in carbon dioxide.

Fastidious: *precise nutritional and environmental requirements for growth and survival*

Agar

In a broth culture, bacteria diffuse throughout the entire solution. Adding *agar,* a seaweed product, to the broth causes it to solidify to the consistency of gelatin. On a solid medium, bacteria grow in *colonies,* masses or clones of bacteria, visible to the naked eye.

Using a solid medium dispensed in a **Petri dish,** the laboratorian can determine the appearance of the colony with respect to its size, texture, color, and shape to help identify the organism.

Types of Culture Media

Culture media may be divided into the following categories:

- Selective media
- Isolation media
- Enrichment media
- Maintenance media
- Differential media

Depending on the needs of the physician, the type of specimen, the area of the body from which the specimen was obtained, and the tentative diagnosis, one or more of these media types will be inoculated by a knowledgeable bacteriologist for culturing the specimen. Media selection for bacteriologic studies is beyond the scope of this text.

BACTERIAL CULTURING

Culturing bacteria entails establishing a microbial population on a suitable medium that can support its growth and reproduction. Medical bacteriology consists of establishing microbial growth from a clinical specimen (throat culture, wound exudate, urine, blood, etc.) in order to identify a suspected pathogen. Microbiologists culture bacteria for one or more of the following reasons:

- To identify a particular organism
- To establish a diagnosis of infection by determining the number of organisms in a body specimen
- To determine the susceptibility of a pathogen to a particular antibiotic using sensitivity testing

The growing or culturing of bacteria from biologic specimens is important in diagnosing and treating disease conditions.

Pure Culture

Since pathogens are frequently associated with normal flora in many biologic specimens, it is often necessary to separate or isolate the pathogen from the flora. This means physically separating microorganisms from each other so that individual bacterial cells are segregated and allowed to form a clone or colony of a single microbial type on a Petri dish. This clone or colony is called a *pure culture* since each cell is genetically the same. Each individual bacterial cell from a pure culture will appear and react in the same manner, a feature that facilitates identifying the bacteria. Without a pure culture, erroneous identification will result.

In the streak plate method for isolation, the laboratorian uses an inoculating loop or needle to spread the bacterial specimen (inoculum) across a solid medium in a defined pattern (Fig. 22–2). By flaming the loop periodically during the streaking, the number of viable organisms decreases. Ideally, individual bacteria will be deposited over a portion of the medium and each bacterial cell will give rise to an isolated colony (Fig. 22–3).

The ability to isolate a pure culture relies on the fact that bacteria reproduce by the process of **binary fission.** In each generation the total number of cells doubles, that is, 1, 2, 4, 8, 16, and so forth. In time, the once invisible bacterium has reproduced sufficiently that the total number of cells present appears as a colony or clone of the original cell.

Types of Streak Patterns

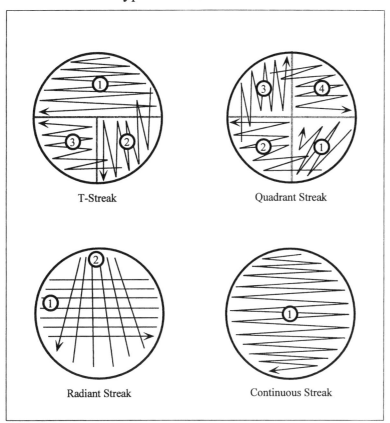

Figure 22–2 Various streaking patterns used to isolate colonies. The inoculating needle is flamed at each change in direction.

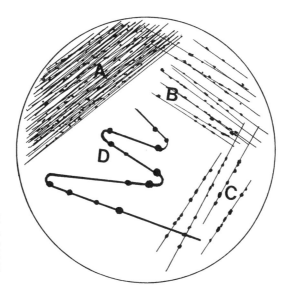

Figure 22–3 Agar plate showing isolated colonies. *(A)* Area A shows no isolated colonies. *(B)* Area B shows a thinning in the number of microorganisms. *(C)* Area C shows several isolated colonies. *(D)* Area D shows a few isolated colonies.

Once a pure culture is obtained, a number of laboratory methodologies may be used to identify the type of bacteria in the pure culture.

METHODS OF IDENTIFICATION

Identification of a bacterial species often relies on one or more of the following laboratory techniques:

- Directly observing the bacteria using the microscope to determine morphology and staining characteristics
- Biochemical reactions
- Serologic methods (discussed in Chapter 24)
- Inoculating a test animal (infrequently performed in medical microbiology)

BACTERIAL MORPHOLOGY AND STAINING CHARACTERISTICS

A prepared smear of bacteria provides the opportunity to observe size, distribution, cellular features, and staining characteristics of bacteria. Each of these features can provide valuable information as to the identity of the organism. Individual bacterial cells have one of three general shapes: sphere, rod, or spiral. Figure 22–4 illustrates these three general shapes and their subtypes.

Spherical bacteria are known as *cocci* (singular, coccus), a Latin word that means "berry." Cocci are able to assume a variety of arrangements depending on the method in which the cells divide. A knowledge of these arrangements can help in identifying an unknown organism because certain groupings may be characteristic of a specific genus. Among the most common arrangements for cocci are:

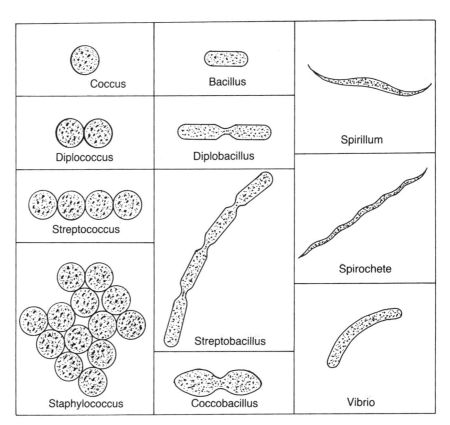

Coccus

Bacillus

Diplococcus

Diplobacillus

Spirillum

Streptococcus

Streptobacillus

Spirochete

Staphylococcus

Coccobacillus

Vibrio

Figure 22–4 Bacterial shapes and arrangements.

- Diplococci—pairs of cocci
- Streptococci—chains of four or more cocci
- Staphylococci—irregular grapelike clusters of cocci

Rodlike organisms are called *bacilli* (singular, bacillus). Bacilli have a greater range in size than the cocci. Some have blunt ends, while others have tapered ends. Some bacilli appear broad and oval, closely resembling cocci; accordingly, they are called *coccobacilli.* Although bacilli may occur singly, in pairs *(diplobacilli)*, or in short or long chains *(streptobacilli)*, bacterial arrangement is usually not a distinguishing feature for identifying bacilli.

The spiral bacteria include three types of organisms. The *vibrios* resemble curved rods or commas; the *spirilla* (singular, spirillum) resemble rigid spirals or corkscrews; and the *spirochetes* resemble spirals and move by flexing and wiggling.

Biochemical Testing

Bacteria are frequently identified by their metabolic activities. This method of identification is called *biochemical testing*. Various sugars may be added to the basic medium along with chemical indicators to determine if and how a species of bacteria uses a particular sugar in metabolic reactions. Other substances such as nitrates, gelatin, amino acids, starches, and fats can also be added to basic media to identify differences in metabolic activity. By observing changes in these additives, the metabolic capabilities of the bacteria are identified. Using various media, the laboratorian determines the nutrients used and waste products produced by the organism. These findings are called *metabolic characteristics.*

COLONY COUNT

A *colony count* determines the number of bacteria present in a specimen. It is commonly used to diagnose urinary tract infections (UTIs). Urine is normally sterile in the bladder but frequently picks up normal flora as it passes from the body. Because all voided urine samples contain some bacteria, a physician usually diagnoses a UTI based on the number of bacteria present in the sample. A fresh urine specimen from a healthy individual collected by a clean-catch technique (Chapter 7) usually contains fewer than 10,000 bacteria per mL. Concentrations of bacteria greater than 100,000 per mL in a clean-catch specimen may indicate infection. When the number of bacteria falls between these two figures, the results are inconclusive and it is necessary to obtain another sample of urine from the patient and retest it.

Clinical Comment: Urinary Tract Infections

A number of factors predispose the urinary tract to infection. Urine provides abundant nutrients that support microbial growth. Any time urine is not completely voided from the bladder but accumulates for long periods of time, there is a chance that a UTI will develop. UTIs are common in women and young girls because the urethra is relatively short (1.5 inches compared with 8.0 inches for males) and the urethral opening lies in close proximity to the vagina and rectum, both of which contain large numbers of normal flora. Serologic tests show that most bacteria responsible for a UTI are derived from the patient's own intestinal tract.

Physicians often request a colony count when the results of the nitrite and leukocyte reaction on the reagent are positive to confirm bladder infections.

A bladder infection is almost always caused by a single bacterial strain, rarely more than one. If more than two different types of bacteria are present, the sample is probably contaminated and another sample from the patient should be retested.

Method

A colony count is based on the assumption that each viable organism in a sample will give rise to a single colony of bacteria. By culturing a measured amount of a specimen and counting the colonies that grow after an incubation period, the number of organisms in the sample can be determined. Manufacturers produce a variety of products for POL use that provide quantitative or semiquantitative methods for determining bacterial colony counts. One product provides a kit that contains a paddle impregnated with media. The paddle is dipped into the urine specimen and later observed for colony growth. The kit contains certificates that verify quality control requirements. Most colony count kits available for POL use are deemed moderate complexity tests.

QUALITY CONTROL

When microbiology testing is undertaken in physicians' offices, quality control must be maintained. Media are especially vulnerable to unwanted changes that negatively influence the results of microbial testing. Follow these guidelines regarding media handling and storage:

- Store media in accordance with the manufacturer's directions.
- Do not use media that exceed the expiration date.
- Inspect all media on arrival and before use. Notify the manufacturer and do not use the media for testing if any of the following characteristics are noted:
  - Cracks in the Petri dishes or media
  - Lumpy or uneven filling of the Petri dish
  - Hemolysis on sheep's blood agar plates
  - Discoloration of the media
  - Contamination
  - Evidence of freezing
  - Bubbles in the media
- Test the medium with a known organism to ensure that it is able to support the growth of the intended organism. (Many producers of bacterial media perform this test before shipping media to customers.)
- Maintain all records on media used for testing.

SUMMARY

In order to treat a patient properly, the physician may need to identify the pathogen causing the disease. Identifying bacterial strains generally begins with preparing a direct smear to observe morphology, staining characteristics, and cellular structures. Further identification involves performing biochemical tests using various media. Other methods for identification include serologic tests and animal inoculations.

Because a great amount of interpretive judgment is needed for bacterial identification, most specimens are sent to referral laboratories. Medical assistants help in specimen collection, processing, and transport (Chapter 9). They should know all specimen requirements before beginning any procedure. If specimens are not properly obtained, the results may be invalid.

Questions

Name _____ Date _____

1. Name and briefly describe the microorganisms associated with human disease.

2. What are normal flora; which body sites contain flora, and when do they cause disease?

3. What are bacterial media? What are some of the components of media?

4. What is agar and when is it used?

5. Briefly describe the proper procedure for flaming an inoculating loop or needle using a Bunsen burner.

6. What is a pure culture? How is it obtained?

7. Why is it necessary to isolate a pure culture from a biologic specimen before identification of the bacterial strain?

8. List two methods used to identify bacteria and briefly describe them.

9. Briefly describe the general morphologic types of bacteria.

10. What is a colony count? What type of sample is needed? How is it performed?

Bacterial Smear Preparation and Gram Stain

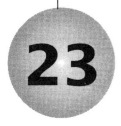

LEARNING OBJECTIVES

On completing this chapter, you will be able to:

COGNITIVE OBJECTIVES
- List five reasons for preparing a bacterial smear.
- List several morphologic characteristics that are used to identify bacteria.
- Give three characteristics of a properly prepared bacterial smear.
- List the reagents in the Gram stain and give the resulting color obtained for gram-negative and gram-positive organisms at each step of the procedure.
- Explain why the Gram stain is important in clinical medicine.

PSYCHOMOTOR OBJECTIVES
- Prepare a bacteriologic smear following the Terminal Performance Objective presented in this chapter.
- Gram stain a prepared smear following the Terminal Performance Objective presented in this chapter.

AFFECTIVE OBJECTIVES
- Recognize the importance of carefully handling any microbial specimens obtained in the physician's office.
- Recognizing that patient specimens may inadvertently infect coworkers, carefully follow all OSHA guidelines regarding cleanup and disposal of organisms.

The most common procedure performed in a bacteriology laboratory is the Gram stain. This procedure requires a well-made bacterial smear for the accuracy of the Gram stain reaction. Medical assistants frequently prepare bacterial smears and Gram stain the slides. The actual "reading" of the slides and interpretation of the results are undertaken by the physician or specially trained personnel.

Preparing a bacterial smear involves transferring bacteria to a glass slide and readying it for staining and microscopic examination. Physicians and microbiologists use bacterial smears to:

Morphologic characteristics: *size, shape, and arrangement*

- Demonstrate **morphologic characteristics**
- Determine staining characteristics
- Diagnose by direct smear
- Demonstrate the purity of a culture
- Determine appropriate media for culturing

In some physicians' offices, smears are prepared on uncentrifuged urine specimens. The finding of bacteria on the smear following a Gram stain is suggestive of a urinary tract infection. Smears are also prepared in some POLs in suspected cases of nonspecific vaginitis in female patients and genital discharge in male patients.

THE BACTERIAL SMEAR

Morphologic Characteristics

The morphologic characteristics important for identifying bacteria include:

- Shape—whether the bacteria are cocci, bacilli, or spirilla
- Arrangement—how the bacteria are grouped together
- Structural features—such as flagella, capsules, and spores

Chapter 22 discussed the classification of bacteria by shape and arrangement (see Fig. 22–4).

Other identifying features (Fig. 23–1) associated with bacteria include:

- *Flagella,* whiplike projections used for locomotion
- *Capsules,* outer coverings or coats
- *Spores,* inert stage of some bacteria.

Pathogenicity: *the ability to cause disease*

Whether an organism has flagella, and where and how they are positioned on the cell, can help to identify a bacterium. Capsules protect the organism from phagocytosis. These coats are also associated with **pathogenicity.** When the coat is removed, most bacteria lose their ability to cause disease. With the proper staining procedures, capsules are visible during microscopic observation. Their presence helps in identification.

Vegetative: *the growing or reproducing phase of a bacterium*

Some bacteria produce spores as a protection against a hostile environment. Spores are resistant to heat, cold, chemicals, and dry conditions. When the environment again becomes benign, spores revert to the **vegetative** form and are capable of reproduction. Spores are believed to be the most resistant form of life.

Staining to demonstrate bacterial structures such as flagella, capsules, and spores is somewhat complicated and not generally performed in POLs. However, medical assistants should know these important structures and the functions they provide.

Staining Characteristics

The bacterial smear provides an opportunity to observe the staining affinity of microorganisms. Classification of bacteria depends, to a great extent, on the Gram stain reaction. Other specialized stains, especially acid-fast stain, assist in classifying and identifying bacteria.

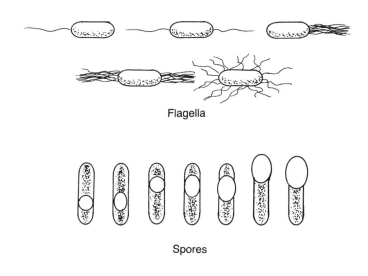

Flagella

Spores

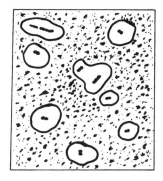

Figure 23-1   Characteristic features of some bacteria include flagella, spores, and capsules.

Capsules

Diagnosis by Direct Smear

A direct smear is one made from a clinical specimen, rather than from media after it has been inoculated with the specimen. In some cases an experienced physician can diagnose a disease by examining a direct smear after taking into consideration a complete clinical picture. The presence of certain bacteria from a specific body site sometimes gives sufficient evidence of a particular disease, and immediate treatment may be undertaken. For example, a preliminary Gram stain report showing gram-negative diplococci within polymorphonuclear cells from an urethral discharge of a symptomatic male is strongly suggestive of gonorrhea and treatment can begin immediately. It is always necessary to confirm any diagnosis made by direct smear with follow-up laboratory testing.

Culture Purity and Appropriate Media

The bacterial smear helps to establish the purity of a culture. A pure culture shows bacterial cells with the same general morphology and staining characteristics. A pure culture is usually required if other bacterial tests are ordered. Finally, the bacterial smear may be used to determine appropriate culture media and determine what further testing may be required to identify an organism.

Types of Specimens

A bacterial smear may be made from three different types of specimens: a broth culture, a colony growing on a solid medium, or a clinical specimen (uncentrifuged urine, wound exudate, urethral discharge, etc.).

In a broth culture, bacteria are in solution. Some bacteria disperse throughout the entire tube. Some grow primarily at the bottom of the tube, and others grow at the top, depending on their affinity for oxygen. When preparing a smear, it is always necessary to disperse bacteria so that the culture appears homogenous before removing any bacteria.

Most bacteria require a supply of environmental gases in order to survive. The plastic caps inverted over culture tubes protect against contamination but do not tighten securely. They allow oxygen from the atmosphere to enter the tube. Therefore, do not invert or shake broth cultures when redispersing the organisms. Instead, hold the tube between the palms of your hands and roll it back and forth until all the bacteria are evenly dispersed throughout the medium. Commercially prepared media have screw caps; these must remain loose after inoculation for gas exchange.

When preparing a smear from a broth culture, a minimum two loopfuls of broth culture are needed to obtain sufficient organisms for observation. When growth is scanty, a larger sample is required.

When preparing a smear from a solid agar medium, "pick" a very small amount of bacteria from an isolated colony using an inoculating needle or loop. Remember, preparing a smear from a colony of bacteria produces a smear that is very concentrated. Beginning students frequently use too much bacteria when making a smear from a colony.

After removing a small amount of bacteria from an isolated colony, suspend the organisms in a loopful of distilled water that you have previously placed on a clean glass slide. Because bacteria tend to cling to each other when growing in colonies, gently "stir" the organisms into the water and continue to rotate the needle until you see a very slight cloudiness in the drop of water.

The third type of smear is one that is made directly from a clinical specimen. Frequently the specimen is collected using a sterile swab, but some specimens are collected using a sterile syringe, especially in a deep wound in which **obligate anaerobic bacteria** are often found.

Direct smears are frequently prepared to determine some sexually transmitted diseases (STDs), especially gonorrhea in male patients. The presence of gram-negative diplococci (GNDC) in pus cells in a urethral discharge from a male patient is suggestive of gonorrhea. Because of normal flora present in the vaginal tract, the presence of GNDC in exudate of a female is not diagnostic. A culture or other testing procedures must be performed to diagnose gonorrhea in the female patient.

A smear from a clinical specimen should be made immediately. Any delay may cause erroneous results. When both a culture and a Gram stain are requested from the same specimen, the culture is inoculated *before* the Gram stain is prepared.

Obligate anaerobic bacteria: *bacteria that must not be exposed to atmospheric oxygen or death will result*

BACTERIAL SMEAR PREPARATION

Liquid Culture Media

With a wax pencil, draw a circle in the center of the underside of a clean glass slide. This provides a target and makes it easier to find the organisms when observing the smear using the microscope. Gently rotate the broth culture tube between the palms of the hands to disperse the organisms. The medium should have a homogenous appearance before removing any bacteria. Use aseptic technique for removing the specimen from the broth culture. Hold the culture tube in the nondominant hand and the loop in the dominant hand. Grasp the cap using the baby finger and palm of the dominant hand. Flame the mouth of the culture tube by briefly passing it through the flame of the Bunsen

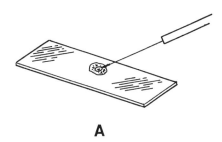

A

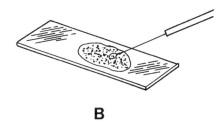

B

Figure 23–2 Preparation of a smear from a liquid culture medium. *(A)* Place 2 or 3 loopfuls of inoculum on a glass slide. *(B)* Spread the inoculum over a large area of the slide using the inoculating loop. *(C)* Allow the slide to air-dry.

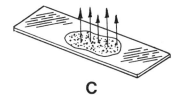

C

burner. Insert a sterile loop into the culture and remove a loopful of inoculum. Reflame the mouth of the tube. Replace the cap and return the culture tube to the rack. Transfer the inoculum to the glass slide above the circle and gently rotate the loop until the sample covers the entire circle. Use a circular motion as you spread the sample on the slide. This helps to disperse the bacteria on the slide. Reflame the loop making sure there is no spattering of the organism. Remember to place the loop in the cone of the Bunsen burner flame to heat-kill the bacteria, before placing the loop in the blue part of the flame.

   Repeat this entire procedure, because you need at least two loopfuls of broth culture to ensure that enough bacteria are present to facilitate finding them with the microscope. In a broth culture showing very little bacterial growth, you may need as many as three or four loopfuls of inoculum to prepare a good smear. Flame the loop each time you enter the broth so that you do not introduce contaminating bacteria to the culture. Allow the slide to air-dry (Fig. 23–2).

Solid Culture Media

When preparing a smear from a solid culture medium, select a single isolated colony growing on a Petri dish. A Petri dish is correctly positioned when the media side of the Petri dish is uppermost and sits on the lid.

   Use a wax pencil to draw a target circle on the underside of a clean glass slide to facilitate finding the organisms when using the microscope. Place a loopful or two of distilled water in the center of the circle. The water is used to disperse a small sample of inoculum. Follow aseptic technique when you remove inoculum from the Petri dish. Flame the inoculating loop or needle and allow it to cool momentarily. Lift the media side of the

Petri dish and locate an isolated colony. Next remove a very small amount of the colony using a sterile loop or needle. Close the Petri dish. Using a circular motion, mix the inoculum in the water. You should see a very slight **turbidity.** The beginning student often uses too much culture, causing atypical staining reactions and morphologic features. Reflame the inoculating loop in the manner described previously. Remember, moist inoculum on a loop may spatter live bacteria into the air. Allow the slide to air-dry.

> **Turbidity:** *slight cloudiness*

Clinical Specimen

Direct microscopic examination of a Gram-stained smear from a clinical specimen (urethral, nasopharyngeal, wound, etc.) often provides preliminary identification of an organism. Physicians generally collect most microbial specimens from their patients. Occasionally the laboratorian collects throat cultures. Throat culture collection is described more fully in Chapter 9.

Use only sterile swabs to collect any clinical specimen for bacterial studies. Swabs collected for diagnosis of gonorrhea should be inoculated to the medium immediately by the person collecting the specimen, then the smear should be made. In a clinic setting the physician performs these tasks in the examination room. Make sure the medium is at room temperature before inoculation.

Roll the swab over the center of the slide, but do not go over the same area twice (Fig. 23–3). Be sure a rolling motion is used. The smear must not be so thick that the presence of pus cells interferes with the proper interpretation of the reading, or so thin that false negatives occur. Allow the slide to air-dry.

Handle all specimens carefully. Show concern for fellow employees and patients. Wipe specimen containers with a disinfectant and keep lids securely in place to protect others against exposure to potential pathogens. Incinerate or autoclave contaminated material after cleanup. When in doubt, check OSHA requirements.

HEAT FIXING

Slides that are prepared for staining must withstand several rinsings during the staining procedure without the loss of organisms. *Heat fixing* is a procedure that partially **Coagulates** bacterial protein, causing the bacteria to cling to the slide. Once they are heat fixed, you can stain them without the loss of the organism.

> **Coagulates:** *gels or solidifies*

After the slide is completely dry, quickly pass it through the flame of the Bunsen burner two or three times, smear side up. Slide forceps should be used for this procedure. Overexposure to heat distorts the bacterial cells and often alters staining reactions. Underexposure to heat fails to coagulate sufficient bacterial protein, and organisms will be washed off the slide during the staining process.

Some POLs are not equipped with gas outlets for Bunsen burners. In an alternate method, apply ethyl alcohol to the slide and let it air-dry. Again, bacterial protein partially coagulates, causing bacteria to adhere to the slide.

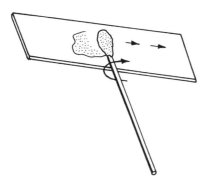

Figure 23–3 Preparation of a slide from a clinical specimen collected using a sterile swab.

THE PROPERLY MADE BACTERIAL SMEAR

A properly prepared smear should withstand one or more washings during staining without dislodging the organisms from the slide. The smear should also show accurate morphology and staining features. A smear that is too thick shows atypical staining and morphology. If the smear is too thin, meaningful data are lost. Finally, in a properly made bacterial smear there should not be excessive distortion or shrinking of the organisms.

STAINING

Three major types of stains are used in the study of microorganisms: *simple stains, special stains,* and *differential stains.* Simple stains reveal size, shape, and arrangement of bacteria after cell division. Special stains are used for observing capsules, flagella, spores, and certain internal cellular details. Differential stains reveal chemical differences in bacterial structures.

The Gram stain, developed in 1884 by a Danish physician, Hans C. J. Gram, is perhaps the most important stain used in bacteriology. This stain divides true bacteria into two physiologic groups, gram-positive and gram-negative. The staining differences of these two groups reflect a fundamental difference in the chemical composition of the cell wall. Many other properties of the bacteria correlate with the chemical structure of the cell wall. Knowing the staining characteristics of an organism provides considerable information about the bacteria, including the selection of an antibiotic.

Almost all bacteria have a surrounding wall composed of a compound called **peptidoglycan.** In gram-positive bacteria, the peptidoglycan wall is very thick. Gram-negative bacteria have a very thin peptidoglycan layer. However, gram-negative bacteria have thick layers of lipoprotein and lipopolysaccharides that surround the thin peptidoglycan layer. These lipoprotein and lipopolysaccharide layers are not found in the gram-positive bacteria.

> **Peptidoglycan:** *a chemical structure found in the walls of bacteria*

The Gram Stain Procedure

OVERVIEW

In the Gram stain procedure four reagents are applied to the slide, one at a time. The end result is that gram-positive organisms show a dark purple color and the gram-negative organisms show a pink or red color. The steps in the procedure include:

- Staining a heat-fixed bacterial smear with crystal violet (also known as gentian violet), coloring all bacterial cells purple
- Applying Gram's iodine, which acts as a **mordant,** firmly attaching the crystal violet to the peptidoglycan
- Decolorizing the smear with ethyl alcohol, removing crystal violet from the cells that do not have thick walls of peptidoglycan (gram-negative cells)
- Flooding the smear with a counterstain (usually safranin), which dyes the decolorized gram-negative cells a contrasting color (pink or red)

> **Mordant:** *a substance that hardens or binds*

After the final water rinse, blot the slide dry using **bibulous** paper. Examine the slide using the oil-immersion lens. The microscopic examination of the slide will enable the observer to distinguish between gram-positive (purple) and gram-negative (pink or red) cells.

> **Bibulous:** *possessing the ability to absorb*

DETAILED INSTRUCTIONS

Place a heat-fixed bacterial smear on a staining rack and flood it with gentian violet or crystal violet (Fig. 23–4). Allow it to stand for 60 seconds. Wash the dye off using a wash bottle or a gentle flow of water from a tap. Do not pour the stain off the slide, but wash it

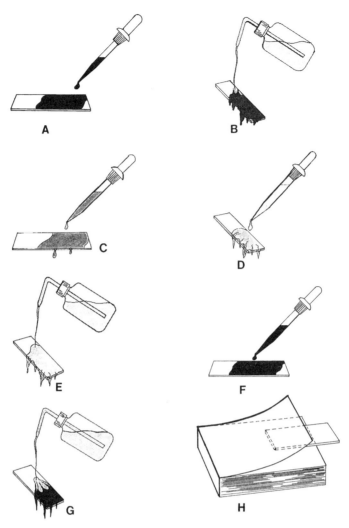

Figure 23–4 Steps in the Gram stain procedure. *(A)* Cover the smear with crystal violet for 1 minute. *(B)* Hold slide at a 45° angle and wash off crystal violet with flowing water. *(C)* Apply Gram's iodine to the smear for 1 minute. *(D)* Hold slide at 45° angle and allow 95% ethyl alcohol to flow over the slide until purple color no longer flows from the slide (usually less than 15 sec). *(E)* Immediately stop decolorization by allowing water to flow over the slide. *(F)* Cover the smear with safranin for about 1 minute. *(G)* Hold slide at a 45° angle and wash off safranin. *(H)* Blot slide with bibulous paper.

off with flowing water. This decreases the precipitation of stain on the slide. Next, flood the smear with Gram's iodine for 60 seconds. The violet dye and the iodine form a dye-iodine complex that is retained by gram-positive organisms (those with thick walls of peptidoglycan) during the decolorizing procedure. Decolorize the smear by letting 95 percent alcohol run over the slide that is held at about a 45° angle, until the violet stain no longer flows from the slide, usually less than 15 seconds. A thick smear requires longer decolorization than a thin smear, so the time needed for decolorization varies. The ethyl alcohol acts as a decolorizer, removing the dye-iodine complex from the gram-negative organisms (those with thin cell walls containing lipoproteins and lipopolysaccharides). This is the most critical step of the staining procedure. Excessive decolorizing strips the dye-iodine complex from the gram-positive organisms; not decolorizing enough leaves the dye-iodine complex in the gram-negative organisms. Both errors yield incorrect results. The beginning student may have difficulty in properly performing this step of the Gram stain. However, with practice the student can quickly master the procedure.

Decolorization is stopped by the addition of water to the slide. This must be done as soon as the violet dye no longer flows from the slide. Stop decolorization by thoroughly rinsing the slide with water. Flow water over the slide, which is still held at a 45° angle.

Note: In clinical settings, acetone or acetone-alcohol is often substituted for ethyl alcohol. Because of the speed at which acetone and acetone-alcohol decolorize, the beginning student should use 95 percent ethyl alcohol, at least until the Gram stain skill is mastered.

Gram Stain Reaction

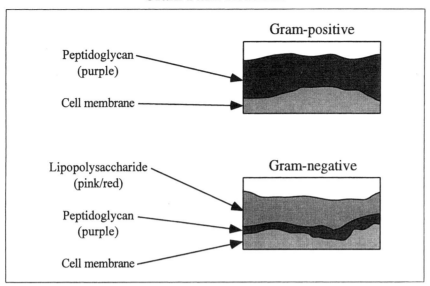

Figure 23–5 Gram-positive organisms have a large layer of peptidoglycan, which retains crystal violet after decolorization. Gram-negative organisms have only a very thin layer of peptidoglycan. The lipopolysaccharide layer retains safranin and appears pink/red after the Gram stain procedure.

The last step in the Gram stain technique is counterstaining. Flood the slide with safranin stain for 60 seconds. The gram-negative bacteria are stained with the safranin and appear pink or red, while the gram-positive organisms retain the purple color (Fig. 23–5).

Wash off the counterstain with water by allowing it to flow over the slide. Blot with bibulous, or blotting, paper. Use only gentle pressure so you do not break the slide or dislodge the organisms.

You can purchase commercial kits for the Gram stain. Processing times vary depending on manufacturer. Always read package inserts and follow directions. Table 23–1 summarizes the appearance of gram-positive and gram-negative organisms after each step of the Gram stain.

Quality Control

You can purchase commercial slides for quality control. One end of the quality control slide contains smears of a known gram-positive organism and a known gram-negative organism. The other end of the quality control slide has spaces for smears of bacteria whose Gram reaction is not known. Since the laboratorian applies the Gram stain to the entire slide at the same time, reagents and technique can be evaluated for correctness. When the known gram-positive organism stains purple and the known gram-negative organism stains red, the laboratorian can assume that the results of the Gram reaction of the unknown organism are accurate.

Table 23–1 **Colors in Gram Stain Procedure**

Reagent	Gram-Positive Organism	Gram-Negative Organism
Crystal violet	Purple	Purple
Gram's iodine	Purple	Purple
Ethyl alcohol	Purple	Colorless
Safranin	Purple	Red

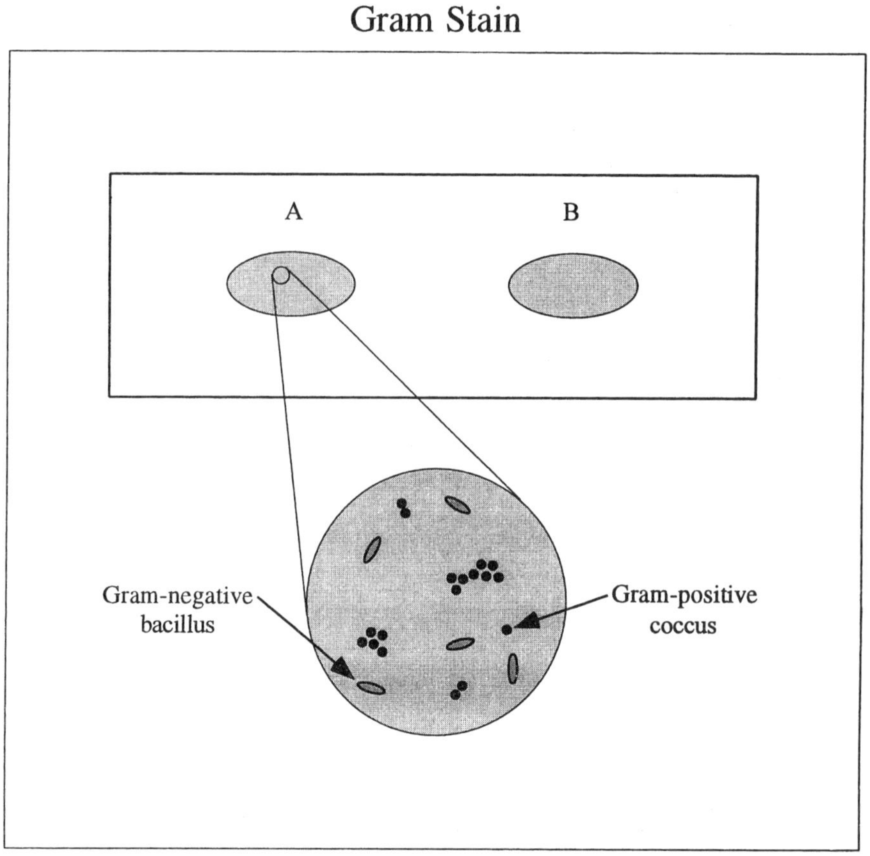

Gram Stain

Figure 23-6 Enlarged section of the Gram stain control. Gram-negative (pink/red) bacillus and gram-positive (purple) coccus indicate that the staining procedure is in control.

Some medical offices or clinical laboratories prepare an in-house control slide by making a smear of a known gram-positive organism and a known gram-negative organism. To do this, prepare a mixed smear of *Escherichia coli* (gram-negative, i.e., pink or red rod) and *Staphylococcus aureus* (gram-positive, i.e., purple cocci) by mixing two loopfuls of each organism in the same area of the slide. Observe the control area of the slide after staining. If you observe gram-negative rods and gram-positive cocci, then you can assume that the Gram staining procedure and reagents for the clinical specimen were correct (Fig. 23-6).

SUMMARY

Preparing a bacterial smear entails transferring bacteria to a glass slide and preparing it for staining and microscopic examination.

Microbiologists observe shape, arrangement, structural features, and staining characteristics in order to identify bacteria. Observing smears also helps to determine the purity of a culture or to select the type of medium for culturing. Occasionally a tentative diagnosis can be made from a direct smear of a clinical specimen.

Three types of specimens are used to prepare smear, a broth culture, a solid medium culture, and a clinical specimen. Slides are heat fixed before staining. Smears must be totally dry before heat fixing.

Three major types of stains are used in bacteriology: simple stains, special stains, and differential stains. Gram stain is the most important differential stain used in bacteriology. It differentiates bacteria with walls that contain thick layers of peptidoglycan (gram-positive) from bacteria with walls that contain a minimum of peptidoglycan (gram-negative). This distinction is most important in the treatment of patients with bacterial infections, because antibiotic selection depends on whether the infectious organism is gram-positive or gram-negative.

Because there is always a chance that pathogens are present, always use care when collecting and processing clinical specimens.

PATIENT EDUCATION

• No particular patient education is required.

TECHNICAL CONSIDERATIONS

• Old cultures produce unreliable results for morphology and staining characteristics.
• Thick smears, especially some species of *Neisseria,* may falsely appear gram-positive.
• Cultures older than 24 hours give unreliable Gram-stain reactions, especially gram-positive organisms such as *Staphylococcus* or *Bacillus.*

SOURCES OF ERROR

• Decolorizing is the most critical step in the Gram stain. Excessive decolorizing or not decolorizing enough can produce erroneous results.

Procedure with Rationale

Bacterial Smear Preparation

EQUIPMENT AND SUPPLIES

Hand soap	Bunsen burner and flint lighter
Latex gloves	Inoculating loop or needle
Petri dish containing nonpathogenic	Slide forceps
bacteria	Distilled water
Clean slide	Surface disinfectant
Permanent marker or wax pencil	Biohazard container

Assemble equipment.

Wash hands with soap and water. Follow the OSHA Standard for this procedure.

Using a permanent marker or wax pencil, draw a circle on the underside of the slide approximately the size of a nickel and identify the slide using appropriate labeling. *The circle acts as a target to help in locating the bacteria when viewing the slide using the microscope.*

Using the flint lighter, light the Bunsen burner and adjust the flame. A small, clear cone should be visible in the center of the blue flame.

Place two or three loopfuls of distilled water on the unmarked side of the slide in the center of the circle.

Flame the inoculating loop in the clear central cone, then in the blue area of the Bunsen burner flame until the entire wire glows red. *The clear cone heat kills bacteria and keeps moist inoculum from spattering. The blue area of the flame incinerates any remaining material and sterilizes the loop or needle by incineration. Follow this procedure each time you flame the loop.*

After the inoculating loop has cooled for about 5 seconds, lift the media side of the Petri dish with the nondominant hand and observe for an isolated colony.

Lightly touch the inoculating loop to one isolated colony. *Take only a small amount of culture since large amounts of bacteria mask staining results and morphology.*

Immediately return the media side of the Petri dish to the lid. *Do not expose media to the air any longer than required to remove bacteria.*

Immerse the tip of the inoculating loop containing the bacterial sample in the water drop on the slide and gently rotate the loop or needle until the bacteria are evenly dispersed within the circle and you see a slight turbidity.

Flame the loop using proper technique.

Let the slide air-dry. *Failure to allow the slide to air-dry will result in "boiling" of the bacteria during heat fixing, producing gross distortion of the bacterial cells.*

Using the slide forceps, heat fix the slide by passing it quickly through the flame of the Bunsen burner about three times. *The fixation process coagulates some of the bacterial protein, causing the bacteria to adhere to the slide, so that they are not washed away during the staining procedure.*

Clean work area following laboratory protocol.

Remove gloves and wash hands with soap and water.

Procedure with Rationale

Gram Stain

EQUIPMENT AND SUPPLIES

Hand soap	Wash-water bottle with distilled water
Latex gloves	Microscope
Gram stain kit	Immersion oil
Heat-fixed bacterial smear with control organisms	Bibulous paper
	Stopwatch
Staining rack	Surface disinfectant
Slide forceps	

Assemble equipment.

Wash hands with soap and water. Follow the OSHA Standard for this procedure.

Place slide on staining rack.

Flood slide with crystal violet or gentian violet stain for 1 minute. *Use plenty of stain to avoid drying since this deposits precipitate on the slide.*

Hold the slide at about a 45° angle and rinse using the wash-water bottle or a gentle flow of water from the tap. *This avoids precipitation of the stain on the slide.*

Drain off the water and flood with Gram's iodine for 1 minute.

Holding the slide at about a 45° angle, decolorize using 95 percent ethyl alcohol. Let the alcohol run down the slide while observing the removal of the purple dye. When dye is no longer observed, the decolorizing is complete. Time cannot be specified but is usually less than 15 seconds. *Thicker smears require more decolorizing time than thinner smears.*

Quickly stop decolorization by flooding the slide with water. *The water bottle must be immediately at hand so that decolorization is stopped promptly.*

Using safranin, flood slide with stain for 1 minute.

Rinse the slide with water by holding it at a 45° angle.

Blot the slide dry using bibulous paper. *Do not rub the slide with bibulous paper since this dislodges the organisms from the slide.*

Examine the controls with the oil-immersion lens of the microscope. Gram-positive organisms should appear purple and gram-negative organisms should appear pink or red. *This verifies the accuracy of the stain and the procedure.*

Record results of the controls.

Interpretation of the Gram stain of the test organism is performed by a qualified microbiologist or medical technologist. Record the results of the test organism as directed.

Clean work area following laboratory protocol.

Remove gloves and wash hands with soap and water.

Questions

Name _____ Date _____

1. Give five reasons for preparing bacterial smears.

2. What characteristics constitute a properly prepared bacterial smear?

3. What three types of specimens are used to make bacterial smears?

4. Give an example of a direct smear from a body specimen used in clinical practice.

5. What is heat fixing? What is the proper technique for heat fixing?

6. List the reagents of the Gram stain in sequence and give the function of each.

7. What is the most critical step of the Gram stain? How is it performed?

8. Regarding peptidoglycan, what is the difference between a gram-positive and gram-negative organism, and how does this relate to the Gram-stain characteristics?

Terminal Performance Objective

Bacterial Smear Preparation

Given the necessary equipment, you will prepare a bacterial smear suitable for staining from a solid media culture within 10 minutes. This procedure must be performed to include all critical steps. Your instructor will determine whether your slide is suitable for staining based on microscopic inspection.

INSTRUCTOR'S EVALUATION FORM

Name _____ Date _____

+ = SATISFACTORY   ✓ = UNSATISFACTORY

_____ Assemble equipment.

_____ Wash hands with soap and water. Follow the OSHA Standard for this procedure.

_____ Using a permanent marker or wax pencil, draw a circle on the underside of the slide approximately the size of a nickel and identify the slide using appropriate labeling.

_____ Using the flint lighter, light the Bunsen burner and adjust the flame. A small, clear cone should be visible in the center of the blue flame.

_____ Place two or three loopfuls of distilled water on the unmarked side of the slide in the center of the circle.

_____ Flame the inoculating loop in the clear central cone, then in the blue area of the Bunsen burner flame until the entire wire glows red.

_____ After the inoculating loop has cooled for about 5 seconds, lift the media side of the Petri dish with the nondominant hand, and observe for an isolated colony.

_____ Lightly touch the inoculating loop to one isolated colony.

_____ Immediately return the media side of the Petri dish to the lid.

_____ Immerse the tip of the inoculating loop containing the bacterial sample in the water drop on the slide and gently rotate the loop or needle until the bacteria are evenly dispersed within the circle and you see a slight turbidity.

_____ Flame the loop using proper technique.

_____ Let the slide air-dry.

_____ Using the slide forceps, heat fix the slide by passing it quickly through the flame of the Bunsen burner about three times.

_____ Clean work area following laboratory protocol.

_____ Remove gloves and wash hands with soap and water.

_____ The procedure was completed within 10 minutes.

_____ The bacterial slide was suitable for staining.

Final Competency Evaluation

____ SATISFACTORY   ____ UNSATISFACTORY

Comments:

Instructor _____ Date _____

Terminal Performance Objective

Gram Stain

Given the necessary equipment, you will perform a Gram stain on a prepared smear having appropriate controls. The stained slide must be suitable for evaluation for a Gram-stain reaction by a qualified microbiologist within 10 minutes. You must accurately record the results of the controls. Your instructor will determine if you have properly performed the Gram stain based on microscopic inspection.

INSTRUCTOR'S EVALUATION FORM

Name _____ Date _____

+ = SATISFACTORY   ✓ = UNSATISFACTORY

_____ Assemble equipment.

_____ Wash hands with soap and water. Follow the OSHA Standard for this procedure.

_____ Place slide on staining rack.

_____ Flood slide with crystal violet or gentian violet stain for 1 minute.

_____ Hold the slide at about a 45° angle and rinse using the wash-water bottle or a gentle flow of water from the tap.

_____ Drain off the water and flood the slide with Gram's iodine for 1 minute.

_____ Holding the slide at about a 45° angle, decolorize using 95 percent ethyl alcohol. Let the alcohol run down the slide while observing the removal of the purple dye. When dye is no longer observed, the decolorizing is complete. Time cannot be specified but is usually less than 15 seconds.

_____ Quickly stop decolorization by flooding the slide with water.

_____ Using safranin, flood the slide with stain for 1 minute.

_____ Rinse the slide with water by holding it at a 45° angle.

_____ Blot the slide dry using bibulous paper.

_____ Examine the controls with the oil-immersion lens of the microscope. Gram-positive organisms should appear purple and gram-negative organisms should appear pink or red.

_____ Record results of the controls.

RESULTS GRAM-POSITIVE CONTROL: _____.

RESULTS GRAM-NEGATIVE CONTROL: _____.

_____ Interpretation of the Gram stain of the test organism is performed by a qualified microbiologist or medical technologist. Record the results of the test organism as directed.   RESULTS: _____.

_____ Clean work area following laboratory protocol.

_____ Remove gloves and wash hands with soap and water.

_____ The procedure was completed within 10 minutes.

_____ The Gram stain reaction was correct.

_____ The results were properly recorded.

Final Competency Evaluation

_____ SATISFACTORY   _____ UNSATISFACTORY

Comments:

Instructor _____ Date _____

Introduction to Immunology

LEARNING OBJECTIVES

On completing this chapter, you will be able to:

COGNITIVE OBJECTIVES

- List and describe the body defenses against infectious diseases.
- List and briefly describe the three major features of the adaptive immune system that cause it to differ from other host defense mechanisms.
- Differentiate cell-mediated immunity from humoral immunity.
- Briefly describe antibody titer and its relationship to the course of a disease.
- List and briefly describe the immunologic techniques used for diagnostic purposes in the medical laboratory.

The body has several defenses to protect itself against the entry of potentially lethal microorganisms or other foreign substances. Collectively, these defenses are called **immunity.** Those that are present at birth or established immediately after birth constitute the **nonspecific** immunity of the body. The immunity that develops slowly over time makes up the **adaptive** or specific immunity of the body. Despite the trillions of microorganisms that we encounter daily, most of us remain in good health almost all of our lives. This is primarily due to the watchful surveillance of the immune system.

> **Immunity:** *the state of being free from the possibility of acquiring an infectious disease*

> **Nonspecific:** *lacking uniqueness or individuality*

> **Adaptive:** *the ability to adjust or modify*

> **Pathogens:** *organisms capable of causing disease*

NONSPECIFIC IMMUNITY

The nonspecific, or innate, protective defenses of the body include the following:

- *Normal flora:* harmless microorganisms that inhabit surfaces of the body that may otherwise be colonized by **pathogens** (Chapter 22)

- *Anatomic barriers:* skin, mucous membranes, tears, gastric juice, and other body fluids that act as physical barriers or chemical deterrents hindering pathogens from gaining entry into the body
- *Inflammation:* a response that controls or arrests the spread of infection and accelerates the healing process (Chapter 14)
- *Phagocytic cells:* mainly neutrophils and **mononuclear phagocytes** that wander throughout the body seeking out and engulfing foreign material (Chapter 14)

Mononuclear phago-cytes: *monocytes and macrophages*

These defenses are called nonspecific because they do not differentiate or identify the various types of foreign material that attempt to invade the body. No endeavor is made by them to "customize" their method of protection. All potential pathogens are treated the same way. The response by the nonspecific immune system is general and predictable, and not dependent on the nature of the invading organism. On rare occasions, an invading pathogen successfully gains entry to the body and begins to establish a disease condition. When this occurs, the highly specific adaptive immune system is activated, and final destruction of the pathogen is imminent.

SPECIFIC IMMUNITY

Antibodies: *glycoprotein products of B cells that have the ability to react with the antigen that caused their formation*

The adaptive immune system is blood-based and composed primarily of two types of white blood cells: *T cells* (T lymphocytes) and *B cells* (B lymphocytes). The B cell response involves the production of highly unique proteins called **antibodies.** The T cell response involves the production of proteins called **cytokines.**

Cytokines: *cell secretions that act upon neighboring cells; method used by cells to "communicate" with each other*

CHARACTERISTICS OF THE ADAPTIVE IMMUNE RESPONSE

The immune system is able to respond to a virtually infinite variety of **antigenic challenges** by eliminating them from the body, destroying them, or neutralizing their pathogenic effects. This response exhibits three distinct characteristics not possessed by any other host defense. They are as follows:

Antigenic challenges: *exposure of an organism to an unknown antigen*

- Recognition
- Specificity
- Memory

Recognition

The immune system has the ability to distinguish "self" from "nonself." In other words, it is capable of recognizing what belongs in the body and what does not belong. When the immune system encounters nonself, it begins to undertake a series of activities designed to rid the body of the alien material. Any foreign substance capable of causing such a response is called an *immunogen* (antigen).

The immune system learns to identify self from nonself during fetal development, when it somehow makes an inventory of body cells and begins to recognize its own tissue. Any immune cell that reacts with the tissue of the host is selectively eliminated. From birth to death, the watchful immune system continually surveys body tissues for viruses, bacteria, and foreign substances. It also checks for cancer cells and other body cells that have been altered by viruses. Even though cancer cells and virus-altered cells belong to the host, they are usually so different in their behavior and membrane chemistry that they appear like an immunogen to the ever-watchful immune system.

Specificity

The response of the immune system to an antigen is highly specific. In other words, the attack used to rid the body of the immunogen is "customized" depending on the unique features of each particular antigen. Exposure of specific T cells and specific B cells to their corresponding antigen causes them to become *immunocompetent,* that is, committed to the destruction of that particular antigen. This exposure occurs when a **macrophage** ingests an antigen and presents the unique "label" of that antigen, called an *epitope* (antigenic determinant) to its corresponding T cell and B cell. Once the exposure has occurred, the T cell and B cell are referred to as *immunoblasts* or *sensitized lymphocytes.* They will mount a response effective only against the specific antigen that caused them to be formed.

The concept of specificity is analogous to a lock and key. A specific key can open only a specific lock; a specific immune cell can react only with the antigen that caused it to be formed. After T cells and B cells become sensitized to an antigen, they form two major **clones**—*effector cells,* which eliminate the antigen, and *memory cells,* which retain information on the mechanisms used for destruction of the immunogen.

Macrophage: *a highly phagocytic cell arising from a monocyte; often acts as an antigen presenting cell*

Clones: *groups of cells with the same genetic composition descended from a single cell*

Memory

Both memory T cells and memory B cells form as part of the immune response. Memory cells are capable of producing more effector cells at a later time. Long after recovery from the disease, memory cells remain in the body, primarily in the lymphatic system. When the same antigen is again encountered, there is an immediate outpouring of effector cells at a number and rate far greater than occurred during the first encounter. This highly effective reaction called the *anamnestic response* protects the host from a second bout of the disease. Memory cells often remain in the body for long periods of time, sometimes several decades after an exposure to an antigen.

Clinical Comment: Immunity

Immunity relies on the fact that the body is capable of "remembering" the mechanisms it undertook to restore health to the host during an initial encounter with a disease. Once learned, the same procedure can be undertaken again. This happens so rapidly that subsequent exposures do not generally result in the manifestation of the disease. Consequently, when a child develops chickenpox, or other types of diseases, he or she is usually immune from contracting these diseases a second time. Vaccines also provide immunity against a variety of diseases. They are considered "preemptive" strikes because they contain dead or inactivated disease-causing organisms or toxins. If the host becomes ill from the vaccination, the disease is generally very mild with few or no symptoms. However, the memory component of the immune system is firmly set in place. Subsequent exposures to these disease-causing organisms will generally find the child immune.

TYPES OF ADAPTIVE IMMUNE RESPONSES

The immune system consists of two major response categories in the host, the *cellular response* and *humoral response.* In both instances the response is characterized by recognition, specificity, and memory. The kind of immunity developed against an antigen, however, depends on which cell type or combination of cells is able to recognize and respond to the presence of the antigen. When T cells respond as the main defense system, a form of immunity known as *cellular immunity* results. When B cells respond as the principal defense, the form of immunity that develops is known as *humoral* or *antibody immunity.*

Although each of these reactions is identified singly, there is a great deal of interaction between them because the two responses always work together.

Cellular Response

Mediated: *coordinated and synchronized*

The cellular response is **mediated** by T cells. These cells originate in the bone marrow but immediately migrate to the thymus gland where they are processed to respond to specific antigens. Binding sites for a specific antigen develop on the surface of the T cells. When T cells are released into the circulatory system, they are referred to as virgin cells. On exposure to their specific antigen by an **antigen presenting cell (APC),** usually a macrophage, they differentiate into subsets and begin to proliferate. The major T effector cell used for destruction of the immunogen is the cytotoxic (killer) T cell. This cell lyses body cells that appear "different" from the host, including cells infected with viruses. It also lyses body cells that have changed so drastically that they are no longer recognized as self. This feature is especially important in the destruction of potentially malignant cells, which may cause cancer if they are not destroyed.

Antigen presenting cell (APC): *cells that break down antigens and display their fragments on the surface receptors*

The cytotoxic T cell also produces cytokines. These chemical messengers coordinate immune activities between the nonspecific and specific defenses of the body. The killer T cells and B cells are assisted in their efforts to destroy antigens by a subset called *helper T cells.* The *suppressor T cells,* another major subset, "turn off" the immune response when the antigen is no longer a threat. Finally, a subset of *memory T cells* develops for protection against subsequent antigenic encounters (Fig. 24–1).

Cellular Immunity

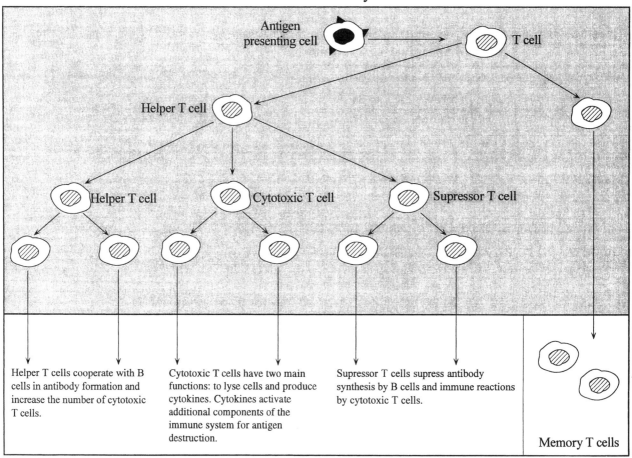

Figure 24–1 Cellular immunity.

Clinical Comment: AIDS

The virus that causes *acquired immune deficiency syndrome* (AIDS) is the *human immunodeficiency virus* (HIV). It attacks the helper T cells, which are essential to the function of both B cells and T cells. The loss of helper T cells ultimately shuts down the entire adaptive immune system. The patient is no longer able to ward off disease. Even the microorganisms that are normally "friendly" become a threat to the life of the patient. AIDS is one of the most devastating diseases known to humans. There is no cure, and there is virtually no hope of an effective HIV vaccine for years to come. Early diagnosis is essential, because medications are available that slow down the progression of the disease or help to ward off some of the opportunistic infections associated with the disease.

Approximately 70 to 80 percent of the circulating lymphocytes are T cells. They are especially effective against intracellular antigens including viruses and bacteria, malignant cells, and foreign tissue (transplants).

Humoral Response

The second type of immunologic response, humoral immunity, is mediated by B cells. These cells originate in the bone marrow and are processed there to develop receptors for a specific antigen. The effector B cells are plasma cells that produce antibodies (Fig. 24–2). Antibodies are released into circulation and are carried throughout the entire body. When antibodies combine with their corresponding antigen they form an antigen-antibody complex. The antibody can destroy the antigen directly by:

- Inactivating it
- Enhancing inflammation
- Activating **complement,** which initiates a variety of destructive activities against the antigen
- Tagging the antigen for phagocytosis, a process called *opsonization*

Complement: *a group of plasma proteins that participate in antigen-antibody reactions such as lysis*

B cells are chiefly responsible for protecting against extracellular bacteria, extracellular viruses, toxins, and parasites.

During the initial period of infection, when the antigen is trying to establish a foothold in the host, the number of antibodies specific for the antigen is nonexistent or very low. As the infection runs its course, the antibody **titer** elevates. Tracking the titer in a patient helps the physician diagnose a disease and follow its course and the effectiveness of the treatment. For example, if an early serum sample shows a very low or nonexistent titer against a certain antigen (e.g., measles) and a sample taken 2 weeks after the onset of symptoms shows an appreciable rise in the titer of measles antibody, the disease was indeed measles.

Titer: *a semiquantitative measure of the concentration of antibodies present in serum*

CHARACTERISTICS OF ANTIGENS

Chemically, the vast majority of antigens are proteins, but some are large polysaccharides. The more common antigens include toxins, foreign tissue, microbial proteins (bacterial, viral, fungal, and parasitic), and allergens (dust, pollen, mold, animal dander). Occasionally, the body fails to properly identify its own tissue, causing the immune system to produce antibodies against its own tissue cells. This is referred to as an *autoimmune disease.*

In order for any substance to act as an antigen, it must be relatively large in size and possess at least two specific regions on its surface called *determinant sites,* or epitopes, where antibodies can attach (Fig. 24–3).

Humoral Immunity

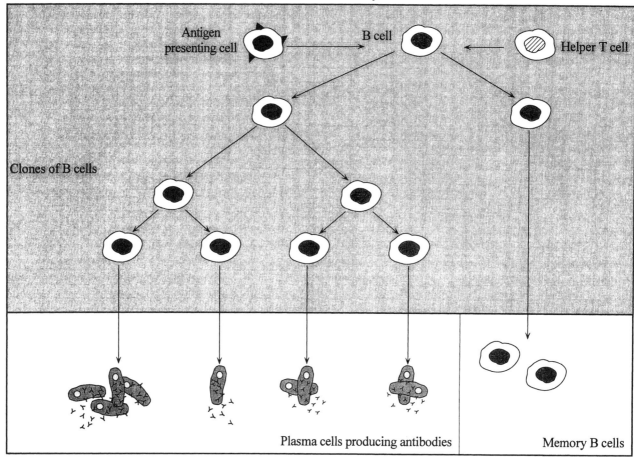

Figure 24–2 Humoral immunity.

CHARACTERISTICS OF ANTIBODIES

All antibodies belong to a group of proteins called *globulins*. Because they are involved in immune reactions, they are called *immunoglobulins* (Ig). Five types of immunoglobulins have been identified, IgG, IgA, IgM, IgD, and IgE. Table 24–1 summarizes information on the different types of immunoglobulins.

Antigen–Antibody Complex

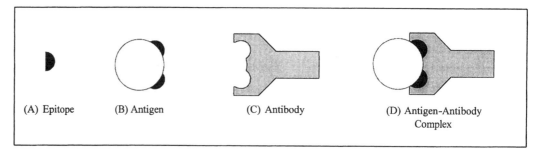

Figure 24–3 Antigen-antibody complex. *(A)* An epitope is the unique "label" of an antigen. *(B)* To act as an antigen, a substance must have two epitopes or binding sites. *(C)* Antibodies are unique to each antigen. *(D)* An antigen-antibody complex, which fits together like a lock and key. Once the antigen-antibody complex is formed, the antigen is tagged for destruction or elimination.

Table 24–1 ***Immunoglobulins***

Class	Locations	Functions	Increased	Decreased

IgG	Plasma
	Interstitial fluid
	Placenta
		Produces antibodies against
		  bacteria, viruses, and toxins
		Protects neonates
		Activates the complement system
		Is a major factor in secondary
		  (anamnestic) response
			Infections—all types,
			  acute and chronic
			Starvation
			Liver disease
			Rheumatic fever
			Sarcoidosis
			IgG myeloma
				Lymphocytic leukemia
				Agammaglobulinemia
				Amyloidosis
				Toxemia of pregnancy

IgA	Respiratory tract
	Gastrointestinal tract
	Genitourinary tract
	Tears
	Saliva
	Milk, colostrum
	Exocrine secretions
		Protects mucous membranes from
		  viruses and bacteria
		Includes antitoxins, antibacterial
		  agglutinins, antinuclear
		  antibodies, and allergic reagins
		Activates complement through the
		  alternative pathway
			Autoimmune diseases
			Chronic infections
			Liver disease
			Wiskott-Aldrich syndrome
			IgA myeloma
				Lymphocytic leukemia
				Agammaglobulinemia
				Malignancies
				Hereditary ataxia
				  telangiectasia
				Hypogammaglobulinemia
				Malabsorption syndrome

IgM	Serum	Primary responder to antigens
		Produces antibody against
		  rheumatoid factors, gram-
		  negative organisms, and ABO
		  blood group
		Activates the complement system
			Lymphosarcoma
			Brucellosis, actinomycosis
			Trypanosomiasis
			Relapsing fever
			Malaria
			Infectious mononucleosis
			Rubella virus in newborn
			Waldenström's
			  macroglobulinemia
				Lymphocytic leukemia
				Agammaglobulinemia
				Amyloidosis
				IgG and IgA myeloma
				Dysgammaglobulinemia

IgD	Serum Cord blood	Unknown	Chronic infections IgD myeloma	

IgE	Serum
	Interstitial fluid
		Allergic reactions
		Anaphylaxis
		Protects against parasitic worm
		  infestations
			Atopic skin disorders
			Hay fever
			Asthma
			Anaphylaxis
			IgE myeloma
				Congenital
				  agammaglobulinemia

Adapted from Watson, J, and Jaffe, MS: Nurse's Manual of Laboratory Tests, ed 2, FA Davis, Philadelphia, 1995, p 89.

SEROLOGICAL TECHNIQUES

The adaptive immune system is the basis for many diagnostic tests performed in the laboratory. Antigen-antibody reactions may occur in a host as well as in an artificial environment such as a laboratory setting. When a reaction occurs in a host or living organism, it is called an *in vivo* reaction. When the reaction occurs in a laboratory testing environment, it is said to be an *in vitro* reaction. Laboratory tests that rely on antigen-antibody reactions are valuable diagnostic and therapeutic tools. Some of the commonly used immunologic tests are discussed here.

Agglutination

Agglutination is the formation of relatively large, insoluble aggregates consisting of soluble antibodies attached to particles such as bacteria, blood cells, and latex beads (see Fig. 28–1). The most familiar agglutination reaction is the one associated with the identification of the ABO blood group. If the surface of an erythrocyte is coated with an antigen and exposed to the corresponding antibody, a latticelike network forms, causing the cells to agglutinate and fall out of solution. This reaction is visible to the naked eye. A variation of this procedure is the agglutination inhibition test (see Fig. 26–2).

Precipitation

Precipitation is the formation of relatively small, insoluble aggregates following reaction of soluble antibody with soluble antigen. The resulting complex is too large to remain suspended in solution, so it precipitates as an opaque, visible mass or *flocculum*. These reactions are similar to agglutination but less visible, and the amount of antigen and antibody must be controlled for optimum results.

Lysis

Antigen-antibody reactions that lead to lysis of bacterial cells or erythrocytes are valuable in serological testing. In this reaction, plasma protein called *complement* must be present for the reaction to occur. After complement is fixed to the surface of the bacteria or blood cells, the action of the antibody causes lysis of the cells. Lysis is a visible disintegration showing that the antibody and antigen have reacted.

Radioimmunoassay

Ligand: *the molecule that binds to the antibody*

Radioimmunoassays (RIAs) are sophisticated serological tests. A **ligand** (radioactively labeled protein or anti-antibody capable of binding to the target antibody) acts as the indicator. The amount of bound radioactive label is measured to show the concentration of the target antibody (Fig. 24–4).

Enzyme-Linked Immunosorbent Assay

Substrate: *any substance acted upon and changed by an enzyme*

The *enzyme-linked immunosorbent assay* (ELISA) is a highly sensitive test using an enzyme linked to an antibody as the basis for the test. The enzyme is able to produce a reaction that causes a color change when placed with its appropriate **substrate.** The antibody retains its binding sites, which are free to react with antigen that is bound to a microtiter well wall. This is one of the fastest-growing methodologies for detecting microbial organisms (Fig. 24–5).

Principle of
RIA Reaction

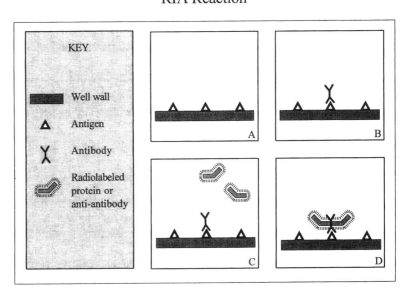

Figure 24–4   Principle of RIA reaction. *(A)* Microtiter well is coated with antigen. *(B)* Antibody specific to the antigen is added. This results in the formation of an antigen-antibody complex. *(C)* A radiolabeled protein or anti-antibody is added as the indicator system. It binds to the antibody of the antigen-antibody complex. *(D)* The amount of bound radioactive material is measured to indicate the concentration of the antibody.

Principle of
ELISA Reaction

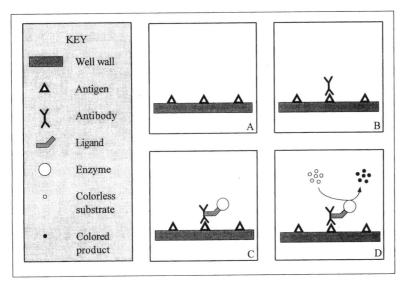

Figure 24-5 Principle of ELISA reaction. *(A)* Microtiter well is coated with antigen. *(B)* Antibody specific to the antigen is added. This results in the formation of an antigen-antibody complex. *(C)* A ligand bearing an enzyme is added as the indicator system. It binds to the antibody of the antigen-antibody complex. *(D)* A colorless substrate of the enzyme is added. The resulting color change is measured to indicate the concentration of the antibody.

Clinical Comment: Immunology

Scientists who first studied antigen-antibody reactions used blood serum (the liquid product of blood after it has coagulated) for their investigations. Because of this, the clinical study of antigen-antibody reactions was called *serology.* Over time, the techniques and methods used in serology were expanded to include whole blood, spinal fluid, synovial fluid, urine, and other body fluids. Today the study of antigen-antibody reactions is called *immunology.*

QUALITY CONTROL

Most immunologic test kits contain both positive and negative controls that must be run daily or when patient testing is performed. Results are recorded on a log sheet. Lot numbers and expiration dates are also recorded as part of the quality control program. Because there are so many types of immunologic tests available for POL testing, it is essential that directions and product inserts be carefully followed. Be sure that specimen collecting and processing follow the requirements of the manufacturer. With most test kits, the reagents must be at room temperature before undertaking testing procedures. Follow all directions meticulously.

SUMMARY

Immunity is the state of being protected from diseases. The body has nonspecific defenses that are present at birth or develop shortly after birth. A highly specific defense system, the adaptive immune system, develops over time as a result of exposures to pathogens. This type of protection is characterized by recognition, specificity, and memory. The immune cells responsible for the adaptive immune response are B cells (humoral response) and T cells (cellular response).

The unique specificity of an antibody for its antigen is the basis for a type of laboratory testing called *immunology.* Immunologic methods are the most effective diagnostic and therapeutic tools in the physician's arsenal of laboratory testing techniques.

More and more tests are being developed that incorporate the principles of immunology. These tests are relatively inexpensive and highly accurate. In addition, they are simple to perform and results are available in only a few minutes.

Questions

Name _____ Date _____

1. Name the nonspecific defenses of the body and briefly describe each.

2. Name the three characteristics of the adaptive immune response and briefly describe each.

3. What is the function of each of the cells associated with cellular immunity?

4. Briefly describe the functions of the effector cells associated with humoral immunity.

5. What is the relationship between titer and the course of a disease?

6. List two characteristics required for a substance to act as an antigen.

7. List the five types of antibodies and briefly tell the function of each.

8. Name and briefly describe five types of immunologic tests.

Streptococci Testing

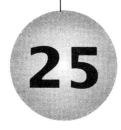

25

Learning Objectives
Cognitive Objectives
Psychomotor Objectives
Affective Objectives

Throat Culture

**Identification of Three Types
of Hemolysis**

Inoculation and Incubation

Rapid Strep Testing

Sensitivity Testing

Method for Culture and Sensitivity

Quality Control

Summary
Patient Education
Technical Considerations
Sources of Error

Procedure with Rationale
Rapid Strep Test

Questions

Terminal Performance Objective
Rapid Strep Test
  ○ Instructor's evaluation form

LEARNING OBJECTIVES

On completing this chapter, you will be able to:

COGNITIVE OBJECTIVES
- Explain the importance of identifying the group A streptococci organisms.
- Identify several diseases caused by group A streptococci organisms.
- Describe three types of hemolysis on a blood agar plate.
- Describe how a sensitivity test is performed and what information is obtained.

PSYCHOMOTOR OBJECTIVES
- Perform a rapid strep test for detection of group A beta-hemolytic streptococci according to the Terminal Performance Objective presented in this chapter.
- Record the results of a rapid strep test for group A beta-hemolytic streptococci.
- Record the results of the positive and negative controls.

AFFECTIVE OBJECTIVES
- Show concern for your coworkers by disposing of the bacterial specimen according to laboratory protocol.
- Assume responsibility for a clean and safe work environment.

Because the signs and symptoms presented by the patient may be vague, a physician often needs to identify a bacterial organism to diagnose and treat an infectious disease. In some cases it is necessary to perform physical, **immunologic,** or chemical tests to identify an infectious organism. Even after you identify an organism, determining whether there is infection may require an understanding of the bacteria that constitute the normal flora found in the specimen. Only a skilled microbiologist can make such an interpretive judgment. The most common pathogenic organism from a throat culture can be identified simply by the way it grows on a particular medium. This is the principle for performing a throat culture using a **blood agar** plate. For a more thorough understanding of culture media, refer to Chapter 22.

Immunologic: *pertaining to immunity to diseases*

Blood agar: *a culture media consisting of sheeps' blood and nutrient agar*

THROAT CULTURE

Physicians request a throat culture to identify the presence of group A streptococci as well as other pathogens that may be found in the throat. Streptococci are a group of gram-positive bacteria that produce many different diseases. Some of these diseases are mild, but many are very serious and may cause lasting problems. Many strains of pathogenic streptococci often colonize areas of the body including the upper respiratory tract, gastrointestinal tract, and the female genitourinary tract. They do not cause disease unless the immune system is compromised or injury or disease allows these organisms to enter the bloodstream or sterile body sites.

Some of the diseases caused by streptococci organisms include pneumonia, meningitis, **sepsis,** bacterial endocarditis, **streptococcal pharyngitis, cellulitis,** wound infection, and **abscesses** in internal organs.

Sepsis: *a condition resulting from the presence of microorganisms or their poisonous products in the bloodstream*

Streptococcal pharyngitis: *an inflammation of the pharynx caused by streptococci; "strep throat"*

Cellulitis: *inflammation of cellular or connective tissue, spreading through the tissue*

Abscess: *a localized collection of pus in any part of the body*

Clinical Comment: Bacterial Endocarditis

Endocarditis is an infectious bacterial inflammation of the inner lining of the heart. It is usually confined to the external lining of the valves, but may infect the lining of the heart's chambers. Treatment for bacterial or infectious endocarditis is by intravenous antibiotic therapy for at least 4 weeks. During the therapy the patient is placed on bed rest to reduce the workload of the heart. Because congestive heart failure can be a complication of endocarditis, the patient is watched for any signs or symptoms of disturbance of the heart's pumping action.

A commonly used classification of streptococci is based on the work of Dr. Rebecca Lancefield, a U.S. bacteriologist, who identified specific carbohydrate or protein antigens in the cell walls of the streptococci organisms. She classified the strep organisms into groups A through G depending on the immunologic reaction of the carbohydrate or protein antigen found in the various groups of streptococci. Originally her idea of identification was based on a beta-hemolytic reaction when these organisms were streaked on a blood agar plate. Later groups H through O and two other hemolytic groups, alpha hemolysis and gamma hemolysis, were added to her system.

Streptococci in group A (beta hemolytic) are of particular concern in clinical practice. Group A streptococci are often called *pyogenes,* a term that means pus producing. Group A strep can cause secondary infections, two of which are very serious, acute rheumatic fever and glomerulonephritis. Acute rheumatic fever often causes valvular heart disease with serious lifelong consequences for the patient. With glomerulonephritis, the glomerular membrane is affected and kidney function is temporarily lost.

Clinical Comment: Rheumatic Fever

Sequelae: *morbid secondary conditions following a primary condition that was less serious*

Rheumatic fever is a systemic, febrile disease that is inflammatory in nature and progressive in severity, duration, and **sequelae.** It is often followed by serious heart and kidney disease. After a streptococcal infection the patient experiences the sudden occurrence of fever and joint pain. This is the most common onset of rheumatic fever. Other symptoms include fever, migratory polyarthritis, pain upon motion, abdominal pain, and cardiac involvement (pericarditis, myocarditis, and endocarditis).

IDENTIFICATION OF THREE TYPES OF HEMOLYSIS

The three types of observable hemolysis on a blood agar plate are:

Alpha hemolysis: Characterized by a narrow zone of green discoloration around the colony. This green color is due to incomplete hemoglobin breakdown. Organisms that cause this greenish color on a blood agar plate are said to belong to the viridans group. Many organisms of the viridans group are normal flora of the throat.

Beta hemolysis: Characterized by a clear or translucent zone around the colony. This clear zone indicates complete destruction of erythrocytes. Beta hemolysis is characteristic of pathogenic organisms, primarily in Lancefield group A, but found also in groups B, C, and G. Group A streptococci completely hemolyze erythrocytes when cultured on blood agar media. Most other organisms only partially hemolyze erythrocytes or cannot hemolyze erythrocytes at all.

Gamma hemolysis: No hemolysis evident. This indicates that the organisms of the colony are incapable of lysing erythrocytes; consequently, there is no observable change in the blood agar surrounding the colony.

INOCULATION AND INCUBATION

Clinics and hospitals frequently use an elaborate system for isolating and identifying group A beta-hemolytic streptococci. However, some POLs use a technique that relies on the fact that group A streptococci infections show abundant growth of beta-hemolytic gram-positive cocci with **growth inhibition** around a bacitracin disk.

Group A beta-hemolytic streptococci are differentiated from groups B, C, and G by using an impregnated disk containing **bacitracin.** This disk is placed on the blood agar plate at the time of inoculation. After 24 hours of incubation, if you observe beta hemolysis along with the failure of bacteria to grow around the bacitracin disk, then the identification is assumed positive for group A beta-hemolytic streptococci (Fig. 25–1).

Growth inhibition: *no growth of organism surrounding the bacitracin disk*

Bacitracin: *an antibiotic whose action is similar to penicillin*

Group A Strep

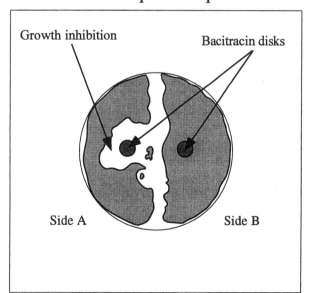

Growth inhibition

Bacitracin disks

Side A

Side B

Figure 25–1 Side A shows beta hemolysis with growth inhibition using a bacitracin disk and is characteristic of group A streptococci. Side B shows no growth.

The method for inoculation and incubation follows: Cover the entire surface of a blood agar plate with **inoculum** by rolling the swab over the entire surface of the medium. Be sure that as much of the specimen is plated on the medium as possible. You do not need to isolate pure colonies. Dispose of the swab in a biohazard container. Using sterile forceps, place a bacitracin disk where the inoculum is heaviest, that is, where the inoculum was first applied to the media surface. Place the blood agar plate in an incubator at 37°C for 24 hours.

After incubation, examine for beta hemolysis by holding the plate to a light source. Colonies of group A beta-hemolytic streptococci are pinpoint size, about 0.5 mm in diameter, translucent to slightly opaque. If the plate shows abundant growth of beta-hemolytic gram-positive cocci with growth inhibition of the organism around the bacitracin disk, then this is presumptive evidence of group A beta-hemolytic streptococci and medical treatment is required.

If only a few isolated colonies show beta hemolysis, the test is inconclusive. When this occurs, prepare a pure culture taken from the plate and inoculate it on a fresh blood agar plate. Refer to Chapter 22 for preparing a pure culture.

When you reculture, streak the new plate *confluently,* that is, totally filling the agar plate in one streak. Place a bacitracin disk in the first streaked area. After incubation at 37° for 24 hours, read the culture in the same manner as the original culture.

RAPID STREP TESTING

A quicker method of testing for group A beta-hemolytic streptococci is the rapid strep test manufactured by various companies. Because it does not require a 24-hour incubation period, this test gives a diagnosis within a short period. Having immediate results is an advantage, because the physician can begin antibiotic therapy before the patient leaves the office. Because **strep throat** is a common ailment of children and young adults, the pediatrician is at a distinct advantage with early diagnosis. Undiagnosed group A beta-hemolytic streptococci can result in chronic kidney disease. If the rapid strep test results are negative, a second throat culture test is performed to ensure accurate identification of any pathogens.

The rapid strep test does not require any sophisticated equipment. The laboratorian is responsible for the proper collection of the throat sample and for following the manufacturer's instructions for the rapid strep test.

Examples of rapid strep tests are Abbott's Testpack Plus Strep A (OBC) with onboard controls and Testpack Plus, STREP A OIA by BioStar, Inc., and Directigen[123] Group A Test by Becton Dickinson (Fig. 25–2).

SENSITIVITY TESTING

Sensitivity testing, also called *susceptibility testing,* determines the **bactericidal** effects of various antibiotics on bacteria. Some bacteria, especially the gram-positive organisms responsible for strep throats, are not easily destroyed by antibiotics. One reason for this is that prolonged use of antibiotics by the patient causes bacteria to develop a resistance to the killing effects of antibiotics. The initial use of an antibiotic destroys only the weakest members of the bacterial strain, and a more potent or longer dosage of the antibiotic may be required to destroy the heartier organisms. If they are not destroyed, the heartier organisms may remain dormant in the patient and later resurface and cause another more serious infection. The second infection may be difficult to cure because of the resistance the bacteria have developed to the antibiotic. When septic sore throat does not respond to traditional antibiotic therapy, the physician will request a culture and sensitivity test (C&S).

Antigen Extraction

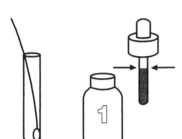

A

Place a **DispensTube** device in the designated area of the work station.

Place a swab into the **DispensTube** device.

Reagent 1-
Fill the dropper to the calibrated line and dispense into the DispensTube device.

NOTE: The **Control +** and **Control -** may be used in place of a swab.

After shaking or vortexing thoroughly, add two drops of **Control +** or **Control -** to the **DispensTube** device.

Add extraction reagent and mix thoroughly.

Alternate Procedure: If desired, add **Reagent 1** to the **DispensTube** device using calibrated dropper as described. Immediately place swab into the **DispensTube** device containing **Reagent 1**.

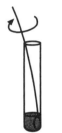

B

Rotate the swab **thoroughly for several seconds** so that it becomes saturated.

C

Reagent 2-

Hold the swab shaft to the side or elevate swab from the **DispensTube** device.

Add 2 drops directly into the DispensTube device

The color of the solution should turn to yellow.

Mix **Reagents 1** and **2** by rolling the swab against the side of the **DispensTube** device and squeezing the swab through the tube several times so that the liquid is expressed from the swab and reabsorbed.

Caution: Assay performance depends upon thorough antigen extraction.

Allow the swab to remain in the fluid at room temperature for 1 minute, but no longer than 30 minutes.

Figure 25–2 Procedure for performing the Directigen$_{123}$ Group A Strep Test. (Courtesy Becton Dickinson Microbiology Systems, Cockeysville, Md.)

Continued

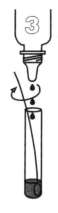

D

Reagent 3-
Hold the swab shaft to the side or express the liquid from and momentarily elevate the swab from the **DispensTube** device.

Add 3 drops directly into the DispensTube device.

The color of the solution should change to pink.

Mix the liquid as described in step C. In exceptional cases, a specimen may not change to pink. If this occurs, add 1 additional drop of **Reagent 3**.

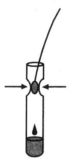

E

Roll the swab against the wall of the **DispensTube device and thoroughly squeeze** the swab between the flexible sides to remove as much liquid as possible.

Discard the swab in a receptacle for microbiological waste.

The pink solution can be held up to 24 h at room temperature before testing, without affecting test results.

Color Development

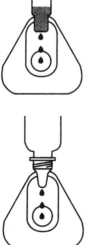

1

Insert a tip into the **DispensTube device**.

Dispense 3 drops in rapid succession onto the ColorPAC membrane.

Allow to completely absorb.

Proceed immediately to step 2.

2

Reagent 4-
Mix thoroughly.

Add 3 drops in rapid succession onto the ColorPAC membrane.

Allow to completely absorb.

Proceed immediately to step 3.

Figure 25–2 *Continued*

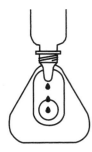

Reagent 5-
Mix thoroughly.
Add 3 drops onto the ColorPAC membrane.
Allow to completely absorb.

RESULTS

Immediately read the results in a well-lighted area as color intensity may change over time. Record the test results.

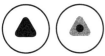

Positive

Positive Test: A pink triangle **of any intensity** appears on the **ColorPAC** membrane, indicating group A streptococcal antigen has been detected. The background area should be white to light pink.

A pink dot will simultaneously appear in the center of the triangle, unless obscured by an intense positive reaction.

Negative

Negative Test: No pink triangle is visible indicating a presumptive negative result, i.e. group A *Streptococcus* antigen was not detected in the specimen. A pink dot appears on the **ColorPAC** membrane and the background area should be white to light pink, indicating proper performance of antigen detection reagents.

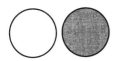

Uninterpretable

Uninterpretable Test: The test is uninterpretable if neither a pink dot nor a triangle is visible.

Any result which obscures the visualization of the control dot and triangle should be regarded as uninterpretable.

If the test is uninterpretable, a new specimen should be obtained and tested using a new **ColorPAC** device.

Example 1   Example 2

Quality Control:
Each **Directigen**₁₋₃ Group A Strep **ColorPAC** device contains two built-in controls. The appearance of a pink control dot provides an internal positive antigen control (Example 1) that validates the immunological reactivity of the device, proper detection reagent function, and assures that the correct detection procedure was followed. The membrane area surrounding the triangle is the internal negative membrane control (Example 2) for the device. The lack of any color development in this area indicates that the detection procedure has been performed correctly.

Liquid Positive (**Control +**) and Negative (**Control -**) controls are also supplied with each kit. These controls are provided in order to monitor

Figure 25-2 *Continued*

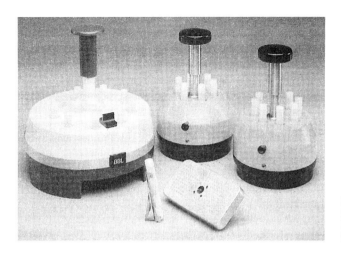

Figure 25–3 Dispensing system for antibiotic sensitivity disks. (Courtesy Becton Dickinson Microbiology Systems, Cockeysville, Md.)

METHOD FOR CULTURE AND SENSITIVITY

Using a pure culture of the pathogen, streak the inoculum on a blood agar plate as described in Chapter 22. Place impregnated disks of various antibiotics on the plate using aseptic technique (Fig. 25–3). Incubate for 24 hours. If the pathogen is resistant to the antibiotic, it will grow to the edge of the disk. An area of no growth around the disk indicates that the antibiotic is effective in inhibiting the pathogen's growth or destroying it. When this happens, the pathogen is said to be sensitive or susceptible to the antibiotic. The clear zone surrounding the disk is called an *inhibition zone*. The pathogen is considered more sensitive when the inhibition zone is large. Charts that interpret zone size are available from the manufacturer of the impregnated disks. Use them when you interpret or record results (Fig. 25–4).

In determining organism sensitivity, the concentration of the pathogen, the concentration of the antibiotic-impregnated disks, and the size of the zone surrounding the colonies are carefully controlled. Sensitivity testing is rarely performed in a POL. How-

Antibiotic Sensitivity

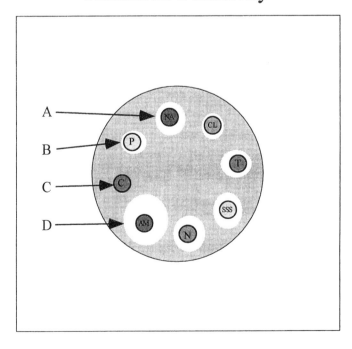

Figure 25–4 Antibiotic sensitivity (susceptibility) test. *(A)* Moderately sensitive. *(B)* Slightly sensitive. *(C)* Resistant. *(D)* Highly sensitive.

ever, you should understand the theory because you may be required to read the results of the laboratory reports and explain them to patients.

QUALITY CONTROL

Quality control presents difficulties in microbiologic testing because of the qualitative interpretation of the results. There are no "normal values" in microbiology in terms of numbers or types of bacteria. For example, there is no set normal for the types or numbers of normal flora in the throat. The areas of quality control that are essential in streptococci testing include the following:

- Proper specimen collection and processing
- Proper storage of reagents and controls
- Maintaining equipment (refrigerators, incubators, autoclaves, etc.)
- Ordering, storing, and maintaining media

When you perform streptococci testing in a POL, dispose of bacterial specimens in a biohazard container. Maintain a clean and safe work environment by cleaning counters according to laboratory protocol. Report and properly record all results and record the positive and negative controls in the log book with the date and lot number of the kit.

SUMMARY

The culturing of bacteria is an important aspect of the diagnostic evaluation of diseased states. Three methods of identifying infectious organisms in the POL include physical findings, immunologic studies, and chemical testing. The laboratorian is responsible for collecting and preparing specimens for streptococci testing. All specimens for culturing must be collected in a manner that prevents contamination of the environment and the specimen.

PATIENT EDUCATION

- Explain all procedures to the patient.

TECHNICAL CONSIDERATIONS

- When collecting specimens for bacterial studies, use aseptic technique.
- Consult the manufacturer's instructions for the proper procedure for the rapid strep test.

SOURCES OF ERROR

- When obtaining a throat culture for the rapid strep test, do not touch the teeth, gums, tongue, or cheeks during the procedure.
- Observe strict adherence to the time recommended by the manufacturer of the product used.
- Bring all kit reagents to room temperature before performing the test.
- Do not use the kit beyond the expiration date.
- Do not mix reagents from kits of different lot numbers.
- Do not mix reagent bottle caps.
- Do not smoke, eat, or drink in areas where specimens or kit reagents are being handled.

Procedure with Rationale

Rapid Strep Test for Group A Beta-Hemolytic Streptococci
EQUIPMENT AND SUPPLIES

Hand soap	Rapid strep test kit
Latex gloves	Surface disinfectant
Culturettes or sterile swabs	Biohazard container
Tongue depressor	

Assemble equipment.

Wash hands with soap and water. Observe the OSHA Standard for this procedure.

Identify and explain the procedure to the patient and ask for cooperation. *Make sure the patient is seated.*

Place the tongue depressor on the back of the throat and ask the patient to say "ahh." *Saying "ahh" forces the uvula up and exposes the back of the throat.*

Observe the oropharynx and tonsillar area for white patches or crypts. *White patches and crypts are usually productive for streptococci organisms and must be swabbed when obtaining the culture.*

Using a rotating motion, swab the back of the throat and the tonsillar area, including any crypts or patchy areas. *Do not touch the tongue, teeth, or cheeks with the swab, because of normal flora contamination.*

Label the specimen, including name, date, and type of specimen.

Perform the rapid streptococci test according to the manufacturer's directions. Identify limitations and sources of errors of the kit.

Record the results of the rapid streptococci test as positive or negative.

Record the results of the positive and negative controls. *Using positive and negative controls provides a measure of quality control of the test kit.*

Dispose of the tongue depressor and swabs in a biohazard container.

Clean work area following laboratory protocol.

Remove gloves and wash hands with soap and water.

Questions

Name _____ Date _____

1. What medium is used for throat cultures and why?

2. Why is it important to correctly identify the presence of group A streptococci?

3. Describe hemolysis of group A beta-hemolytic streptococci.

4. What is a bacitracin disk and how is it used?

5. Briefly describe the rapid strep test and tell why its use is preferred in the pediatrician's office laboratory.

6. What is a sensitivity test, and how is it interpreted?

Rapid Strep Test for Group A Beta-Hemolytic Streptococci

Given the necessary equipment, you will be able to perform a rapid strep test according to the manufacturer's directions. Record your results of the test and the positive and negative controls. This procedure must be completed within the time recommended by the manufacturer of the kit with the degree of accuracy defined by your instructor.

INSTRUCTOR'S EVALUATION FORM

Name _____ Date _____

+ = SATISFACTORY   ✓ = UNSATISFACTORY

_____ Assemble equipment.

_____ Wash hands with soap and water. Observe the OSHA Standard for this procedure.

_____ Identify and explain the procedure to the patient and ask for cooperation.

_____ Place the tongue depressor on the back of the throat and ask the patient to say "ahh."

_____ Observe the oropharynx and tonsillar area for white patches or crypts.

_____ Using a rotating motion, swab the back of the throat and the tonsillar area, including any crypts or patchy areas.

_____ Label the specimen, including name, date, and type of specimen.

_____ Perform the rapid streptococci test according to manufacturer's directions.

_____ Record the results of the rapid streptococci test.

RESULTS: _____ .

_____ Record the results of the positive and negative controls.

RESULTS: _____ .

_____ Dispose of the tongue depressor and swabs in a biohazard container.

_____ Clean work area following laboratory protocol.

_____ Remove gloves and wash hands with soap and water.

_____ The procedure was completed within the recommended time.

_____ The results of the test were acceptable to your instructor.

_____ The results were properly recorded.

Final Competency Evaluation

_____ SATISFACTORY   _____ UNSATISFACTORY

Comments:

Instructor _____ Date _____

Pregnancy Testing

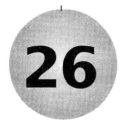

26

Learning Objectives
Cognitive Objectives
Psychomotor Objectives
Affective Objectives

Specimen Collection for Pregnancy Testing

Pregnancy Testing Methods
Enzyme Immunoassay
Agglutination Inhibition

Pregnancy Test Results

Quality Control

Summary
Patient Education
Technical Considerations
Sources of Error

Procedure with Rationale
Rapid Slide Pregnancy Test

Questions

Terminal Performance Objective
Rapid Slide Pregnancy Test
○ Instructor's evaluation form

LEARNING OBJECTIVES

On completing this chapter, you will be able to:

COGNITIVE OBJECTIVES
- Describe the formation of human chorionic gonadotropin.
- Describe specimen collection for pregnancy testing.
- Explain the proper handling of the specimen.
- Describe the enzyme immunoassay techniques used for detecting human chorionic gonadotropin.
- Explain the agglutination inhibition principle for detecting human chorionic gonadotropin.
- List the clinical conditions other than pregnancy that produce human chorionic gonadotropin.

PSYCHOMOTOR OBJECTIVES
- Perform a rapid slide test for human chorionic gonadotropin following the Terminal Performance Objective presented in this chapter.
- Record the results of rapid slide test for human chorionic gonadotropin.
- Record the results of the positive and negative controls.

AFFECTIVE OBJECTIVES
- Show concern for laboratory personnel by following laboratory protocol for disposing of urine specimens.
- Maintain a safe environment for the safety of your coworkers and yourself.

Testing for pregnancy is a simple procedure that uses in vitro antigen-antibody reaction to determine the presence of *human chorionic gonadotropin* (hCG or HCG). HCG is a hormone that is secreted in large amounts by the placenta during **gestation**. It is produced by the chorionic villi of the developing placenta and appears in the serum and urine of pregnant women. The level of hCG reaches a peak between the 50th and 80th days of gestation and then begins to decline, disappearing within a few days after **parturition**.

> **Gestation:** *the length of time from conception to birth*

> **Parturition:** *the birthing process*

SPECIMEN COLLECTION FOR PREGNANCY TESTING

For all hCG testing, use a first morning urine specimen because it is more concentrated and contains higher levels of hCG than random specimens. The urine specimen must be fresh. Since detergents can interfere with results, collect urine specimens in a disposable urine container. When this is not practical, use a clean, well-rinsed container without any chemical residue. A dirty container, or one that contains residue, is the most common source of error in POLs when urine is brought to the office.

Before performing the test for hCG, screen the urine for the presence of hematuria, bacterial contamination, and proteinuria. Do not use urine specimens containing blood, large amounts of protein, or excessive bacterial contamination since they may produce invalid results. Collect another sample of urine specimen for more accurate testing.

HCG deteriorates during storage without appropriate refrigeration. Perform the test as soon as possible, preferably within 1 to 2 hours of collection. If necessary preserve the specimen by refrigeration at 2°C to 8°C. For storage longer than 24 hours and up to 6 months, freeze the specimen (−20°C). To thaw a frozen specimen, place it in a 37°C water bath. Mix the thawed specimen and remove excessive sediment by centrifuging it and decanting the supernatant prior to testing. Do not refreeze samples.

PREGNANCY TESTING METHODS

The two methods used for the detection of hCG are a modified enzyme immunoassay test and the agglutination inhibition test. Both methods adopt the use of antigen-antibody reactions for identifying the hCG. Refer to Chapter 24 for a thorough understanding of the antigen-antibody complex formation, enzyme immunoassay testing, and agglutination.

Enzyme Immunoassay

The enzyme immunoassay (EIA) is designed to detect hCG in serum and urine. Most pregnancy tests are a modification of the EIA principle known as solid-phase or membrane EIAs. Antibodies and other reagents are immobilized in an absorbent membrane enclosed in a plastic case. When the specimen is added to the membrane it migrates through the membrane and comes in contact with the reagents. This results in a color reaction visible to the eye (Fig. 26–1).

Sensitivity: *a term used in assessing the value of a diagnostic test, procedure, or clinical observation*

EIAs are designed to selectively identify hCG in both serum and urine with a high degree of **sensitivity**. Levels of hCG as low as 25 mIU/mL will be detected in serum or urine. Because **ectopic pregnancies** or spontaneous abortion produce low levels of hCG, EIAs are important for clinical evaluation of these conditions.

Ectopic pregnancy: *implantation of the fertilized ovum outside of the uterine cavity*

Examples of the rapid slide tests for hCG using modified enzyme immunoassay are Clearview HCG II and HCG DUO by Wampole Laboratories; TestPack Plus hCG Urine and TestPack hCG-Combo, Abbott Laboratories.

Agglutination Inhibition

As explained in Chapter 24, agglutination occurs when a specific antibody unites with antigen coated with particulate matter. An agglutination inhibition test is designed so that agglutination appears in the sample only when the antigen being tested is absent. Therefore, the slide pregnancy test is designed so that no agglutination will occur if hCG is present in the sample.

Antiserum: *serum that contains antibodies for a specific antigen; may be of human or animal origin*

UCG-SLIDE TEST by Wampole Laboratories is a two-step procedure. The test contains two reagents: (1) **antiserum** reagent (anti-hCG serum) and (2) antigen reagent (hCG-coated latex suspension). The anti-hCG serum is made from the serum of rabbits injected with purified hCG. The rabbit develops hCG antibodies called anti-hCG.

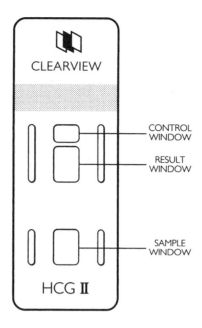

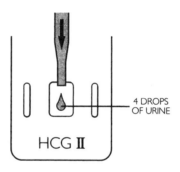

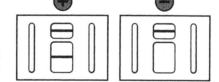

Figure 26–1 Procedure for performing Clearview HCG II enzyme immunoassay pregnancy test. (Courtesy Wampole Laboratories, Cranbury, NJ.)

First, mix a urine sample with the antiserum reagent. If the sample contains hCG antigen, it combines with the anti-hCG antibody, forming an antigen-antibody complex.

Next, add antigen reagent, which consists of hCG-coated latex particles. If hCG *was* present in the sample, it has already combined with the anti-hCG (first reagent). Therefore, no antigen-antibody reaction occurs when the hCG antigen-coated latex particles (second reagent) are added to the sample. In other words, agglutination is inhibited, *no* agglutination occurs, and the test result is positive.

If hCG is not present in the sample, the anti-hCG (first reagent) is free to react with the hCG on the latex particles (second reagent). The antigen-antibody reaction causes the latex particles to agglutinate. In other words, agglutination occurs and the test result

Principle of Agglutination Inhibition Test

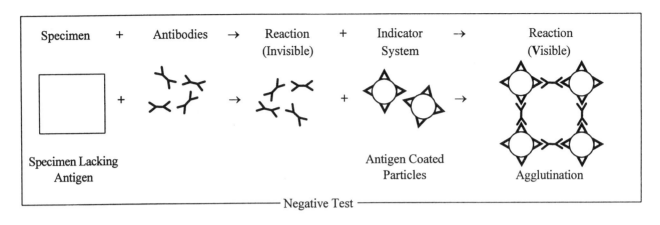

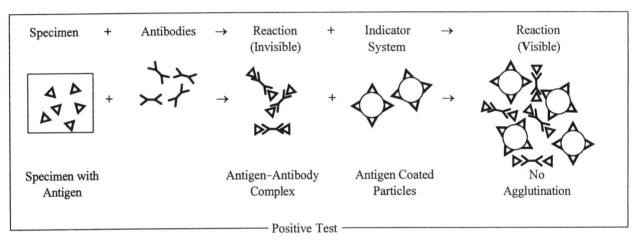

Figure 26-2 Illustration showing the principle of agglutination inhibition test for hCG.

Human Chorionic Gonadotropin
(hCG)

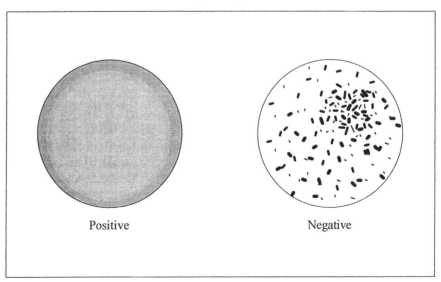

Figure 26-3 Human chorionic gonadotropin test and results using agglutination inhibition. No agglutination is positive; agglutination is negative.

is negative. Figure 26–2 illustrates the reactions that lead to both positive and negative results, and Figure 26–3 illustrates the results as they appear on the slide.

PREGNANCY TEST RESULTS

A positive test result does not always indicate pregnancy. Some diseases may cause a positive test result in the absence of pregnancy. False-positive and false-negative results also occur in tests of specimens from individuals taking a variety of drugs. The presence of interfering substances (e.g., hematuria, proteinuria, and bacterial contamination) may give false results.

Clinical Comment: Trophoblastic Diseases

Urine specimens from patients with **trophoblastic** diseases such as *choriocarcinoma, hydatid mole*, or malignant tumors of the ovaries or testes can secrete HCG. Choriocarcinoma is a malignant neoplasm of trophoblastic cells formed by abnormal growth of the placental epithelium without producing chorionic villi. Hydatid mole is a degenerative process in the chorionic villi, which produces benign cysts and rapid growth of the uterus with hemorrhage.

Trophoblastic: *pertaining to the outer layer of the developing embryo*

As with all diagnostic tests, the physician evaluates pregnancy test results in terms of the total clinical profile of the patient. If results are questionable, that is, the test agglutinates only slightly, the test should be repeated. This can be done immediately with a more sensitive test or with a fresh sample taken 1 or 2 days later when the concentration of hCG should be greater.

Another consideration for interpretation of hCG results is the stage of the pregnancy. In a normal pregnancy, hCG increases rapidly with time. Levels of hCG double approximately every 2 days. In an ectopic pregnancy, hCG levels typically increase at a slower rate. Ectopic and other abnormal pregnancies may produce too little hCG to be detected by the rapid slide method. With early spontaneous abortion, hCG levels first rise and then begin to decline (Fig. 26–4).

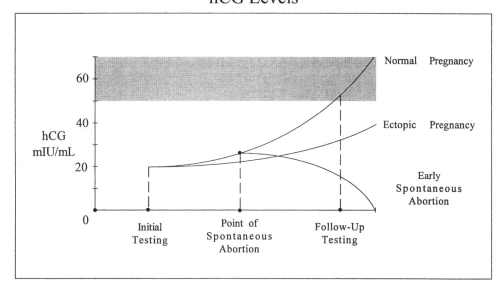

mIU = milli International Unit (¹/₁₀₀₀ of an IU)

Figure 26–4 Typical patterns of hCG activity. Normal pregnancy: hCG levels double approximately every 2 days. Ectopic pregnancy: hCG typically increases at a slower rate. Early spontaneous abortion: hCG first rises and then begins to fall.

QUALITY CONTROL

When doing a urine pregnancy test, use one sample each of a known positive and a known negative hCG urine sample. Record the results of the controls in a daily log with expiration date and lot numbers of reagents used.

The reagents of some test kits must be stored at 2°C to 8°C and brought to room temperature before using. In other test kits the reagents are stored at room temperature. Read package inserts carefully. Collect and store urine specimens to ensure all aspects of quality control.

If glass slides are used, wash them each time with detergent. Thoroughly rinse with tap water, and wipe with lint-free tissue to avoid spotting. Since detergents may interfere with testing, rinsing is a critical step. Follow the product insert exactly for quality assurance in testing.

Properly dispose of the urine specimen according to your laboratory protocol. Disposing of the urine specimen properly shows concern for your safety and the safety of your coworkers. Clean the work area with 10 percent bleach and maintain a safe environment by washing the work station after each use.

SUMMARY

Rapid slide tests for pregnancy are useful in determining whether hCG is present in the urine. The presence of hCG may indicate pregnancy or it may assist in the diagnosis of trophoblastic diseases, such as hydatidiform mole and choriocarcinoma, or malignant tumors of the ovaries or testes. The proper use of positive and negative controls in conjunction with this test should ensure that the testing procedure is accurate.

PATIENT EDUCATION

- The patient must be instructed to collect a first morning sample in a clean and well-rinsed container, free of detergents or other chemicals.
- Document in the patient's chart that the patient was properly instructed in the collection of the urine specimen.

TECHNICAL CONSIDERATIONS

- Depending on the test kit used, the rapid slide test for pregnancy may be designed to test serum and urine or only urine. Check the manufacturer's brochure.
- Use positive and negative controls when testing all specimens.

SOURCES OF ERROR

- The most accurate test results are obtained from specimens of patients who are not on drug therapy.
- Bring all reagents to room temperature if necessary.
- The presence of interfering substances (e.g., hematuria, proteinuria, and bacterial contamination) may give false results depending on the kit used.
- Store all reagents according to manufacturer's recommendations.
- The reagents of the rapid slide test kit can be damaged by bacterial growth or by extremes of temperatures during transit and storage.
- Make sure the antigen reagent is well mixed before using.
- Do not interchange reagents of one kit with those of another kit.
- Using outdated reagents may give inaccurate results.
- Traces of detergent or previous specimens on test slide may invalidate the results.

Procedure with Rationale

Rapid Slide Pregnancy Test

EQUIPMENT AND SUPPLIES

Hand soap	High-intensity lamp
Latex gloves	Timer
Urine specimen	Surface disinfectant
Positive and negative urine controls	Biohazard container
UCG-SLIDE TEST Pregnancy kit	

Assemble equipment.

Wash hands with soap and water. Observe the OSHA Standard for this procedure.

UCG-SLIDE TEST

Bring all specimens and reagents to room temperature before beginning the test. *If specimens and reagents are not at room temperature, the test may be invalid.*

Using the special slide and the disposable pipette provided with the kit, place one drop of urine into the center circle of the glass slide.

Place one drop of positive control into the left circle and one drop of negative control in the right circle of the slide.

Add one drop of the antiserum reagent directly on the urine and control samples. Do not touch the samples with the pipette of the antiserum reagent. *Touching the samples will result in contamination of the antigen reagent.*

Add one drop of well-mixed antigen reagent directly on the urine-antiserum specimen. Do not touch the sample with the pipette. *Touching the samples will result in contamination of the antigen reagent.*

Mix the urine, antiserum reagent, and the antigen reagent together with separate stirrers for each test by spreading the mixture over the entire circle. Discard the stirrers in a biohazard container.

Rock slide gently and slowly for 2 minutes and immediately observe for agglutination. Use a direct light source when observing agglutination. Read and record results. *Read within 2 minutes after rocking begins or the sample may dry, causing erroneous results.*

Read the positive and negative controls and log your results.

Clean work area following laboratory protocol.

Remove gloves and wash hands with soap and water.

Questions

Name _____ Date _____

1. What is hCG? Where is it formed? When is it at its peak level in pregnancy?

2. Briefly describe the test principle of the pregnancy slide test for detection of hCG.

3. Name the two methods most frequently used to test for hCG and give a brief description of them.

4. Describe the results of the rapid slide test for hCG.

5. Name the clinical conditions other than pregnancy that produce hCG.

6. Name the substances that may interfere when testing for hCG.

Terminal Performance Objective

Rapid Slide Pregnancy Test

Given the necessary equipment, you will be able to perform a rapid slide test for pregnancy. Record the results and the positive and negative controls. This procedure must be performed within 5 minutes to a level of accuracy specified by your instructor.

Infectious Mononucleosis Testing

27

Learning Objectives
Cognitive Objectives
Psychomotor Objectives
Affective Objectives

Nature of the Disease
Symptoms
Treatment

Rapid Slide Test for Infectious Mononucleosis

Method for Performing the Rapid Slide Test

Interpreting Test Results

Quality Control

Summary
Patient Education
Technical Considerations
Sources of Error

Procedure with Rationale
Rapid Slide Test for
  Infectious Mononucleosis

Questions

Terminal Performance Objective
Rapid Slide Test for
  Infectious Mononucleosis
  ○ Instructor's evaluation form

LEARNING OBJECTIVES

On completing this chapter, you will be able to:

COGNITIVE OBJECTIVES
- Describe the condition known as infectious mononucleosis.
- List the symptoms of infectious mononucleosis.
- Explain the treatment for infectious mononucleosis.
- Describe the rapid slide test for infectious mononucleosis.

PSYCHOMOTOR OBJECTIVES
- Perform a rapid slide test for infectious mononucleosis that meets the Terminal Performance Objective presented in this chapter.
- Record the results of rapid slide test for infectious mononucleosis.
- Record the results of the positive and negative controls.

AFFECTIVE OBJECTIVES
- Show concern for laboratory personnel by following laboratory protocol for disposing of blood and decontaminating the work area.
- Care for your coworkers by maintaining a safe and clean environment.

Infectious mononucleosis (IM) is an acute infectious disease. Patients who have IM often have enlarged lymph nodes and a marked increase of atypical lymphocytes in the blood *(lymphocytosis)*. A virus called Epstein-Barr is the causative agent for IM.

IM may be transmitted by direct oral contact, and for this reason it is often called the "kissing disease." It occurs more frequently in the spring of the year and affects primarily children and young adults. IM usually occurs early in life with no recognizable disease. When the primary infection is delayed until young adulthood and adolescence, there is a 50 percent chance that it will occur with the classic clinical symptoms associated with IM.

NATURE OF THE DISEASE

Heterophile antibodies: *characteristic antibodies of the IgM classification found in 90 to 95 percent of adolescents and 50 percent of children with infectious mononucleosis*

Patients infected with the Epstein-Barr virus produce **heterophile antibodies.** These antibodies, classified as IgM, are usually present in the body by the 6th to 10th day after the onset of illness. Most patients have a detectable level of heterophile antibody within 3 weeks of infection. Occasionally, a patient with clinical symptoms of IM will take 3 months to develop a detectable level of heterophile antibody. Some patients remain negative for heterophile antibody even when clinical symptoms and hematological evidence of IM are present. The level of antibody activity is not correlated with the severity of the disease or the degree of lymphocytosis.

Symptoms

Symptoms occur after an incubation period of 1 week to several weeks. The most frequent symptoms are sore throat, fever, and headache. Severe weakness, mental and physical fatigue, and symptoms typical of influenza are common. Skin rashes may also occur.

Physicians diagnose IM on the basis of immunologic test results, a marked increase in the number of lymphocytes in the blood, enlarged lymph nodes, and possibly an enlarged spleen. The lymph nodes and spleen may remain enlarged for some time after other symptoms have disappeared. Involvement of the liver occurs in about 10 percent of all cases of IM, and jaundice may be a side effect of liver involvement. In rare cases the heart, lungs, and central nervous system may be affected or the spleen may rupture.

Clinical Comment: Infectious Diseases

Infectious mononucleosis is difficult to diagnose because infectious diseases such as influenza, rubella, and hepatitis have clinical symptoms that mimic IM. The rapid slide test alone should not be used to diagnose IM. The final diagnosis also depends on clinical findings and hematology reports.

Treatment

Vaccine: *a suspension of infectious agents, or a part of them, given for the purpose of developing resistance to a specific infectious disease*

Bed rest is especially important in the early stages of the disease or later if the liver becomes involved. At this time there is no immunization, but a **vaccine** is being developed that is expected to provide immunity to this disease.

RAPID SLIDE TEST FOR INFECTIOUS MONONUCLEOSIS

Many companies manufacture a rapid slide test for IM based on agglutination principles. Mono-Latex and Mono-plus are manufactured by Wampole Laboratories; Cards O.S. and Concise Plus Mono Tests by Quidel; Color Slide II Mononucleosis Test by Seradyn; and BBL Monoslide Test by Becton Dickinson. Consult the manufacturer's brochure to determine the type of specimen necessary for testing. Refer to Chapter 8 for specimen collection.

Since the heterophile antibody of IM is relatively stable, uncontaminated specimens of serum or plasma can be stored at 2°C to 8°C for 3 days. If the specimen needs prolonged storage, freeze the specimen. Serum or plasma samples should be clear and particle-free. Do not use contaminated or grossly hemolyzed specimens, which may indicate that the specimen has been exposed to adverse temperatures, improper handling, or contamination.

METHOD FOR PERFORMING THE RAPID SLIDE TEST

The slide test for IM is actually a test to demonstrate the presence or absence of the heterophile antibodies. You can detect these antibodies with the Mono-Latex test in a single-step agglutination reaction. The Mono-Latex test reagent consists of a mononucleosis antigen obtained from bovine cell membranes attached to latex particles.

The Mono-Latex test procedure consists of adding one drop each of positive control and negative control and 50 µL of patient specimen to the appropriate circles etched on the slide provided with the test. After gently mixing the vial, add one free-flowing drop of Mono-Latex Reagent Latex to each circle. Be sure not to touch the dropper of the bottle to the specimen and controls. Mix the contents of each circle with a different stirrer, covering the entire area of the circle. Rotate the slide at room temperature for 2 minutes (Fig. 27–1).

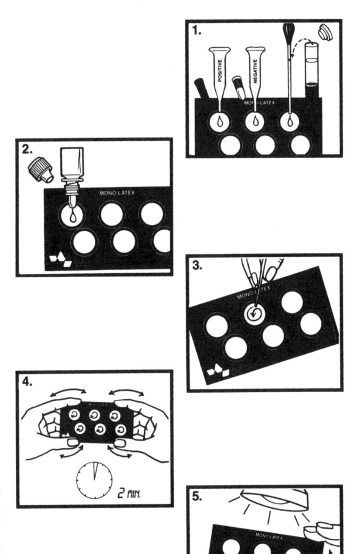

Figure 27–1 Mono-Latex test procedure. *(1)* Place positive and negative controls into the appropriate labeled circles. *(2)* Dispense reagent latex to each circle. *(3)* Mix contents of each circle thoroughly, covering the entire area. *(4)* Rock slide by hand in a circular motion. *(5)* After 2 minutes, immediately observe for agglutination. (Courtesy Wampole Laboratories, Cranbury, NJ.)

Infectious Mononucleosis

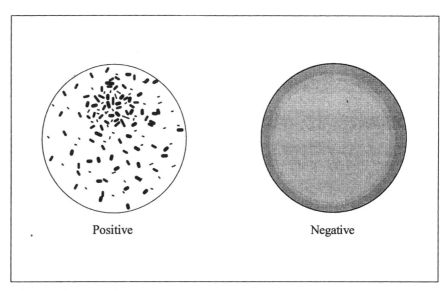

Positive   Negative

Figure 27–2   IM slide test results. Agglutination is positive; no agglutination is negative.

INTERPRETING TEST RESULTS

The Mono-Latex reagent will agglutinate in the presence of heterophile antibody. Observe for visible agglutination of the latex particles within 2 minutes of rotation. If there is agglutination, the test is positive; if there is no agglutination, the test is negative. Agglutination that appears after a 2-minute reading time is not to be interpreted as a positive result for the heterophile antibody (Fig. 27–2).

QUALITY CONTROL

It is important to follow the manufacturer's instructions in order to maintain quality control. Do not use reagents after their expiration dates. If refrigeration is necessary, be sure to bring the reagents to room temperature and mix them thoroughly before adding them to the sample to be tested. Be sure that glass slides are completely clean before using them.

To ensure that the test kit is functioning properly, use both positive and negative controls each time a specimen is tested. Record the results in a permanent log with the date of expiration and lot numbers of reagents. If the manufacturer's insert is followed exactly, the test results should be reliable.

Maintain a safe and clean laboratory by disposing of the test specimens into a biohazard container and decontaminate the work area. Specimens are potentially infectious; handle with appropriate precautions.

SUMMARY

The rapid slide tests for IM heterophile antibody are useful for determining the presence or absence of the specific IM antibody. Demonstration of the presence of this antibody assists the physician in diagnosing IM. Besides the immunologic testing, the clinical findings of enlarged lymph glands or enlarged spleen and the hematology report of lymphocytosis confirm the IM diagnosis.

Using positive and negative controls when testing for heterophile antibodies ensures the accuracy of the testing procedure and contributes to quality assurance in the medical office.

PATIENT EDUCATION

- No special preparation of the patient is required prior to specimen collection.

TECHNICAL CONSIDERATIONS

- Serum, plasma, or whole blood may be tested for IM depending on the kit used.
- Use positive and negative controls when testing all specimens.
- Follow the manufacturer's recommendation for timing the test.

SOURCES OF ERROR

- Contaminated or grossly hemolyzed specimens or specimens that have been exposed to adverse temperatures or improper handling may produce inaccurate results.
- Improperly cleaned glass slides may interfere with results.
- Reagents not thoroughly mixed or brought to room temperature may alter test results.
- Not using reagents before their expiration date may produce inaccurate results.

Procedure with Rationale

Rapid Slide Test for Infectious Mononucleosis

EQUIPMENT AND SUPPLIES

Hand soap	Serum or plasma sample
Latex gloves	Timer
Mono-Latex slide test or other slide test kit for IM	Surface disinfectant
	Biohazard container

Assemble equipment.

Wash hands with soap and water. Observe the OSHA Standard for this procedure.

Bring the specimens and reagent to room temperature.

Place the glass slide on a flat surface under a direct light source.

Place one free-falling drop of well-mixed positive control and negative control into the appropriate labeled circles.

For each specimen, fill a capillary tube supplied in the kit with serum or plasma up to the marked line. Squeeze the capillary bulb to deliver 50 µL of specimen into the center of the appropriate circle. Use a fresh capillary pipette to deliver each test specimen.

Dispense one drop of thoroughly mixed reagent latex on top of the specimen and controls. Be sure to use a free-falling drop created by holding the dropper bottle vertically and gently squeezing. Do not touch the tip of the reagent latex bottle to the test specimens or controls. *Touching the test specimens and controls will result in contaminating the reagent latex.*

Mix the contents of each circle thoroughly with a different disposable stirrer, covering the entire area of the circle. *Using a new stirrer for each circle will avoid cross-contamination of samples.*

Immediately rock the slide by hand in a circular motion or on a serological rotator for 2 minutes.

After 2 minutes, immediately observe for agglutination and record results. A light held over the slide will improve the readability of the test. The test must be read at 2 minutes. *If the test is not read at 2 minutes, the results are invalid.*

Read the positive and negative controls and record your results.

Clean work area following laboratory protocol.

Remove gloves and wash hands with soap and water.

Questions

Name _____ Date _____

1. What is infectious mononucleosis (IM)? What is the causative agent for IM?

2. What are heterophile antibodies?

3. At what stage of infection is the heterophile antibody of IM demonstrated?

4. List the symptoms of IM.

5. What is the treatment for IM?

6. List four sources of error that may interfere with accurate results when testing for IM.

Terminal Performance Objective

Rapid Slide Test for Infectious Mononucleosis

Given the necessary equipment, you will be able to perform a rapid slide test for IM following manufacturer's directions. Record the results of the test and the positive and negative controls. This procedure must be completed within 10 minutes with the degree of accuracy defined by your instructor.

INSTRUCTOR'S EVALUATION FORM

Name _____ Date _____

+ = SATISFACTORY   ✓ = UNSATISFACTORY

_____ Assemble equipment.

_____ Wash hands with soap and water. Observe the OSHA Standard for this procedure.

_____ Bring the specimens and reagents to room temperature.

_____ Place the glass slide on a flat surface under a direct light source.

_____ Place one free-falling drop of well-mixed positive control and negative control into the appropriately labeled circles.

_____ For each specimen, fill a capillary tube with serum or plasma up to the marked line. Squeeze the capillary bulb to deliver 50 μL of specimen into the center of the appropriate circle. Use a fresh capillary pipette to deliver each test specimen.

_____ Dispense one drop of thoroughly mixed reagent latex on top of the specimen and controls.

_____ Mix the contents of each circle thoroughly with a different disposable stirrer covering the entire area of the circle.

_____ Immediately rock the slide by hand in a circular motion or on a serological rotator for 2 minutes.

_____ After 2 minutes, immediately observe for agglutination and record results.

RESULTS: _____.

_____ Read the positive and negative controls and record your results.

RESULTS: _____.

_____ Clean work area following laboratory protocol.

_____ Remove gloves and wash hands with soap and water.

_____ The procedure was completed within 10 minutes.

_____ The results obtained were accurate to the level specified by your instructor.

_____ The results were properly recorded.

Final Competency Evaluation

_____ SATISFACTORY   _____ UNSATISFACTORY

Comments:

Instructor _____ Date _____

Rheumatoid Arthritis Testing

28

Learning Objectives
Cognitive Objectives
Psychomotor Objectives
Affective Objectives

Nature of the Disease
Rheumatoid Factor
Symptoms
Treatment

Method for Performing the Rapid Slide Test

Interpreting Test Results

Quality Control

Summary
Patient Education
Technical Considerations
Sources of Error

Procedure with Rationale
Rapid Slide Test for
    Rheumatoid Arthritis

Questions

Terminal Performance Objective
Rapid Slide Test for
    Rheumatoid Arthritis
    ○ Instructor's evaluation form

LEARNING OBJECTIVES

On completing this chapter, you will be able to:

COGNITIVE OBJECTIVES
- Describe the condition known as rheumatoid arthritis.
- List the symptoms of rheumatoid arthritis.
- Explain the treatment for rheumatoid arthritis.
- Describe a rapid slide test for rheumatoid arthritis.

PSYCHOMOTOR OBJECTIVES
- Perform a rapid slide test for rheumatoid arthritis using the Terminal Performance Objective presented in this chapter.
- Record the test results of the rapid slide test for rheumatoid arthritis.
- Record the results of the positive and negative controls.

AFFECTIVE OBJECTIVES
- Show concern for your coworkers by following laboratory protocol for disposing of the test specimens.
- Protect your laboratory personnel by maintaining a safe and clean laboratory environment.

Rheumatoid arthritis (RA) is a chronic **systemic** disease characterized by inflammatory changes occurring throughout the body's **connective tissue.** RA affects joints and related structures and results in crippling deformities. It is classified as a *collagen* disease. Collagen is a fibrous, insoluble protein found in the connective tissue, including skin, bone, ligaments, and cartilage. Collagen represents about 30 percent of the total body protein.

Systemic: *pertaining to a whole body rather than to one of its parts*

Connective tissue: *tissue that supports and binds other tissues and parts*

389

NATURE OF THE DISEASE

The specific cause of RA is unknown, but it is generally believed that the pathological changes in the joints are related to an antigen-antibody reaction. Some researchers believe RA to be an **autoimmune disease.** Others contend that the disease may be due to infection by an undefined virus or some other microorganism. Another theory holds that RA is a genetic disorder, in which one inherits a predisposition to the disease. Physical and emotional stress may have some effect in the beginning of **acute** attacks.

Rheumatoid Factor

Most of the patients afflicted with RA produce autoantibodies called *rheumatoid factor* (RF). They are autoantibodies of the IgM classification and are usually present in the serum of 70 to 80 percent of adults with RA (see Table 24–1). This RF is formed when the immune system encounters an **aberrant** antibody (IgG), which has been altered in such a way that it is no longer recognized as an antibody. The RF reacts with the aberrant IgG to produce an antigen-antibody (immune) complex. These complexes migrate to connective tissue throughout the body, causing tissue destruction.

We do not fully understand how the aberrant IgG becomes **antigenic.** Perhaps the IgG is altered by a virus. The altered IgG is called an *autoantigen* because it is produced by the host and causes the production of antibodies. The IgM (rheumatoid factor) reacts with the aberrant IgG to form antigen-antibody complexes called *autoantibodies.*

Symptoms

The onset of RA is gradual with only mild symptoms in 75 percent of the cases. Early symptoms include malaise, fever, weight loss, and morning stiffness of joints. One or more joints may become swollen, painful, and inflamed. Some patients experience only mild episodes of acute symptoms with long periods of remission between attacks.

Acute attacks of arthritis may develop during the most productive years of adulthood. In the majority of cases onset occurs between the ages of 20 to 40. Men and women are afflicted equally, but three times as many women as men manifest symptoms severe enough to require medical attention. The disease may also affect infants.

For the most part, the typical patient experiences increasingly severe and frequent attacks with deformity and cartilage damage of the joints due to the immune complexes. Also, there is **atrophy** of the surrounding muscles, bones, and skin. Remissions and **exacerbations** continue throughout the disease.

Treatment

There is no specific therapy for RA. Bed rest is recommended with at least 10 to 12 hours of sleep to allow the body's natural defenses to work against inflammation. Aspirin (acetylsalicylic acid) is most effective when given at high dosage to relieve the symptoms of swelling and pain, but may cause stomach upset or other gastrointestinal side effects. Other nonaspirin, anti-inflammatory drugs, such as ibuprofen and indole derivatives, may be effective. Physicians may also use corticosteroids, but only for short-term therapy to reduce the immune reaction.

Intra-articular injection of cortisone helps treat painful and acute inflammation of the joints. This local treatment is temporary and lasts only 2 to 3 weeks. It permits the patient to remain ambulatory. Local use of cortisone does not cure the disease process or prevent its progression.

Exercise and physiotherapy are important in maintaining a range of motion of affected joints. Passive exercise helps to prevent contracture during the inflammatory period. When inflammation has subsided, physicians recommend active exercise for muscle strength and range of motion. Surgical procedures, such as arthroplasty and total hip replacement, may be effective.

Autoimmune disease: *disease in which the body produces antibodies against its own cells and tissues*

Acute: *having rapid onset, severe symptoms, and a short course; not chronic*

Aberrant: *abnormal, atypical, and varying from the usual*

Antigenic: *capable of producing an antibody*

Atrophy: *a decrease in size of an organ or tissue*

Exacerbation: *an increase in the severity of a disease or any of its symptoms*

Principle of Latex Agglutination
for Rheumatoid Factor

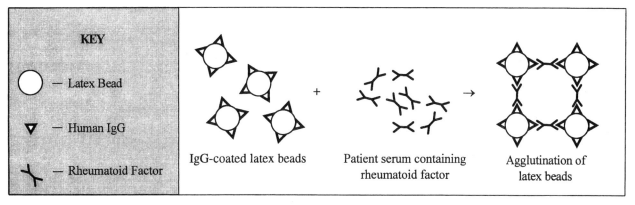

Figure 28-1 Principle of latex agglutination test for rheumatoid factor. Rheumatoid factor in patient's serum reacts with the latex particles coated with human IgG to cause agglutination.

METHOD FOR PERFORMING THE RAPID SLIDE TEST

RFs are not specific for RA but are not usually elevated in other forms of arthritis. They are helpful in diagnosing and investigating the disease process. Very high RF titers might indicate a poor prognosis with severe joint disease and probable systemic complications.

The rapid slide test provides a simple, rapid qualitative method for detecting RF in serum. The rapid slide test reagent consists of small latex particles coated with specially treated human immunoglobulin (IgG). When a serum specimen containing RF is mixed with the reagent, a visible agglutination reaction develops (Fig. 28-1).

Available RF kits are the Rheumaton and Rheumatex by Wampole Laboratories, Rfscan Latex by Becton Dickinson, and SeraTest RF Latex by Seradyn, Inc. With the exception of Rheumaton, these kits provide coated latex particles, positive and negative control sera, and buffer and other material necessary to perform the tests. The Rheumaton kit consists of sheep erythrocytes sensitized with rabbit gamma globulin for the determination of RF in serum and **synovial fluid.** It has positive and negative sera.

Synovial fluid: *clear lubricating fluid secreted by the synovial membrane of a joint*

INTERPRETING TEST RESULTS

Nearly all patients with RA, and those with inflammatory diseases such as **Felty's** or **Sjögren's syndrome,** may show positive results for RF. Positive specimens readily show visible agglutination with the rapid slide test reagent. Negative specimens show no agglutination or a finely granular pattern (Fig. 28-2).

Felty's syndrome: *chronic rheumatoid arthritis associated with splenomegaly, neutropenia, and anemia and thrombocytopenia*

QUALITY CONTROL

To ensure quality control, use positive and negative controls with each specimen tested with the rapid slide test. The positive control shows agglutination and the negative control shows no agglutination.

Using positive and negative controls will confirm that the reagents are working properly. Record the results of positive and negative controls in a permanent log with the expiration date and lot number. Follow product inserts exactly for quality assurance in testing for RA.

Sjögren's syndrome: *an immunologic disorder with rheumatoid arthritis occurring in postmenopausal women*

Rheumatoid Arthritis Slide

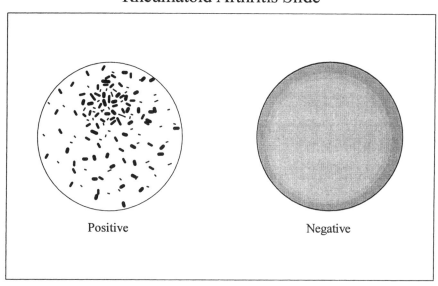

Positive   Negative

Figure 28-2 Rheumatoid arthritis slide agglutination results. Agglutination is positive; no agglutination is negative.

If there is any variance in the results obtained with the controls, examine the procedure and check the reagents for expiration dates. Improper storage of reagents can affect the quality of the test. The reagents are stable when stored as directed. However, the reagents in rapid slide test kits can be damaged by extremes of temperature. Do not interchange reagents among kits.

Maintain a clean and safe laboratory by disposing of the test specimens into a biohazard container. Disinfect the area by following laboratory protocol.

SUMMARY

The rapid slide test for RA is helpful in determining the RF present in the majority of patients afflicted with the disease. Patients with RA produce antibodies that react with the aberrant IgG to form immune complexes. These complexes are responsible for the destruction of the connective tissue found mostly in joints.

PATIENT EDUCATION

- No special preparation of the patient is required prior to specimen collection.

TECHNICAL CONSIDERATIONS

- Use positive and negative controls for this test.
- Use only serum or synovial fluid for this procedure.
- Glass slides are recommended when testing RF with the Rheumaton and Rheumatex test kits.

SOURCES OF ERROR

- Using specimens showing gross hemolysis, **lipemia,** or turbidity may yield incorrect results.
- Never interchange reagents from different kits.
- Maintain reagents at the temperature recommended by the manufacturer of the kits.
- Bring all reagents to room temperature prior to use.
- When using glass slides, wash each time with detergent, rinse several times with tap water, and wipe with lint-free tissue to avoid spotting.

Lipemia: *pertaining to fats or fatlike substances*

Procedure with Rationale

Rapid Slide Test for Rheumatoid Arthritis
EQUIPMENT AND SUPPLIES

Hand soap	Timer
Rheumaton or any other rapid slide test	Surface disinfectant
Serum specimen	Biohazard container
Latex gloves	

Assemble equipment.

Wash hands with soap and water. Observe the OSHA Standard for this procedure.

Allow the reagents and serum to reach room temperature before testing.

Place glass slide or card provided with the kit on a flat surface under a direct light source.

Fill capillary pipette provided to the mark with serum and dispel the serum into the center of the middle section of the etched slide or vacant circle on the card.

Using the droppers provided with the controls, place one drop of positive control and one drop of negative control in the appropriate test circles.

Add one free-falling drop of well-mixed reagent to each section of the slide. *The reagent must be well-mixed prior to use to resuspend cells or test results may be inaccurate.*

Using a clean, disposable stirrer for each mixture, mix each sample by spreading uniformly over the entire section. *Using a clean, disposable stirrer for each mixture prevents contamination of the samples.*

Rock the slide gently with rotary motion for the time recommended by the manufacturer. Immediately observe for agglutination and record your results. Record agglutination as positive. Record no agglutination as negative. *Failure to read the results at the end of the specified time may invalidate the results.*

Read the positive and negative controls and record your results.

Clean work area following laboratory protocol.

Remove gloves and wash hands with soap and water.

Questions

Name _____ Date _____

1. What is rheumatoid arthritis? What is the cause of this disease?

2. What is an autoimmune disease?

3. What are rheumatoid factors? Where are they found?

4. Name the symptoms of rheumatoid arthritis.

5. List various treatments for rheumatoid arthritis.

6. Name the two syndromes other than rheumatoid arthritis that exhibit rheumatoid factors.

Terminal Performance Objective

Rapid Slide Test for Rheumatoid Arthritis

Given the necessary equipment, you will be able to perform a rapid slide test for RA following the manufacturer's directions. Record the results of the test and the positive and negative controls. This procedure must be completed within 10 minutes with a level of accuracy specified by your instructor.

INSTRUCTOR'S EVALUATION FORM

Name _____ Date _____

+ = SATISFACTORY   ✓ = UNSATISFACTORY

_____ Assemble equipment.

_____ Wash hands with soap and water. Observe the OSHA Standard for this procedure.

_____ Allow the reagents and serum to reach room temperature before testing.

_____ Place glass slide or card provided with the kit on a flat surface under a direct light source.

_____ Fill capillary pipette provided to the mark with serum and dispel the serum into the center of the middle section of the etched slide or vacant circle on the card.

_____ Holding the dropper perpendicular, place one drop of positive control and one drop of negative control in the appropriate test circles.

_____ Add one free-falling drop of well-mixed reagent to each section of the slide.

_____ Mix with a disposable stirrer, spreading each mixture over the entire section.

_____ Rock slide gently with rotary motion for recommended time. Immediately observe for agglutination and record your results.   RESULTS: _____.

_____ Read the positive and negative controls and record your results.

RESULTS: _____.

_____ Clean work area following laboratory protocol.

_____ Remove gloves and wash hands with soap and water.

_____ The procedure was completed within 10 minutes.

_____ The results obtained were accurate to the level specified by your instructor.

_____ The results were properly recorded.

Final Competency Evaluation

_____ SATISFACTORY   _____ UNSATISFACTORY

Comments:

Instructor _____ Date _____

OSHA Precautions in Collection of Specimens*

Certain pathogenic microorganisms can be found in the blood and other body fluids of infected individuals. These pathogens can be transmitted to uninfected individuals from infected individuals. OSHA has developed standards and guidelines for employees who are at risk for exposure to blood and other infectious materials. All blood and potentially infectious material are to be considered infectious regardless of the perceived status of the source client. The most significant pathogens that require preventive measures are the hepatitis B virus (HBV) and human immunodeficiency virus (HIV). OSHA Standards require that universal precautions guidelines, developed by the Centers for Disease Control (CDC) in Atlanta, Georgia, be observed at all facilities.

BASIC RULES OF UNIVERSAL PRECAUTIONS

- The purpose of universal precautions is to prevent or minimize exposure to blood-borne pathogens.
- Approach *all* clients as if they are HIV- or HBV-infectious.
- Universal precautions apply to tissues, blood, and other body fluids containing visible blood.
- Approach *all* blood, body fluids, and tissues as if they are HIV- or HBV-contaminated.
- Approach *all* needles and sharps as if they have been contaminated with HIV or HBV.
- Blood is the single most important source of HIV, HBV, and other blood-borne pathogens in the workplace.
- Universal precautions also apply to tissues, semen, vaginal secretions, cerebrospinal fluid, synovial fluid, pleural fluid, pericardial fluid, and amniotic fluid.
- Universal precautions do not apply to feces, nasal secretions, breast milk, sputum, sweat, tears, urine, and vomitus unless they contain visible blood.
- Precautions do not apply to saliva, except in dentistry.
- Anticipate the kind of client contact and use appropriate personal protective equipment.

*From Watson, J, and Jaffe, MS: Nurse's Manual of Laboratory and Diagnostic Tests, ed 2, 1995, pp 967–969, FA Davis, Philadelphia, with permission.

- Know the limitations of the personal protective equipment being used, when it can protect and when it cannot.
- Do not recap needles.
- Do not break or otherwise manipulate needles.
- Place contaminated sharps in puncture-resistant containers.
- Wash hands immediately after contamination or removing gloves.
- Universal precautions do not eliminate the need for other category-specific or disease-specific isolation precautions, such as enteric precautions for infectious diarrhea.

HAND PROTECTION

- Wash hands before and after contact with any client whether gloves are worn or not.
- Wash hands before and after a procedure is performed whether gloves are worn or not.
- Always wear gloves when obtaining, handling, or testing specimens (body fluids, excretions, secretions) or touching any items or articles exposed to substances with contamination potential.
- Change gloves between clients or when soiled or torn.
- Wash hands or any skin or mucous membrane area immediately following contact with blood, body fluids, or any potentially infectious material; flush with water or wash with soap and water as soon as is feasible following the contact.
- Gloves are not to be washed or decontaminated for reuse.

PERSONAL PROTECTION

- Anticipate splashing of blood or body fluids, and attempt to eliminate or minimize spills or splashes.
- Wear disposable gown, apron, or lab coat when in contact or potentially in contact with blood or other infectious materials.
- Wear mask, eye protection (goggles with solid side shield), or chin-length face shield, as indicated, to protect skin, eyes, and mouth from contact with splashes, sprays, splattering, or droplets of potentially infectious body fluids.
- All garments contaminated by blood should be removed immediately; garments and protective equipment that are worn should be removed and disposed of properly prior to leaving work.
- Wearing apparel that is contaminated with blood or body fluids should be placed in a waterproof labeled bag in a designated area.

NEEDLES AND SHARPS

- Contaminated needles and other sharps should not be bent, recapped, removed, sheared, or purposely broken; in cases where there is no alternative to removal or recapping a needle, a mechanical device or one-handed technique should be used.
- In cases where a needle puncture accidentally occurs, report immediately for further evaluation and counseling.
- Discard used disposable needles, syringes, and other sharps in puncture and leakproof containers marked with a biohazard label; the articles should be discarded as soon as feasible following use.
- Discard reusable sharps in a color-coded, labeled container for decontamination.

- Never reach into the container of used needles or sharps.
- Replace containers when they are three-quarters full; close the full container and place in a designated area.

SPECIMENS

- Gloves should *always* be worn when collecting, handling, and testing specimens that are or have a potential to be contaminated with infectious microorganisms.
- Gloves should *always* be worn when collecting blood specimens, as all specimens are assumed to contain potentially infectious material.
- Avoid accidental sticks from needles when obtaining blood samples.
- Mouth pipetting of blood or other potentially infectious materials is prohibited.
- Always use disposable supplies to collect specimens when possible.
- Specimens of blood or other potentially infectious materials should be placed in a container and then in a biohazard bag that prevents leakage during the collection, handling, processing, storage, and transport of the specimens.
- Containers should be labeled or color-coded. If the outside of the primary container is contaminated, it should be placed in a secondary container that is puncture-resistant.
- Specimens that are to be transported outside of the facility are to be labeled with a biohazard sticker on the container.
- All microbiologic waste such as cultures and stocks of etiologic agents must be steam-sterilized in the lab prior to transport.
- All anatomic pathology wastes are placed in a color-coded bag or lined box prior to transport by housekeeping.
- All blood product containers are placed in a bag within a biohazard-labeled container.
- Cleanse any spills of body fluids during collection or handling by wiping with paper toweling first, then washing with soap and water, and then washing with a disinfectant solution.

B

Abbreviations in Clinical Medicine

a	arterial		F	Fahrenheit
aPTT	activated partial thromboplastin time		f	fasting
			FBS	fasting blood sugar
A/G	albumin-globulin ratio		fL	femtoliter
AHF	antihemophilic factor		g	gram
B	blood		GC	gonococci, gonorrhea
baso	basophil		GI	gastrointestinal
BP	blood pressure		GNDC	gram-negative diplococci
bp	boiling point		GTT	glucose tolerance test
BUN	blood urea nitrogen		GU	genitourinary
c	capillary		Hb, Hgb	hemoglobin
C	Celsius, centigrade		HBV	hepatitis B virus
CBC	complete blood count		HCG, hCG	human chorionic gonadotropin
cc, cm^3	cubic centimeter			
CDC	Centers for Disease Control		HCl	hydrochloric acid
CF	complement fixation		Hct	hematocrit
cm	centimeter		HDL	high density lipoprotein
CO	carbon monoxide		HIV	human immunodeficiency virus
CO_2	carbon dioxide			
C & S	culture and sensitivity		HPF, hpf	high power field
CSF	cerebrospinal fluid		Ig	immunoglobulin, antibody
d	24 h; day		IM	infectious mononucleosis
Diff	differential blood count		IU	international unit
DNA	deoxyribonucleic acid		IV	intravenous
EIA	enzyme immunoassay		IVP	intravenous pyelogram
EMB	eosin-methylene blue		kg	kilogram
Erc	erythrocyte		LDL	low density lipoprotein
ESR	erythrocyte sedimentation rate		Lkcs	leukocytes
			LMP	last menstrual period
E.U.	Ehrlich units		LPF, lpf	low power field

m	meter
MCH	mean corpuscular hemoglobin
MCHC	mean corpuscular hemoglobin concentration
MCV	mean corpuscular volume
mg	milligram
mEq	milliequivalent
mL	milliliter
MLT	medical laboratory technician
mm	millimeter
mm^3	cubic millimeter
MT	medical technologist
NaCl	sodium chloride, saline
nm	nanometer
O.D.	optical density
P	plasma
pg	picogram
pH	symbol denoting acidity and alkalinity
PKU	phenylketonuria
PMN	polymorphonuclear neutrophil
Pt	patient
PT	prothrombin time
PTT	partial thromboplastin time
qns	quantity not sufficient
RBC	red blood cell, erythrocyte
RES	reticuloendothelial system
RF	rheumatoid factor
RNA	ribonucleic acid
S	serum
S.I.	le Système International d'Unités (International System of Units)
sp. gr.	specific gravity
Staph	*Staphylococcus*
stat	immediately
STD	sexually transmitted disease
Strep	*Streptococcus*
TNTC	too numerous to count
μ	micro
U	urine
UA	urinalysis
UTI	urinary tract infection
v	venous
VLDL	very low density lipoprotein
WBC	white blood cell, leukocyte

APPENDIX

Reference Ranges

REFERENCE RANGES—BLOOD

Bilirubin, mg/dL × 17.10 = μmol/L

Conventional Units, mg/dL		SI Units, μmol/L
Total bilirubin		
Newborn	2.0–6.0	34.2–102.6
48 h old	6.0–7.0	102.6–119.7
5 days old	4.0–12.0	68.4–205.2
1 mo to adult	0.3–1.2	5.1–20.5
Indirect bilirubin (unconjugated, prehepatic)		
1 mo to adult	0.3–1.1	5.1–18.8
Direct bilirubin (conjugated, posthepatic)		
1 mo to adult	0.1–0.4	1.7–6.8

Bleeding Time

Method	Value
Duke	1–3 min
Ivy	3–6 min
Template	3–6 min

Blood Glucose, mg/dL × 0.0555 = mmol/L

Conventional Units, mg/dL		SI Units, mmol/L
Whole blood		
Children	50–90	2.8–5.0
Adults	60–100	3.3–5.5
Serum or plasma		
Children	60–105	3.3–5.8
Adults	70–110	3.9–6.1

Urea Nitrogen, mg/dL × 0.3570 = mmol/L

Conventional Units, mg/dL		SI Units, mmol/L
Serum or plasma	6–20	2.1–8.2

Cholesterol (Total), mg/dL × 0.02586 = mmol/L

Conventional Units, mg/dL		SI Units, mmol/L
Desirable level	Less than 200	Less than 5.2
Borderline high	200–239	5.2–6.2
High	240 or higher	6.2 or higher

Complete Blood Count

	Red Cell Count	
	Conventional Units, millions of cells/mm³	SI Units, cells × 10¹²/L
Newborn	4.8–7.1	4.8–7.1
Adult male	4.6–6.2	4.6–6.2
Adult female	4.2–5.4	4.2–5.4

	Hematocrit, % × 0.01 = fraction of 1.00	
Newborn	44–64	0.44–0.64
Adult male	40–54	0.40–0.54
Adult female	38–47	0.38–0.47

	Hemoglobin, g/dL × 0.6206 = mmol/L	
	g/dL	mmol/L
Newborn	14–24	8.7–14.9
Adult male	13.5–18	8.4–11.2
Adult female	12–16	7.4–9.9

Cell Indices

	MCV μm³ × 1.0 = fL	
	μm³	fL
Newborn	98–108	98–108
Adult male	80–94	80–94
Adult female	81–99	81–99

	MCH pg × 0.06206 = fmol	
	pg	fmol
Newborn	32–34	2.0–2.1
Adult	27–31	1.7–1.9

	MCHC g/dL 3 0.6206 5 mmol/L	
	g/dL	mmol/L
Newborn	32–33	19.9–20.5
Adult	32–36	19.9–22.3

White Blood Count

	Conventional Units, cells/mm³	SI Units, cells × 10⁹/L
Newborn	9,000–30,000	9.0–30.0
Adult	5,000–10,000	5.0–10.0

Differential

Cell Type	Conventional Units		SI Units, cells × 10⁹/L
	Percentage, %	Absolute, cells/mm³	
Neutrophils	54–62	3000–5800	3.0–5.8
Bands	3–5	150–400	0.2–0.4
Eosinophils	1–3	50–250	0.05–0.25
Basophils	0–0.75	15–50	0.01–0.05
Monocytes	3–7	300–500	0.3–0.5
Lymphocytes	25–33	1500–3000	1.5–3.0

Platelet Count

Platelets, Cells/mm³ 5 Cells 3 10⁹/L

Conventional Units, cells/mm³	SI Units, cells × 10⁹/L
150,000–350,000	150–350

Erythrocyte Sedimentation Rate

	Wintrobe, mm/h	Westergren, mm/h	Cutler, mm/h
Males:			0–8
<Age 50 yr	0–7	0–15	
>Age 50 yr	5–7	0–20	
Females:			0–10
<Age 50 yr	0–15	0–20	
>Age 50 yr	25–30	0–30	

	Landau Micro Method	Smith Micro Method
Children:		
Newborn–2 yr	1–6	0–1 (newborn)
4–14 yr	1–9	3–13

Glucose Tolerance Test, mg/dL × 0.0555 = mmol/L

Time After Carbohydrate Challenge, h	Conventional Units, mg/dL	SI Units, mmol/L
Whole blood		
½	<150	8.3
1	<160	8.9
2	<115	6.4
3	Same as fasting	Same as fasting
Serum or plasma		
½	<160	8.9
1	<170	9.4
2	<125	6.9
3	Same as fasting	Same as fasting
Urine	Negative throughout test	

Heterophile Antibody (Infectious Mononucleosis)

Male and female	Negative

Human Chorionic Gonadotropin (HCG)

Nonpregnant	< 3 mIU/mL
Pregnant	
8–10 days	5–40 mIU/mL
1 mo	100 mIU/mL
2 mo	100,000 mIU/mL
4 mo to term	50,000 mIU/mL

Lipoprotein Composition

	Triglyceride, %	Cholesterol, %	Phospholipid, %	Protein, %
Chylomicrons	85–95	3–5	5–10	1–2
VLDL	60–70	10–15	10–15	10
LDL	5–10	45	20–30	15–25
HDL	Very little	20	30	50

Partial Thromboplastin Time

Male and female	30–45 sec

Activated Partial Thromboplastin Time

Male and female	35–45 sec (may vary depending on laboratory)

Prothrombin Time

Male	9.6–11.8 sec
Female	9.5–11.3 sec

Rheumatoid Factor

Male and female	Negative

Serum Creatine, mg/dL × 76.25 = μmol/L

	Conventional Units, mg/dL	SI Units, μmol/L
Male	0.1–0.4	7.6–30.5
Female	0.2–0.7	15.3–53.4

Serum Creatinine, mg/dL × 88.4 = μmol/L

	Conventional Units, mg/dL	SI Units, μmol/L
Children to age 6	0.3–0.6	26.5–53.0
Children 6–18	0.4–1.2	35.4–106
Adults		
Male	0.6–1.3	53.0–114.9
Female	0.5–1.0	44.2–88.4

Serum Proteins

Age	Total Protein, g/dL	Albumin, g/dL	Globulins, g/dL	Gamma Globulins, g/dL
Newborn	5.0–7.1	2.5–5.0	1.2–4.0	0.7–0.9
3 mo	4.7–7.4	3.0–4.2	1.0–3.3	0.1–0.5
1 yr	5.0–7.5	2.7–5.0	2.0–3.8	0.4–1.2
15 yr	6.5–8.6	3.2–5.0	2.0–4.0	0.6–1.2
Adults	6.6–7.9	3.3–4.5	2.0–4.2	0.5–1.6

Albumin/globulin (A/G) ratio 1.5:1–2.5:1

Uric Acid, mg/dL × 59.48 = μmol/L

	Conventional Units, mg/dL	SI Units, μmol/L
Male	4.0–8.5	237.9–505.6
Female	2.7–7.3	160.6–434.2

Urinalysis

Macroscopic	
Color	Pale yellow to amber
Appearance	Clear to slightly hazy
Odor	Mildly aromatic
Specific gravity	1.001–1.035 (usual range, 1.010–1.025)
pH	4.5–8.0
Protein	Negative
Glucose	Negative
Other sugars	Negative
Ketones	Negative
Blood	Negative
Bilirubin	Negative
Urobilinogen	0.1–1.0 Erhlich units/dL (24 h)
Nitrite	Negative
Leukocyte esterase	Negative

Microscopic	
Red blood cells	0–3/hpf
White blood cells	0–4/hpf
Epithelial cells	few
Casts	Occasional hyaline
Crystals	Occasional (uric acid, urate, phosphate, or calcium oxalate)

Symbols for OSHA Bloodborne Pathogen Exposure Controls Applicable to Clinical Procedures

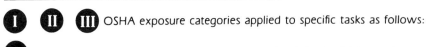 OSHA exposure categories applied to specific tasks as follows:

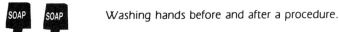 Tasks that involve exposure to blood, body fluids, or tissues, or that carry a potential for spills or splashes. Appropriate protective measures should be used *every time.*

Tasks that involve no exposure to blood, body fluids, or tissues in the normal work routine, but exposure or potential exposure may occur in certain situations. Appropriate protective measures should be used in these situations.

Tasks that involve no exposure to blood, body fluids, or tissues. Appropriate protective measures are *not* necessary.

 Washing hands after a procedure.

 Washing hands before and after a procedure.

 Disposable sharp equipment that must not be bent, recapped, removed, sheared, or purposely broken. Equipment should be disposed of in a rigid, leakproof, puncture-resistant container that is color-coded orange or orange-red or labeled with the orange-red biohazard sign.

 Reusable sharp equipment that must be placed immediately, or as soon as possible, after use into appropriate sharps containers. The containers used to receive contaminated equipment must be puncture-resistant, leakproof, and color-coded orange or orange-red or labeled with the orange-red biohazard sign.

 Face shielding with masks and goggles is required as protection whenever splashes, spray, splatter, or droplets of blood or other potentially infectious materials may be generated and eye, nose, or mouth contamination can reasonably be anticipated.

Protective clothing, such as laboratory coats, gowns, or aprons, is required as protection whenever splashes, spray, splatter, or droplets of blood or other potentially infectious materials may be generated and clothing contamination can reasonably be anticipated.

Biohazard bags must be used to discard materials containing blood or other potentially infectious materials. The bags must be leakproof and color-coded orange or orange-red or labeled with the orange-red biohazard sign.

Decontamination requires using a bleach solution or Environmental Protection Agency–registered germicide. All contaminated work surfaces must be decontaminated after completion of procedures and immediately, or as soon as feasible, after any spill of blood or other potentially infectious materials (as well as at the end of the work shift) if the surface may have become contaminated since the last cleaning.

Gloves must be worn when it is reasonably anticipated that there will be hand contact with blood, other potentially infectious materials, nonintact skin, and mucous membranes. Gloves are not to be washed or decontaminated for reuse and are to be replaced as soon as practical when they become contaminated, or if they are torn or punctured or their ability to function as a barrier is compromised. *Utility* gloves may be decontaminated for reuse provided that the glove is intact and able to function as a barrier. *Examination* gloves are used for nonsterile procedures. *Sterile* gloves are used for minor surgery and other sterile procedures.

From Frew, MA, Lane, K, and Frew, D: Comprehensive Medical Assisting: Competencies for Administrative and Clinical Practice, ed 3, 1995, FA Davis, Philadelphia, with permission.

1990 DACUM
Analysis of the Medical
Assisting Profession

1.0 Display profession-alism	1.1 Project a positive attitude	1.2 Perform within ethical boundaries	1.3 Practice within the scope of education, training, and personal capabilities	1.4 Maintain confidentiality	1.5 Work as a team member	1.6 Conduct one-self in a courteous and diplomatic manner	1.7 Adapt to change
2.0 Communicate	2.1 Listen and observe	2.2 Treat all patients with empathy and impartiality	2.3 Adapt communi-cation to individual's abilities to understand	2.4 Recognize and respond to verbal and nonverbal communica-tion	2.5 Serve as liaison between physician and others	2.6 Evaluate understand-ing of communi-cation	2.7 Receive, organize, prioritize, and transmit informa-tion
3.0 Perform administra-tive duties	3.1 Perform basic secre-tarial skills	3.2 Schedule and monitor appoint-ments	3.3 Prepare and maintain medical records	3.4 Apply computer concepts for office pro-cedures	3.5 Perform medical trans-cription	3.6 Locate resources and infor-mation for patients and employers	3.7 Manage physi-cian's pro-fessional schedule and travel
4.0 Perform clini-cal duties	4.1 Apply princi-ples of aseptic tech-nique and in-fection control	4.2 Take vital signs	4.3 Recognize emer-gencies	4.4 Perform first aid and CPR	4.5 Prepare and maintain exami-nation and treat-ment area	4.6 Interview and take patient history	4.7 Prepare patients for pro-cedures
5.0 Apply legal concepts to practice	5.1 Document accu-rately	5.2 Determine needs for documen-tation and reporting	5.3 Use appro-priate guidelines when releasing records or information	5.4 Follow estab-lished policy in initiating or terminating medical treatment	5.5 Dispose of con-trolled sub-stances in com-pliance with govern-ment regula-tions	5.6 Maintain licenses and accredita-tion	5.7 Monitor legisla-tion re-lated to current health-care issues and practice
6.0 Manage the office	6.1 Maintain the physical plant	6.2 Operate and maintain facilities and equipment safely	6.3 Inventory equipment and supplies	6.4 Evaluate and recommend equipment and supplies for practice	6.5 Maintain liability coverage	6.6 Exercise efficient time man-agement	Supervise* personnel
7.0 Provide instruction	7.1 Orient patients to office policies and pro-cedures	7.2 Instruct pa-tients with special needs	7.3 Teach pa-tients methods of health pro-motion and disease prevention	7.4 Orient and train personnel	Provide* health informa-tion for public use	Supervise* student practicums	Conduct* continu-ing edu-cation activities

1.8	1.9			
Show initiative and responsibility	Promote the profession	Enhance* skills through continuing education		

2.8	2.9	2.10	2.11	
Use proper telephone technique	Interview effectively	Use medical terminology appropriately	Compose written communication using correct grammar, spelling, and format	Develop* and conduct public relations activities to market professional services

4.8	4.9	4.10	4.11	4.12	4.13	4.14	
Assist physician with examinations and treatments	Use quality control	Collect and process specimens	Perform selected tests that assist with diagnosis and treatment	Screen and follow-up patient test results	Prepare and administer medications as directed by physician	Maintain medication records	Respond* to medical emergencies
Develop* and maintain policy and procedure manuals	Establish* risk management protocol for the practice						
Develop* job descriptions	Interview* and recommend new personnel	Negotiate* leases and prices for equipment and supply contracts					
Develop* educational materials							

1990 DACUM Analysis of the Medical Assisting Profession Continued

8.0 **Manage practice finances**	8.1 Use manual book-keeping systems	8.2 Implement current procedural termi-nology and ICD-9 coding	8.3 Analyze and use current third-party guidelines for reim-bursement	8.4 Manage ac-counts re-ceivable	8.5 Manage accounts payable	8.6 Maintain rec-ords for accounting and bank-ing pur-poses	8.7 Process employee payroll

*Denotes advanced-level skills. The medical assistant should be able to perform all other skills after completing a CAHEA-accredited program and starting a first job.

Source: The American Association of Medical Assistants, Inc., 20 North Wacker Drive, Suite 1575, Chicago, Illinois 60606. Consultants: Mary Lee Seibert, EdD, CMA, and Patricia A. Amos, MS.

1990 DACUM Analysis of the Medical Assisting Profession Continued

Manage*
    personnel
    benefits and
    records

Index

Page numbers followed by "f" indicate figures; page numbers followed by "t" indicate tables.